Disease and Demography in Colonial Burma

Judith L. Richell

NUS PRESS
SINGAPORE

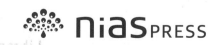

First published in 2006 by:

NUS Press
an imprint of NUS Publishing
National University of Singapore
AS3-01-02, 3 Arts Link
Singapore 117569

Fax: (65) 6774–0652
E-mail: nusbooks@nus.edu.sg
Website: http://www.nus.edu.sg/npu

ISBN 9971-69-301-1

First published in 2006 for distribution in Europe by

NIAS Press
Nordic Institute of Asian Studies
Leifsgade 33, 2300 Copenhagen S
Denmark
Tel: (+45) 3532 9500 Fax: (+45) 3532 9549
E-mail: books@nias.ku.dk
Website: www.niaspress.dk

ISBN 87-91114-70-5

National Library Board Singapore Cataloguing in Publication Data

Richell, Judith L., 1943–1999.
    Disease and demography in colonial Burma/Judith L. Richell. – Singapore:
NUS Press; Denmark: NIAS Press, 2006.
    p. cm.
    Includes bibliographical references and index.
    ISBN: 9971-69-301-1 (NUS: pbk.)
    ISBN: 87-91114-70-5 (NIAS: pbk.)

    1. Demography – Burma – History. 2. Burma – Population – History.
    I. Title.

HB3636.7.A3
304.609591—dc22   SLS2006026798

Typeset by : Scientifik Graphics (Singapore) Pte Ltd
Printed by : Print Dynamic (S) Pte Ltd

Contents

Illustrations

Foreword

The author of this book, Judith Richell, died in 1999, at the age of 56. For some years she had been registered as a doctoral student in the History Department of the School of Oriental and African Studies, University of London, and indeed at the time of her death she was extremely close — a matter of a few weeks — to submitting a completed thesis for examination. Following her death, it was hoped that the university would still allow the thesis to be submitted. But although the authorities were sympathetic, the university's regulations in such sad circumstances are precise, and Judith's work, as a thesis, could proceed no further. The alternative route, then, was to seek a publisher, and it is to the immense credit of NUS Press — in particular its Managing Director, Paul Kratoska, and senior editor, Ms Cheong Yun Wan — that it took on the challenge of producing the book in what were, obviously, exceptional and difficult circumstances. Immense credit is also due to Judith's husband, Peter, who completed the final typescript — what would have been a matter of a few weeks for an author is clearly a much greater task for someone who had not been immersed in the work — and who subsequently dealt with the many queries at the editorial stage. Without Peter, Judith's work would not have been brought to publication.

I have dwelt on this detail not simply from a wish to pay tribute but also because I think it important that the reader of this book should be aware of the circumstances in which it was completed. The fact is that Judith's final adjustments to the typescript would almost certainly have been different, and her responses to editorial issues more informed, despite Peter's heroic efforts. More importantly, the ideas and evidence here have not been subjected to the processes of reflection and expansion that occur in the reworking of a doctoral thesis into a book. That said, this study remains a fine piece of scholarship, and an important contribution to the study of the historical demography of Southeast Asia.

The demographic history of Southeast Asia has two principal distinctive features. In broad terms — the exceptions are Java and the Red River delta in northern Vietnam — the region has had a low average density of population, relative to that found in the neighbouring

ix

India, China, and Japan, and relative to Southeast Asia's vast agricultural potential. On that second comparison, it need only be noted that the Burma delta, the world's single most important exporter of rice in 1900, with annual exports approaching two million tons, was extremely sparsely populated a mere five decades earlier. The second feature is that over the seventeenth and eighteenth centuries, Southeast Asia's population grew extremely slowly, barely perceptibly, but that from the end of the eighteenth century — the precise turning point apparently came at different times in the different parts of the region — there was a pronounced acceleration into the more rapid demographic growth of the nineteenth and twentieth centuries. Those two features — low density, and the acceleration into the modern era — have long attracted scholarly interest. Particularly important early contributions were Wilbur Zelinsky, "The Indochinese Peninsula: A Demographic Anomaly" (*Far Eastern Quarterly*, 9, 1950), and Charles A. Fisher's article "Some comments on population growth in South-East Asia, with special reference to the period since 1830", in C. D. Cowan's edited volume *The Economic Development of South-East Asia* (London: George Allen and Unwin, 1964). But interest in the demographic history of Southeast Asia moved forward decisively in the 1980s with two particularly significant publications. The first was a volume of essays edited by Norman G. Owen, *Death and Disease in Southeast Asia: Explorations in Social, Medical and Demographic History* (Singapore: Oxford University Press, 1987). In terms of approach, the essays ranged widely, from attempts to measure, statistically, morbidity and mortality in parts of the region, to explorations of indigenous attitudes towards illness and healing, to assessments of the impact of government action, or inaction, on mortality in colonial Southeast Asia. The second was Peter Boomgaard's *Children of the Colonial State: Population Growth and Economic Development in Java, 1795–1880* (Amsterdam: Free University Press, 1989). This too took demographic history far beyond statistical calculations, to establish the economic and social contexts for the up-turn in the rate of population growth in nineteenth-century Java.

Judith Richell's research was an important part of that renewed interest in the demographic history of Southeast Asia in the 1980s. Not least, it extended the work, hitherto dominated by Java and the Philippines, to Burma. Judith's interest in Burma — although in very different contexts — had been sparked during her undergraduate years at Hatfield Polytechnic (now the University of Hertfordshire), where she had been taught by Victor Lieberman, now at the University of Michigan, but then in the throes of completing his first major monograph, *Burmese Administrative Cycles: Anarchy and Conquest, c.1580–1760* (Princeton: Princeton University Press, 1984). Colonial Burma was an excellent choice for work in historical demography. The existing writings in this field were extremely thin, and much of the primary research material was easily accessible in London — although it should be added that Judith was able to make a brief research visit to Burma in 1987. The foundation of her study is a highly sophisticated recalculation of the demographic statistics of colonial Burma, primarily between the censuses of 1891 and 1941. But, as with the work by Norman Owen and Peter Boomgaard, it is the contexts that are critical — in Judith's case, the family and childhood, the provision of public health, issues of nutritional levels, and the impact of malaria. This book thus becomes the pivotal, founding contribution to modern scholarship on the history of population, disease, and medical practice in Burma, areas of research that will undoubtedly figure prominently — I am thinking of more recent work by, among others, Monique Skidmore, and Naono Atsuko, author of a recent dissertation on "The State of Vaccination: British Doctors, Indigenous Cooperation, and the Fight Against Smallpox in Colonial Burma" (PhD, University of Michigan, 2005) — in a now greatly reinvigorated Burma studies.

Ian Brown
School of Oriental and African Studies, London

In 1998 when my wife, Judith, was told she was terminally ill, she made great efforts to finalise her research work. Shortly before her death in 1999, she asked me to try to get her work published so that it would be available to others. It gives me great pleasure that, with support from many people, this has now been achieved and I would like to make the following dedication.

To Judith, who wasn't able to see her work published;

to all those who supported Judith in her work to

produce the material in this book,

particularly Professor Ian Brown (School of Oriental and

African Studies, London);

and to the people of Burma.

Peter Richell

Introduction

The subject of this book is an examination of the factors affecting demographic change in Burma between 1852 and 1941. Despite the increasing contemporary interest in the historical demography of the non-European world, few historians have attempted a detailed examination of Burma's population records.[1] Michael Adas' important work of economic and social history, *The Burma Delta*,[2] is primarily a study of the development of rice monocrop agriculture in the delta area of Burma. Although this entails an examination of internal and international migration and some use of population statistics, it is not primarily an analysis of demographic change. James Andrus' *Burmese Economic Life*[3] and John Furnivall's *Colonial Policy and Practice*[4] contain little historical demography. Charles Fisher's work[5] provides some general information on population growth in Southeast Asia, and Irene Taeuber's work[6] contains useful information covering the general problems associated with demographic research and the factors affecting demographic change. Kingsley Davis' book on India and Pakistan[7] is useful because the Indian censuses included Burma from 1872 to 1931. He identified problems with these census results, showed how these can lead to misleading growth rates, and suggested reasons for the fluctuations in the birth and death rates.

Only two scholars have previously explored Burmese demography. They are A. R. Vyatkin,[8] a Russian, whose work is not yet available in an English translation, and R. M. Sundrum, whose paper, "Population Statistics of Burma",[9] contains important historical references.

Many of the early reminiscences and histories of Burma speculate upon the size of the population of Burma, both pre- and post-annexation. The empirical interests of these men, often members of the Indian civil service, are shown in their desire to record and measure all aspects of Burmese life, from mean temperatures to infant mortality. But inevitably their estimates of population prior to British rule rely heavily on a few sources such as the depleted *sit-tan* records and the works of Henry Burney, Michael Symes, Hiram Cox, Henry Yule, Father Sangermano and John Crawfurd.

The work of June and Manning Nash, in the early 1960s, explored, at a local level, the cultural influences of Burmese society and Buddhism on rates of demographic growth. They described a late marriage age, a high percentage of unmarried adults and infrequency of remarriage as contributing to a relatively slow population growth.[10]

A discussion in the *Journal of the Burma Research Society* in 1914 between J. Stuart and Maung Ba Aung also considered the influence of Buddhism as a reason for the relative sparseness of population in Burma.[11] Stuart's views on the lack of cultural emphasis on sons or children in Burmese society are echoed in Nash's comments that "Buddhist values do not extol the family or marriage".[12] When this is considered in conjunction with Nash's description of the strong kinship ties between mother and daughter, and the important social roles of the unmarried, it provides a strong argument for the use of anthropological data in assessing the determinants of fertility.[13]

Three basic factors determine the growth or decline of any population. These are birth rates, death rates, and migration. Changes in these vital rates affect not only the gross numbers but also the structure of the population. For example, the equilibrium between the vital rates affects the age structure of the population, thus determining the number of children under 15 years, the number of men and women of both fertile and economically productive age, and the numbers of those dependent by virtue of longevity. Migration may affect both the gross numbers of the population and its structure, due to the probability of involvement of high numbers of young, adult males. The out-migration of adult males, even if seasonal only, may lower the fertility of women of child-bearing age in that society.

Economic, social and demographic histories are, therefore, inter-twined aspects of a community's development. In Edward Wrigley's words: "The wider value of demographic studies lies in the sensitivity with which a community's demography reflected its economic, social and natural environments. These relationships are two-way. Fertility and mortality were not simply a passive reflection of the general circumstances of a community. They helped in turn to shape those circumstances."[14]

Therefore it is hoped that, in this study of the influences effecting change in the vital rates, some of the links between the cultural, social and economic aspects of Burmese life will become clearer. This will include the degree to which the colonial administration influenced the rise in population under their government. Examination of the bare bones of vital rates, divorced from this economic, social, and environmental background, can become mathematical modelling, which is not the object of this study. Works by Carlo Cipolla, Kingsley Davis and Edward Wrigley provide a useful discussion of the importance of the socio-cultural factors.[15]

1 Numbering the people

Burma is part of mainland Southeast Asia, an area dominated physically by great river systems running roughly in a north-to-south direction, separated by mountain ranges and plateaux. Burma's topography typifies this, as its main features are the Irrawaddy and Chindwin valleys, their surrounding mountain ranges and the Shan Plateau. The horseshoe of mountains, which almost encircles the lowlands of Burma, starts in the extreme southwest as the Arakan Yoma, and divides the Irrawaddy delta and the central plain of Burma from the narrow coastal lowlands of the Sandoway, Kyaukpyu and Arakan districts. This range culminates in Mount Victoria (10,200 feet), and then continues to form the western boundary of Burma as the Chin, Manipur and Naga hills.

The far north of Burma, where the highest mountains are over 19,000 feet, forms the southern fringe of the huge mountain plateau of Tibet. Northeast of Çʻe Burmese border is the range through which the Salween and Mekong rivers flow, before the Salween plunges into Burma and carves its way through the Shan Plateau. The Mekong flows through south Yunnan to form the border between Burma and Laos before flowing east and then south.

In the east of Burma, the mountains of the Shan Plateau rise in places to over 8,000 feet, and provide a sharp physical contrast to the flat, dry and sandy plains of central Upper Burma. These dry plains, with their light soil and rainfall of only 30 to 40 inches a year, nevertheless have historically formed the heartland of the Burmese kingdoms. Despite the low rainfall, the cultivation of wet rice has been practised here from the twelfth century, chiefly in the four irrigated areas of the Lower Chindwin, Taungdwingyi, the Mu River and Kyaukse district.[1]

The central belt of lowland Burma is climatically an intermediate zone linking the high rainfall areas of Lower Burma to the dry central plain of Upper Burma. The amount of rainfall in this belt varies widely; for example, in parts of the western district of Thayetmyo,[2] the landscape is arid, often receiving only 31 inches of rain a year, but in the east, much of the large district of Toungoo has a sub-deltaic climate with twice as much rain per annum.[3]

The deltaic area of Lower Burma has a very low relief and the country is characterised by the intersection of tributary rivers and high rainfall. Much of it is unprotected from the "rainshadow effect", which makes Upper Burma dry, and instead receives at least 100 inches of rainfall per year, with up to 170 inches on the west coast and Mergui Peninsula.[4]

The topography and climate of Burma have helped to determine the settlement patterns and the agriculture and social structure of the population. The central lowlands from Shwebo in the north to the southern deltas have seen civilisations and empires wax and wane. For example, there is descriptive evidence from AD 600 of the Mon people, who were the original builders of the canal systems in the Kyaukse district of Upper Burma, but by the nineteenth century, they were confined to Lower Burma and were partly assimilated by the Burmese, whom they had introduced to Buddhism.[5] The Pyu people, who probably entered Burma from central Asia later than the Mons, left behind their cities, their sculptures and their Buddhism, but no records after AD 1113.[6] Presumably their kingdom was overrun and the people assimilated by the incoming Burmese, who moved down through northeast Tibet into Upper Burma via the Shan Hills.[7]

The more recent history of lowland Burma is concerned with the interplay of Mon, Burmese and Shan power[8] until the last Burmese Konbaung Dynasty was deposed by the invading British in the nineteenth century. Despite the power struggles of the Mon, Burmese and Shan, the three groups had much in common: most of the population was employed in agriculture, they practised wet-rice cultivation and, for the Mon and Burmese in particular, there was the bond of Theravada Buddhism.

The physical characteristics of Burma still largely determined the lives of the people in the period of this study. The high mountains were the home of tribal peoples who practised shifting cultivation and animist religions. The lowland areas were dominated by Burmese and Mon people, who generally favoured settled agriculture and practised Theravada Buddhism. The Shan people of the plateau between central Burma and Thailand fell between these two approximate divisions; most of them, but not all, were Buddhist and cultivated wet rice, but some were much closer to the tribal hillsmen in both belief and social structure.[9]

These are broad generalisations that can of course be challenged by more detailed analysis, but will suffice for this brief introduction. The main hill or tribal groups of Burma, reading from west to east, were the

Chin and Lushai people, the Nagas of northwest Burma, the Kachins and Lisus of northeast Burma and the Was and Palaung people, who lived on parts of the Shan Plateau. South of the plateau and lying broadly between the Sittang and Salween valleys were the Karens. Within these groups were numerous subgroups and sub-cultures, but the main factors determining their difference from the lowland people were ecological and economic; that is, the difference between the cultivation of wet rice through the use of draught animals and the practice of shifting cultivation.[10] Again it must be emphasised that these are broad statements sweeping over intricate and inter-connected systems, ignoring for example the construction of irrigated rice terraces by some Naga and Kachin groups, and the close similarities between some Shan and Kachin tribes.[11]

In addition to the groups already described, other immigrant groups found a home in the lowlands of Burma or the Shan Hills during the British occupation. Two of these groups, the European and Chinese communities, were numerically insignificant but of great economic importance. The Chinese community numbered only 100,000, or 0.7 per cent of the total population, by 1931. The pattern of their settlement can be seen in Appendix 1. There was a concentration of Chinese immigrants in Lower rather than Upper Burma, a ratio of males to females of approximately two to one in 1931, and a steady growtb/in numbers. Many male Chinese married into the Burmese community and established themselves as tradesmen. They were also found working in the mines in the Shan Hills, and later, on the Burma-Yunnan Road.

The reference to the Yunnan Chinese in Appendix 1 is to a small community of Muslim Chinese who fled to northern Burma in 1873 following the defeat of their rebellious sultanate by the Chinese Imperial armies.[12] However, the overall numbers of the combined Chinese population in Burma remained numerically insignificant in the overall population dynamics.

The European community, despite its administrative dominance in the period of the study, remained small, the numbers fluctuating between 0.10 per cent and 0.15 per cent of the total population. Neither this community nor the Chinese community will be examined as autonomous units in the study nor will any attempt be made to extract their data from the figures relating to the population as a whole, as they are statistically negligible.

There was, however, an immigrant community in Burma that was far from negligible in numbers: the Indian community, which was more than a million-strong by 1931. The role and origin of this group has been ably documented and researched,[13] so the discussion of them in this study will be limited to those aspects of their history that bear on the broad demographic issues.

Most of the migrants from India were between 15 and 40 years of age; they were male and unaccompanied by wife or family. The majority were short-term migrants, some staying for one harvest season only, others for two to five years. They worked in the rice mills and in agriculture as seasonal demand for labour rose and fell. The total numbers of migrants in the country rose steadily because, in most years, there were more immigrants from India than returning emigrants. Between 1921 and 1931, there was a net gain of 480,869 immigrants despite the two Depression years of 1930 and 1931, which both showed a net loss.[14]

The majority of this Indian community were either Hindu or Muslim, and their numbers and distribution in Burma are shown in Appendices 2 to 5. There were more than twice as many Hindus as Muslims in Rangoon town, and a high ratio of Hindus persisted in Lower Burma up to the last informative census year of 1931. However it was a different story in Upper Burma, where Hindus and Muslims maintained a rough balance numerically, although they were unevenly distributed geographically.

This disparity between the communities in Upper and Lower Burma reflects employment opportunities and preferences. In Rangoon, for example, where nearly 50 per cent of the population was Indian in 1891, the high number of Hindus is related to the labouring jobs available in the ports, as well as the virtual Indian monopoly of subordinate posts in the colonial administration.[15] The districts of Insein, Pegu and Hanthawaddy each had Indian populations of 40,000 plus by 1931, and this can be seen clearly in Appendix 5, where the numbers are expressed as a percentage of the total populations. These immigrants illustrate the huge demand that existed in colonial Burma for cheap manpower. They worked in the rice mills, the sawmills and on the railways, and responded to the demand for seasonal harvest labour. In 1872, there were 136,500 Indians in British Burma (Lower Burma only); in 1931, there were more than one million in the whole of Burma.

Obviously this immigrant community, unlike the Chinese and European, cannot be ignored in a study of population dynamics. This is not a history of the Indian community in Burma, but due to their large numbers, their involvement in the administration of the sanitary services and the vulnerability of the Indian labourer to disease, later chapters will contain many references to them.

The objective of this first chapter is simple: to establish the number of the Burmese population during the period of the British adminis-tration, specifically the period from 1891 to 1941. Unfortunately, this supposedly simple demographic objective was far from easy in execution. To clarify the somewhat complex explanations, the chapter has therefore been sub-divided into sections, which examine separately the area of the study and how estimates were made of the population of nineteenth-century Burma, and then discuss the census as a source of demographic data. This is followed by separate estimates of population numbers for Upper and Lower Burma and explanations of how these were calculated.

The study area

The term "study area" defines the geographical extent of the territory of Burma selected for this demographic analysis. Its extent and boundaries are shown in Map A. The reasons why the boundaries of the study area are not the same as the political territory of Burma in the period are explained below.

The most important sources for demographic data are census and vital registration records. Both of these sources were introduced by the British administration, but unfortunately were available for limited areas of Burma only, thus making longitudinal analyses of the geopolitical country of Burma very difficult. The population totals by census, the dates on which the census was taken and the approximate areas covered are shown in Table 1.1. This shows a gradual expansion of the area covered by the census, which commenced in 1872 and covered Lower Burma only. The mountain and hill areas, including the Shan Plateau, were not included at all until 1901, and even then the method of data collection was either by a non-synchronous census or by estimation. Some areas, such as the extreme north, or the western part of the Shan states, were still excluded. A glance at Table 1.1, which offers a reassuring picture of expanding population, actually therefore merely offers an illusion of workable data and not a firm statistical base.

The collection of vital registration statistics also started in Lower Burma only and was gradually expanded as the administration annexed Upper Burma. However, the collection of this data was concentrated in the lowland areas, and by 1911, only 82 per cent of the census population was even nominally under vital registration requirements.

Thus the hill and mountain areas of Burma, although fascinating to the anthropologist, offer little encouragement to the historical demographer. It was reluctantly decided that, as these areas lacked basic data, they would have to be discarded from the study.

All of the mountain and plateau country has been excluded from the study area, with the exception of the Pegu Yoma and parts of the

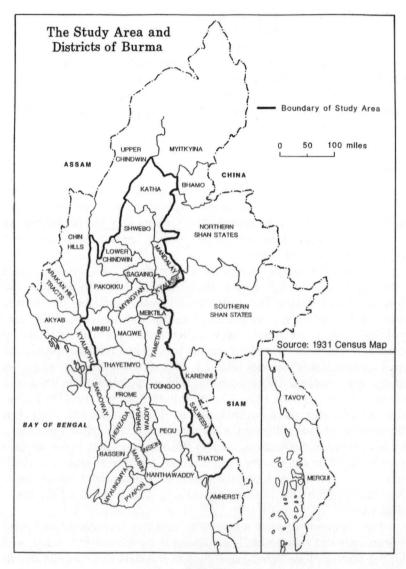

MAP A

Arakan Yoma. The Mergui Peninsula was also excluded, as it had very patchy vital registration, as were areas in which the census was continuously estimated only.

The decision to exclude the districts of Arakan and Kyaukpyu was due to a different problem. Their population is, in many senses, atypical of Burma. Much of the population of Arakan is Muslim, which made

TABLE 1.1

Census of Burma (all figures gross and unadjusted)

Date of Census	Population	Approximate Area	Map
15 August 1872	2,747,148	Lower Burma	B
17 February 1881	3,736,771	Lower Burma	B
26 February 1891	7,605,560	excluding Shan states and hill areas	C
1 March 1901	10,490,624	Burma	D
10 March 1911	12,115,217	Burma	E
18 March 1921	13,212,192	Burma	F
24 February 1931	14,667,146	Burma	G
5 March 1941	16,823,798	Burma	–

it difficult to distinguish between Arakanese Muslims and immigrant Indian Muslims in the census records. Also, these two districts formed the main land route for Indian immigrants to enter Burma, and as there was no check or registration of these newcomers, again it is difficult to distinguish the local population from those who were merely "passing through" at the time of the census.

The areas selected for and excluded from this demographic study are shown in Map A. The study area focuses on the more "Burman peoples" and the territory of the country where agriculture, religion and the structure of society are similar. The majority of the people in the study area practice sedentary agriculture, Theravada Buddhism and have a "Burmese" culture. In addition, the census data and vital registration records are better in the study area than in the discarded districts, were administered over a longer period, and are therefore more suitable for longitudinal population studies.

The British administration introduced the census and the vital registration recording into Lower Burma in the mid-nineteenth century. Although there were, to say the least, major problems with these early records, they served as a prototype and example when Burma, and therefore the study area, was reunited in 1886. The fledgling sanitary services, the collection of vital registration data and the census apparatus had to be extended to Upper Burma following its annexation, but they did not have to be built from scratch as the example already existed in Lower Burma.

In 1891, the first census was taken of both Upper and Lower Burma, which means that data, synchronously obtained, is available for most of the study area. There are specific problems with the 1891 census (which will be discussed later in the chapter), but it remains the first census to cover the major lowland centres of population, and thus provides a starting point for comparative study. The later censuses of 1901, 1911, 1921, 1931 and 1941 all provide data of population numbers in the study area, but each contains its own problems, not the least of which is that each census had a different geographical boundary from the preceding one, making comparative calculations difficult.

The 1891 census therefore provided a starting point for comparative, longitudinal studies, but it was felt that if estimations could be added of the earlier nineteenth-century population of Burma, then this would greatly enhance the usefulness of the study. Many of the early European visitors and emissaries to the Burmese Court had made estimates of the population numbers between 1800 and 1860, and recently, historians have added to these calculations. The arguments for examining these are of course that populations do not appear instantly and therefore the processes that influence population change should be seen, if possible, as part of a long-term and continuous process, as well as short-term response to immediate stimuli.

Estimates of the population of nineteenth-century Burma

The population of Burma was a matter of interest and concern to both Europeans and Burmese officials in the nineteenth century. The problem with the estimates they produced is not the quantity but the quality of the data, and the wide variations in the areas enumerated. The quality and value of the estimations ranges from Henry Burney's careful examination of the *sit-tan* records, which produced a figure for the "Burmese Empire" of 4,200,000 in 1787, to Michael Symes' assessment of "the population of the Burman dominions" as 17,000,000 in 1795, which he thought an underestimate.[16]

What did Symes mean when he referred to the "Burman dominions", or Burney, the "Burman Empire"? Other contemporary commentators wrote about the "Kingdom of Burma"[17] and "Burmah Proper",[18] and the British described Lower Burma (excluding Arakan and Mergui) as Martagan and Pegu after 1855. The task for the demographer is to attempt to define the geographical boundaries behind these loose descriptions and then to put the estimates into comparable groups or tables for examination.

TABLE 1.2

Nineteenth-century Estimates of the Population of Greater Burma or the Burman Empire

Year	Source	Population Numbers
1783	Burney	4.2 million
1795	Symes	17 million
1796	Cox	8 million
1826	Alves	4 million
1826	Burney	4.2 million
1855	Yule	3–3.6 million
1891	Census + estimate for excluded areas	8.8 million

Sources: 1783: Burney, "On the Population of the Burman Empire", p. 22; 1795: Symes, *Embassy to the Kingdom of Ava*, pp. 314–5; 1796: Cox, in Yule, *Mission to the Court of Ava*, p. 287; 1826: Alves, in Burney, "On the Population of the Burman Empire", p. 27; ibid., p. 23; 1855: Yule, *Mission to the Court of Ava*, p. 290.

The sources in Table 1.2 refer to "Greater Burma" or the "Burman Empire", which includes the Shan states, Arakan and Tenasserim, and what were termed "the wild tribes". Three of the sources — Burney, Yule and Alves — have produced broadly similar estimates. As they were all largely drawn from the *sit-tan* records assembled by the Burmese kings in 1783 and 1826, this is hardly surprising. The estimates produced by Symes and Cox lack credibility, as they have little statistical basis.

An examination of the sources relating to "Burma Proper" or the "Kingdom of Burma" still leaves the demographer with few viable sources to work with. Burney produced an estimate of the population of "Burma Proper": the area he defined corresponds closely to the area of the 1891 census, with the exception of the Mergui Peninsula and the districts of Arakan and the Upper Chindwin, which are included in the census but do not form part of his "Burma Proper". This therefore looks quite hopeful, certainly more promising than the figures of Father Sangermano, the Italian priest who lived in Ava and Rangoon from 1783 to 1806. Sangermano estimated the population of what he called the "kingdom" of Burma as 2,000,000.[19] However, the kingdom that he described lay between latitudes 19 and 24 degrees north, which is Upper Burma only, approximately from Prome to Katha, and therefore cannot be compared to either Burney's "Burma Proper" or the 1891 census.[20] Another figure for "Burma Proper" is John Crawfurd's, quoted

TABLE 1.3

Estimates of the Nineteenth-century Population of "Burma Proper"

Date	Source	Population Numbers
1783	Burney	2.2 million
1826	Burney	2.3 million
1826	Crawfurd	2.4 million

Sources: 1783: Burney, "On the Population of the Burman Empire", p. 22; 1826: Burney, ibid., p. 23; 1826: Crawfurd, in Yule, *Mission to the Court of Ava*, p. 288.

in Yule, which again is very much in line with Burney's.[21] This leaves only Burney and Crawfurd's estimates for "Burma Proper" (Table 1.3), all of which are taken from the *sit-tan* records.

Before the figures from Table 1.3 are examined and compared to the 1891 census data, one other possible source of information should be considered. The British Administration produced population returns that were published in the annual reports from 1852 onwards. There are major problems with the use of these figures as demographic data and this will be discussed in more detail later in the chapter. Briefly, the two factors that mitigated against the use of this data are that the figures applied to Pegu and Martaban only and excluded the populations of Arakan, Tenasserim and Upper Burma, and also that the data was produced for the British Administration by the village headmen for capitation tax collection. The administration itself admitted considerable under-enumeration,[22] which is hardly surprising, but is discouraging to the demographer.

To summarise the position: there are estimates for the wider Burman Empire, some of which (Burney, Yule, Alves) were based on the *sit-tan* records, and there are estimates for Burma Proper (Burney and Crawfurd) which are also derived from the *sit-tans*. At the opposite end of the nineteenth century, the 1891 census data is available, the area of which is similar to Burma Proper. Can these figures be used to provide acceptable estimates of population numbers and used to calculate rate of change in the nineteenth century, and if so, how much sceptical analysis or smoothing do they require before they can be used?

The data for the beginning of the nineteenth century will be the first to be considered with the major aim of finding acceptable figures for Burma Proper that can be compared to the 1891 census.

Factors that affected population growth from the 1780s to 1826

The figures for 1783 and 1826 (Tables 1.2 and 1.3) need smoothing as this was a turbulent period in Burma's history, including, for example, the wars with Siam (Thailand) and Maha Bandula's wars in Assam and Cochar in 1820. A "successful" war in Southeast Asia was often marked by the seizure of prisoners for resettlement in the victorious country (for example, the deportation of population from Assam and Cochar to Upper Burma),[23] but this apparent population gain was often more than counterbalanced by losses caused directly or indirectly by unsuccessful wars. The Burmese campaigns in Siam in 1785–86 are estimated to have cost Burma the loss of 80,000 men through death, disease and desertion,[24] but even "successful" wars often cause population displacement and disrupt agriculture, and the resulting death and disease remains unquantified. These factors must be taken into account in the calculations of population change.

Unfortunately for the Burmese, there were two other possible causes of crisis mortality during the period 1783 to 1826 — one documented and one that is probability only. In 1805, famine started in the dry zone of Upper Burma; it reached a peak in 1810 and came to a gradual end between 1812 and 1814, having by then affected most of the country. During the famine period, when "many thousands" were said to have starved to death,[25] the military campaigns against the Thais continued, accompanied by forced levies of men and money. The other possible cause of crisis mortality at this time was cholera, which may have reached epidemic form in Burma between 1818 and 1820. The pandemic started in Bengal in 1817 and was documented in Siam by 1820.[26] Given Burma's close physical proximity to the source of the cholera and the fact that the disease had previously been recorded in the country (by Father Sangermano), it is highly unlikely that Burma escaped the pandemic.[27]

This discussion has suggested that between 1783 and 1826, the Burmese population suffered the depredations of war, famine and disease. Any analysis of population data for that period must also take into account the probable reaction of the Burmese people to this series of crises. The traditional response of the Burmese to heavy demands by the kings for military or crown services was to move away, to become part of an uncontrolled floating population.[28] William Koenig describes the formation of a considerable displaced population by the end of the eighteenth century and the beginning of the nineteenth.[29] This floating population traditionally included necromancers, tattooers, wizards and bandits, and as such would have been beyond the reach of crown services, tax assessments or the *sit-tans*. When Burney did his population calculations for 1783 and 1826, he added an extra ten per cent to the totals to allow for the tradition of under-reporting by the *thugyis*, or headmen, to decrease the tax base.[30] But when the evidence for war, famine, disease and the probable response of the population to these disasters is considered, this addition of ten per cent may be considered too low.

This probability of population moving away from government control may help to explain an apparent anomaly in Burney's figures. He estimated that the population of Greater Burma was 4.2 million and that of Burma Proper 2.2 million, thus locating nearly half the population in the Shan Plateau and upland and mountain areas. It would seem unlikely that this was a normal state of affairs and if these figures are compared, for example to the 1901 census (which records 9 million in the lowlands and 1.5 million in the hills), they would seem improbable. Admittedly the census data is separated from Burney's figures by one hundred years of agricultural development, but even so, the disparity would suggest either under-enumeration in the *sit-tan* lowland areas or a major movement of population away from crown control to the less disturbed hill areas. Koenig referred to a downward demographic trend in the rice-growing centres in Upper Burma,[31] which perhaps may be partly explained by Burney's figures.

The evidence so far would suggest that Burney's figures are both too low, and that the division of population between the hills and lowland areas may be wrong. But instead of discarding these estimates, it might be rational to "smooth" them by adjusting the proportion of the population located in hill and lowland areas. Burney's estimate for Greater Burma put two million of the 4.2 million total population in the hill areas, but given the likelihood of temporary movement to escape famine, war, disease and crown control, it could be suggested that at least one million of this hill population belonged to Burma Proper in more peaceful times. This would suggest an approximate, and probably still underestimated, figure for Burma Proper of 3.3 million at the beginning of the nineteenth century.

It would be helpful if this figure of 3.3 million could be chronologically located or periodised with slightly more precision. Can this be done? Burney's estimates were for 1783 and 1826, based on the *sit-tans* of those dates. Burney noted that the *sit-tan* figures for 1826 showed an increase in the population of "Burma Proper" of only 42,662 from 1783, whereas his estimates from those records put the increase at 100,000, still a slow rate of growth. His explanation for the low growth recorded by the Burmese officials was the unwillingness of provincial officers to report an increase in population, as this would increase their taxable assessment. However, given the probability of

TABLE 1.4
Lower Burma: Selected Population Returns

Date	Population Numbers
1852	718,000
1859	948,731
1864	1,350,989

Sources: 1852: Furnivall, *Colonial Policy and Practice* (1948), p. 59; 1859 and 1864: Economic and Social Board, *A Study of the Economic and Social History of Burma* (1957), p. 5.

high crisis mortality in this period, the rate of population growth may well have been very low or nil. This would suggest that the estimate of 3.3 million for Burma Proper could be appropriate for 1826 and could be used as a starting point for comparison with other nineteenth-century data.

Reliability of population information for nineteenth-century Burma

For the period 1826 to 1900, there are four possible sources of population information: the tax returns from Lower Burma mentioned previously, and three censuses — 1872, 1881 and 1891. Of these sources, only the 1891 census was used in this study, as the quality of the other data and difficulties in using them could not be overcome with any confidence. The reasons for discarding the tax returns and the censuses of 1872 and 1881 will be briefly discussed before an examination is made of the evidence from the 1891 census. The tax returns referred to were population figures contained in the annual reports published by the British Administration from 1852. As mentioned previously, they applied only to Lower Burma, that is, Pegu and Martaban, and excluded Arakan and Tenasserim. Table 1.4 shows extracts from the reports for selected years.

The critical issue is, can any value be put on this data even for the restricted area? The answer would appear to be no. There are good reasons for regarding these figures as gross underestimates of the population. Arthur Phayre, the Commissioner of Pegu, was the most notable of the British administrators who regarded the figures with

scepticism.[32] The population returns were produced for the administration by the local village headmen, who routinely under-reported the
number of tax payers in their circles. This not only protected the people
from the capitation tax, but also provided the headmen with an income
in the form of bribery and gifts. This practice was deeply rooted and
survived the changes imposed by the colonial government. A report of
1899 stated that "a comparison of cropped area totals compiled by
regular settlement officers and local *thugyis* in the Thongwa District
revealed that the latter had under-reported by as much as 75%."[33]

If Burmese headmen under-reported, it was also common for
urbanised Europeans to underestimate peasant populations. Kingsley
Davis described it as a "universal tendency", and further pointed out
that as the figures improved in accuracy, a false impression of rapid
population growth was given.[34] The truth of this was admitted in the
Annual Report of 1864/65, which stated that the recorded population
increase from 948,731 in 1859 to 1,350,989 in 1864 (an incredible 42.4 per
cent) "was mainly due to the increased accuracy of the Returns and
more especially as regards children under ten years of age."[35] It would
seem impossible therefore to unravel this data from underestimation
and illusory population growth rates.[36]

The other major factor in the decision to discard the figures from
these annual reports relates to their restricted geographical area. The
boundary between Pegu and Martaban and the independent Kingdom
of Upper Burma, known as the Allan Line, was not closed. There was
constant ebb and flow of population across the border, and the British
in fact encouraged this movement, as they wanted new settlers to take
up land in Lower Burma. Ideally, the whole area (Lower and Upper
Burma) should be considered as one unit, thus overcoming the problem
of this internal migration. Unfortunately there is no matching data from
the Kingdom. The only way in which corresponding figures for Upper
Burma could be produced is by retrospective calculation from the 1891
census to produce a population figure for 1852. It was decided that this
was too subjective an estimate to be justifiable, so these figures from the
annual reports were noted but discarded.

The censuses of 1872 and 1881 were rejected for very similar
reasons. Upper Burma was not annexed until 1886, and so the two
censuses apply to Lower Burma only; therefore the same problems of
assessing an unquantified internal migration apply. Both censuses
also suffered from under-enumeration, probably to a high degree, but
again unmeasured. This is discussed in more detail later in the chapter
under "The Census as a Source of Demographic Data in Burma".

Discarding the data from the 1852 to 1865 annual reports and the
censuses of 1872 and 1881 leaves no population figures for Burma

Proper or the study area between the estimates for 1826 and the 1891 census figures. However, if the 1891 census could be viewed with some confidence, then it would still be possible to produce an estimate of population change in nineteenth-century Burma. How accurate was the 1891 census? What was the historical background to the enumeration?

Upper Burma was annexed in 1886, and the 1891 census was therefore the first to cover both Upper and Lower Burma. However, the fighting that preceded and followed the annexation required a force of troops and military police whose numbers eventually rose to over 40,000. Many districts, including Yamethin, Katha, Mandalay and the Ruby Mines, were violently disturbed until 1890. In Thayetmyo district, the resistance continued until 1892. The British response to this included the enforcement of the Upper Burma Village Regulations of 1887, which held the village and community responsible for crimes committed within their tract, and permitted movement of whole villages where the authorities decreed it necessary.[37]

The accuracy of the 1891 census must have been affected by this continuing violence and displacement of population, especially in those districts containing or bordering hill country, which was the ideal cover for Burmese guerrillas. The problem though is to try to assess how much higher the under-enumeration of 1891 was compared to the under-enumeration of later censuses; that is, if the degree of miscount was constant, then this would not affect a calculation of population change. A very conservative estimate of this excess under-enumeration might be five per cent, but this is subjective and may well be too low.[38]

Before any adjustment is made to the 1891 census figure for under-estimation, its geographical area should be considered. What this study requires is a census area that is the same as the defined study area, or Burma Proper, so that the population can be compared to the estimate, already obtained, for 1826. In order to achieve that, the combined census populations of the north Arakan, Kyaukpyu, Akyab, Mergui, Tavoy, Amherst and the Upper Chindwin districts (1,250,000) were deducted from the census total of 7,600,000. (No attempt was made in 1891 to enumerate the Shan Plateau or the hill areas.) When these district totals are deducted from the census total, the resulting figure is 6,350,000 for the defined study area. When the absolute minimum of an additional five per cent for under-enumeration is added, then the total is 6,667,500.

The objective of this section of Chapter One was to obtain estimates of the population of nineteenth-century Burma and this has now been achieved for the study area. An estimate of 3.3 million derived from Burney's figures has been accepted for the period 1783 to 1826, assuming a nil or very low growth rate in the intervening period, and there is now an acceptable population estimate for 1891 of 6.6 million, a figure derived from the census. This would produce an average rate of increase per annum (from 1826 to 1891) of just over one per cent (1.07 per cent).

Comparing estimates with those of adjacent countries

Does Burma's average rate of increase seem likely or attainable? The probability of such a growth rate happening in Burma in the nineteenth century can be critically examined in two ways: firstly by considering the history of the area in that period, and secondly by comparing this growth rate to the experience of adjacent countries.

The history of Burma between 1826 and 1891 would suggest that this was an attainable rate of increase. The direct losses from the three Britain–Burma wars do not appear to have been high, although allowance must be made for indirect losses due to dislocation of the population and the destruction of some villages. Albert Fytch, when Deputy Commissioner of Bassein, described the destruction of houses by rebel forces in 1853, and the appointment of a headman "to call the people in from the jungle and settle them down on the old sites of their villages."[39] Despite the wars and the upheavals at the Burmese Court between 1826 and 1853, it seems probable that the Burmese agriculturalist was prospering mildly as there were no major climatic catastrophes in this period. Adas has charted an early and gradual expansion of Burmese agriculture in the delta, and he estimated that 700,000 to 800,000 acres there were under wet-rice cultivation before the British annexation of Pegu in 1852.[40] This desire to migrate and take up new land can be an indicator of population growth, particularly in the absence of the sort of catastrophic events that hindered population growth between 1783 and 1826.

How does the estimated one per cent growth rate for a 65-year period compare to the experience of adjacent countries? Table 1.5 suggests that Burma's estimate is comparable to the existing estimates for the neighbouring countries. All the countries in the table, with the exception of India, show accelerating rates of population growth by the end of the nineteenth century. There are, of course, individual differences; for example, a mortality crisis in the Philippines lowered the rate of growth by 0.3 per cent in the last quarter of the nineteenth century, but even so it remained above the estimate for Burma. However, an acceptance of these different experiences does not alter the overall picture — most of the Southeast Asian countries and Ceylon achieved sustained population growth in the second half of the nineteenth century. To suggest, therefore, that the population of Burma grew at an average rate of one per cent per annum for 65 years is not inconsistent with the

TABLE 1.5

Nineteenth-century Population of South and Southeast Asia

Country	Period and Percentage Growth Rate Per Annum		
Burma	1783–1826 0.0%	1826–1891 1.0%	
Philippines	1591–1817 0.54%	1817–1876 1.54%	1876–1903 1.23%
Malay Peninsula		1830–1900 1.0%	
Java (Peper)		1800–1850 0.5–1.0%	1850–1900 1.55%
Java (Breman)		1800–1850 1.4%	1850–1900 1.7%
Siam		1800–1850 0.05–0.15%	1850–1900 0.2–0.95%
Ceylon		1800–1850 0.5%	1850–1900 1.15%
Indian Sub-Cont.		1800–1850 0.4%	1850–1900 0.43%

Sources: Philippines: Smith and Ng, "The Components of Population Change in Nineteenth-century South-east Asia", p. 241; Malay Peninsula: Dodge, "Population Estimates for the Malay Peninsula in the Nineteenth Century, pp. 453–4; Java: Breman, *Java: Population Growth and Demographic Structure*, p. 302; Java: Peper, "Population Growth in Java in the Nineteenth Century", p. 84; Siam: Sternstein, "The Growth of the World's Pre-eminent 'Primate City'", p. 57; Ceylon: McEvedy and Jones, *Atlas of World Population History*, p. 189; Indian Sub-Cont.: McEvedy and Jones, *Atlas of World Population History*, p. 185.

more general Southeast Asian experience. But it must be emphasised that this was an average rate, and almost certainly not a constant rate.

The population numbers and growth rates estimated for the nineteenth century can now be used as a basis for the more detailed study of the population dynamics between 1891 and 1941. A census was taken in Burma every ten years from 1891, and this material must therefore be a major demographic source.

The census as a source of demographic data in Burma

The census and its importance have already been referred to in "The Study Area" section of this chapter. In this section, an attempt will be made to analyse and evaluate the significance and accuracy of the Burma census for the purpose of this study.

Colonial Burma was ruled by the British as a province of India until the passing of the Government of India Act of 1935. As a province, Burma was included in the Census of India up to and including 1931.

In 1941, an independent Census of Burma was held. This means that a large volume of demographic data exists, as six censuses — from 1891 to 1941 — covered, at a minimum, the study area.

Unfortunately nothing in the study of Burmese historical demography is either simple or straightforward. A closer inspection of the census records reveals major difficulties with each individual census and their comparability with each other. In this section, an analysis will be made of the problems within the records, and this will be followed by three further sections in which data smoothing and calculation is attempted.

The major problems identified for examination include the changing calendar dates of the census and the changes in the geographical areas of the census, which involved both the external and the internal boundaries. The variations and fluctuations in the methods of enumeration used caused great difficulties — some were synchronous, some non-synchronous and in some areas, estimates were used. Another major difficulty that was easily identified but not easily solved was that of migration; there was seasonal migration, internal permanent migration, and of course the massive in-migration from India that could be seasonal, permanent or semi-permanent. Probably the simplest way to examine these problems will be to look at them in turn as a difficulty common to more than one census, rather than somewhat laboriously examine each census in turn. A map series has been included to assist with area and district location.

Before looking at these common problems, it would perhaps be as well to identify an issue that fortunately only arose with the 1941 census; namely, the loss of all the records and data except a single sheet that shows the provisional totals of houses, and numbers of males and females by district only. All the other texts of what was originally a full census were lost in the debacle of the British retreat from the Japanese in 1942. The details of age, for example, so important to a demographer, are gone.

Shifted boundaries and re-assigned districts

When geographical areas and boundaries are changed from census to census, they can make comparative studies almost impossible. No two Burmese censuses covered quite the same geographical area, so direct comparison of population from one census to another was impossible without adjustment of the data. This often required information that was not included in the census. The degree of change on the external boundaries varied, but as a general rule, each census involved an extension of the area surveyed, reflecting what Norman Owen described

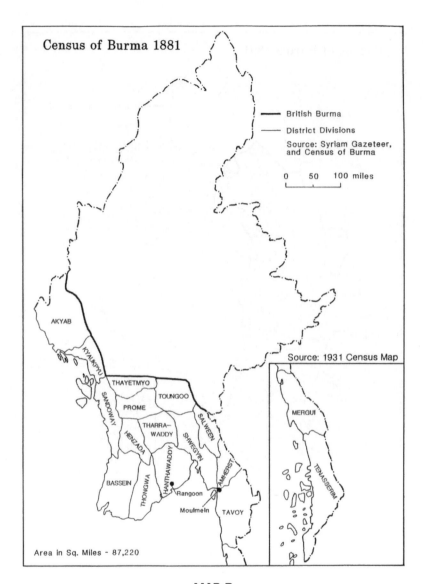

MAP B

as the "administrative migration" of the colonial power.[41] The most extreme example of this is the limitation of the 1872 and 1881 censuses to Lower Burma, and its extension in 1891 to include Upper Burma. This administrative migration is illustrated by the series of Maps B to G, from which it can be seen, for example, that the 1901 census was the first to include most of the Shan states, but that areas in the north and

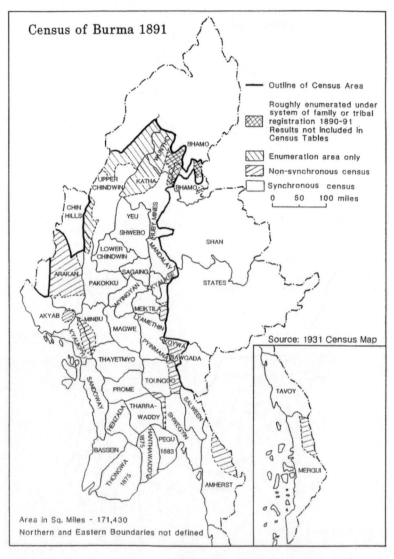

MAP C

east of Burma were omitted. Further reference to the map series will show that the boundaries of these omitted areas were not constant in the subsequent censuses, and that the area enumerated also sometimes shrank and sometimes expanded.

Minor fluctuations of the external boundaries also took place in the south of Burma. For example, in 1921, a full census of the Coco Islands,

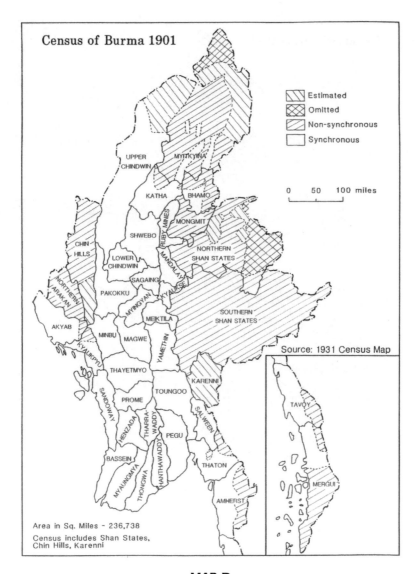

MAP D

part of the Hanthawaddy district, took place for the first time and 46 people were recorded. But in 1941, the boat-living Salons of the Mergui district were omitted from the census although they had been included in 1931. Possibly the Salons were forgotten by a hard-pressed official.

One boundary change that cannot be identified by the map series appeared in the 1931 census. This was the recalculation of the area of

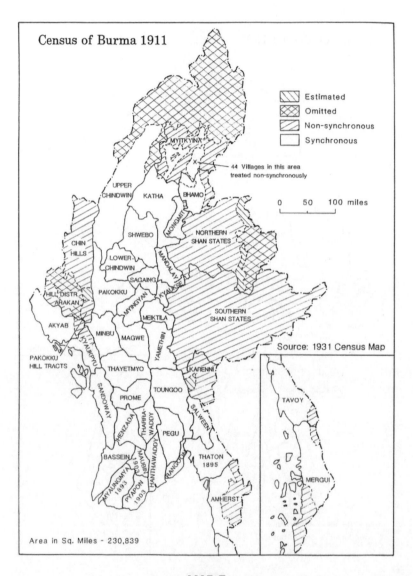

MAP E

all states, districts, townships and tracts, with the result that, in many
cases, the areas shown in the 1931 census were inconsistent with the
areas shown in previous censuses. In some cases, boundary fluctuation
was caused by the considerable natural force of river erosion.

These were relatively minor internal boundary changes compared
to the constant alterations to the administrative units of districts and

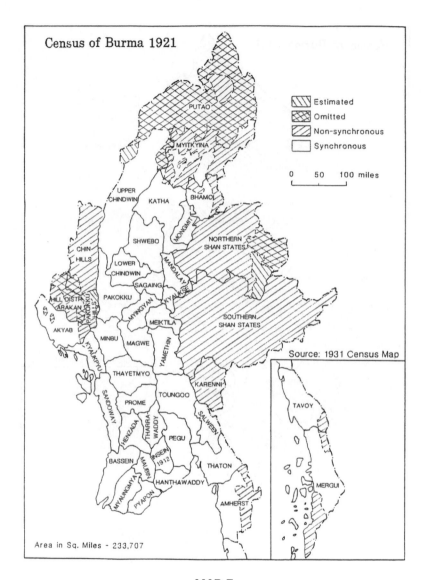

Census of Burma 1921

Estimated
Omitted
Non-synchronous
Synchronous

0   50   100 miles

PUTAO

MYITKYINA

UPPER
CHINDWIN   KATHA   BHAMO

CHIN
HILLS   SHWEBO   MONGMIT   NORTHERN
SHAN STATES

LOWER
CHINDWIN

SAGAING

HILL DISTR   PAKOKKU   MANDALAY   KYAUKSE

ARAKAN

AKYAB   MINBU   MYINGYAN

MEIKTILA   SOUTHERN
SHAN STATES

MAGWE   YAMETHIN

Source: 1931 Census Map

KYAUKPYU   THAYETMYO

KARENNI

SANDOWAY   PROME   TOUNGOO   TAVOY

THARRA
WADDY

HENZADA   SALWEEN

PEGU

INSEIN
1912

BASSEIN   MAUBIN   THATON

MYAUNGMYA   PYAPON   HANTHAWADDY   MERGUI

AMHERST

Area in Sq. Miles - 233,707

MAP F

townships by the colonial government. Most of these changes were in
response to the steady growth of the population, especially in the delta.
As a result, densely populated districts were sub-divided and new
districts formed. A clear example of the multiplication of districts can
be seen by comparing Map B to Maps F and G: where three districts
existed in the delta in 1881, there were six in 1921. This type of boundary

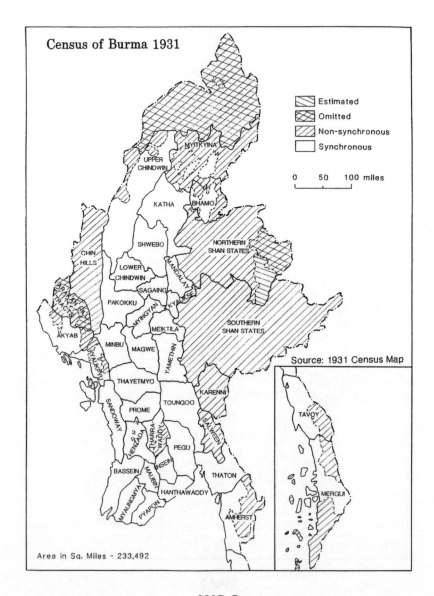

MAP G

change involved the sub-division of districts and the transfer of village tracts and townships, and unfortunately, it was often poorly recorded by the administration. The paucity of these records is most apparent prior to 1900, and the following quotation from the 1881 Census report shows what difficulty the census officials had in trying to trace and confirm detailed boundary alterations between the 1872 and 1881 censuses. (Comparisons were also rendered more difficult by the changes in the Romanisation of place names.)

> The only important changes in the areas of districts which have been made since the Census of 1872 and call for present notice, are the formation in 1875–6 of the Thongwa District from portions of the Bassein, Henzada and Rangoon Districts and the re-erection of Tharrawaddy into a District in 1878 by separation from Henzada with which it had been combined in 1862. In the year 1880 the towns of Rangoon and Moulmein were detached from the surrounding areas and constituted distinct districts. The remainder of the Rangoon District, from which the town was separated, received the title of Hanthawaddy. A few minor changes of area may hereafter require notice, but the want of records of the details of the previous census make it impossible, except in the case of Bassein, to ascertain what was the population in 1872 of the areas which have since been transferred from one district to another, or to effect accurate comparisons in all cases between the populations of 1872 and 1881.

> *Census of British Burma 1881, Report, Vol. 1*, p. 18

The quotation is also useful in demonstrating the complexity of many of the changes that occurred. In a nine-year period, Thongwa was formed from portions of three other districts, and four other major changes occurred to the delta, along with minor changes that the census officials said were insufficiently recorded.

This 1881 census report is also very interesting when considered in conjunction with the report of the 1901 census. In the latter, the administration introduced retrospective adjustment to district population figures published in a previous census, or as they described it, "for changes of jurisdiction so as to show the population, at those dates, of the various Provinces and States as now constituted."[42] If the Census Commissioner had found these boundary changes so poorly recorded in 1881 that he could not make comparisons with 1872, it is difficult to regard as credible adjustments made in 1901 to figures from earlier censuses. The problem of these retrospective adjustments of population can be illustrated by a brief examination of one delta district, Maubin.

Maubin was created as an autonomous district in 1903, when Thongwa district was divided to form two new districts, Maubin and Pyapon. Prior to 1875, Thongwa did not exist but was part of the districts of Rangoon and Henzada. In 1893, the 18-year-old district of Thongwa was itself divided into the two districts, Myaungmya and Thongwa.[43] Therefore Maubin district was formed as the result of four sub-divisions and mergers of districts in a period of 28 years.

In addition to these major changes to Maubin, there were many minor adjustments of territory. For example, when the district was divided in 1903, Kyaiklat township was one of four townships made part of the new Pyapon district, but 22 villages from Kyaiklat were transferred to Maubin township in the Maubin district. At the same time, the Pantanaw township was transferred from Myaungmya district to Maubin district.[44] A further complication is the statement in the 1912 *Burma Gazetteer, Vol. B, Myaungmya District* that 23.09 square miles were transferred from the Einme township of Myaungmya district to Maubin district, a change that is not confirmed by the corresponding *Gazetteer* of Maubin district.[45] Between 1916 and 1918, there were three more transfers of *kwins* across the borders of Myaungmya and Maubin districts, and further transfers of land and population between Myaungmya and Thongwa districts due to river action.[46]

This is a brief history of the boundaries of one delta district, but the complexity of the changes is not unusual. These transfers do, however, suggest that the retrospective adjustments to district populations made by the census officials from 1901 should be treated with extreme caution. On a wider scale, they also illustrate the difficulties demographers face when attempting to use the data for Lower Burma for comparative or longitudinal studies. Unfortunately, these are not the only problems that complicate the analysis of the census; the methodology and effectiveness of the enumeration must also be examined.

Counting heads and making guesstimates

The data for the census in Burma was usually collected synchronously; however, where the administration was over-stretched, the census often took the form of a simple enumeration over a period of a week. In some areas of the country, the population was merely estimated. For example, in the 1901 census, parts of the Upper Chindwin, Pakokku, Bhamo and Myitkyina districts were estimated on the basis of what was thought to be a typical household. This meant that in the Upper Chindwin district, some areas had a synchronous census, some had a non-synchronous one and some areas were estimated, thus making the district totals and comparisons with the 1891 and 1911 censuses suspect.[47]

These problems run right through the census series and were not confined to the hill or rural areas. The report of the 1872 census includes a vivid description of the difficulties the administrators met in Rangoon. The accuracy of the census was undermined by the reluctance of those sections of the Rangoon population termed "coolie classes" to be enumerated. The town magistrate complained of "great want of legal authority" and also that the police had to force entrance to barracks and lodging houses "so dark within" that the accuracy of the count must have been jeopardised. Furthermore, the police and the enumerators were then sent around the town over a period of a week to check the figures.[48] These extended activities took place within a nominally synchronous census.

Nearly 50 years later, the administration was again in difficulty in Lower Burma, this time in the districts of Henzada and Tharrawaddy. In 1931, parts of these districts were subject to a non-synchronous census due to the Saya San Rebellion. Other districts such as Pegu, Pyapon, Insein, Prome and Thayetmyo were also considerably disturbed, with a high probability that the accuracy of the census was damaged in those districts as well.

This discussion of enumeration has focused so far on the methodology used, but the major area of concern is, of course, the accuracy of the final published results. The concern about methodology is only that the most accurate enumerations would probably come from a synchronous census. The historical demographer has no means of making post-enumeration surveys to check the accuracy of the original data,[49] but has to rely on verification through such methods as comparison of data from census to census and consideration of other historical information. How much confidence can be placed in the figures produced by the census series as to the accuracy of the enumeration?

This question has already been partly answered at least. Some general statements can be made: the accuracy of the census probably improved through time as the administration established more thorough control of Burma and became more practised and experienced at the organisation involved. But this assessment also depends on historical factors such as the Saya San Rebellion (1930–32), and the resistance to annexation, which affected the 1891 census. Inaccuracy has a two-fold effect: it obviously distorts population numbers; perhaps more importantly, if it is not constant from census to census, it affects comparative calculation and therefore assessment of population dynamics.

It was suggested earlier in the chapter that a very modest additional five per cent should be added to the population totals for 1891 to allow for under-enumeration. The invasion of Upper Burma occurred in 1885, and the formal annexation was announced on 1 January 1886, but the subsequent guerrilla war lasted, even in parts of the central districts, for six years. Its duration depended on the suitability of the terrain for guerrilla activity and local leadership. The author of the Mandalay *Gazetteer*, H. F. Searle described the "wild" southeast sector of the Mandalay district as troubled in 1890,[50] just prior to the census, and conditions were still described as "abnormal" in 1892.[51]

The unrest was not confined to Mandalay district, but was "a nation wide reaction against foreign rule".[52] It is possible that some of the population might have taken refuge from the military activity by moving to the hills, a traditional response which would have left them outside the 1891 census area. If the population had then moved back and were enumerated in 1901, then this would contribute to an artificially high rate of increase in the ten-year inter-censal period. In some areas, their return was just prior to or coincidental with the census; in the Lower Chindwin district, the population was noted to be returning in the 1890/91 period: "it is an illustration of the rapidity with which population returned after the troubled times of the annexation that the collections from the tax rose for the whole district in that year."[53]

These problems with the 1891 census can only be noted at this stage, but the 1872 census will be firmly discarded due to obvious and gross under-enumeration. It was exceptional in the census series in that the published numbers were based on lists prepared for the annual capitation tax returns, to which the "floating population and others not affected by the capitation tax" were supposedly added.[54] The inadequacy of this arrangement led to the situation commented on by H. L. Eales, the author of the 1891 Census report, who noted that the number of Karens had apparently increased by 56 per cent between 1872 and the next census of 1881! Some acknowledgement of the under-enumeration was conceded in the 1872 Census report, with an admission that the tax returns had been accepted as a census in the Shwegyin and Tenasserim districts, and that in the Karen part of the Amherst district, the census return was actually 2,708 less than the 1872 tax return,[55] a considerable feat given the admitted under-reporting of taxable populations.

Moving dates and migrating people

The 1872 census was also "the odd one out" in terms of the date and season of enumeration, as it was held on 15 August in the wet season. All the other censuses were held in February and March. Unfortunately for the demographer, the dates were not constant but progressed from 17 February in 1881 to 18 March in 1921, and back to 24 February in 1931 (Table 1.1). The 1872 census has already been discarded from this study, so in many ways the specific change of date and season by 1881 is not important, but it can be used to demonstrate the importance of date and seasonality. Two comments from the 1881 Census report will highlight this. The increase in the number of Shans recorded in 1881 was due to the change of the census date, as the Shans come to the lowlands in the dry season to trade, and were thus temporary migrants. The second point was that the 1881 census must have included an estimated 80,000 temporary migrants from Lower Burma and India who were seasonal workers, and therefore unlikely to be in Lower Burma for an August census.

The shift of the census dates mentioned above, from 17 February in 1881 to 18 March in 1921, has a particular significance for the historical demographer of Burma. The success of the agricultural economy of Lower Burma depended to a large extent upon seasonal labour from Upper Burma.[56] These migrant labourers usually returned to their homes in Upper Burma during February or March, but the precise date would obviously vary slightly from year to year as the weather, and therefore crop growths, fluctuated. The "migration" of the census dates also from February to March and back to February means that the number of workers (enumerated) in transit must also have varied from year to year.

The original extent and then the gradual decline of seasonal or permanent migration is shown in Table 1.6, which gives the numbers

TABLE 1.6

Persons enumerated in Lower Burma whose Birthplace was the Dry Zone (by district of origin)

	1		2		3		4		5	
District	1891	%	1901	%	1911	%	1921	%	1931	%
Mandalay	75,171	20	55,000	15	33,000	12	20,000	10	13,000	9
Shwebo	21,820	9	34,000	10	25,000	9	17,000	8	11,000	8
Sagaing	18,583	8	22,000	6	18,000	6	13,000	6+	8,000	6
L Chindwin	26,505	11	28,000	8	2,000	7	12,000	6	9,000	6
Myingyan	43,452	12	44,000	12	33,000	12	21,000	11	16,000	12
Pakokku	31,758	10	34,000	10	26,000	9	18,000	8+	12,000	9
Minbu	41,554	19	44,000	12	28,000	10	15,000	7	8,000	6
Magwe	23,332	11	29,000	8	21,000	7	22,000	10	13,000	9
Kyaukse	2,662	2	3,000	1	1,000	−1	1,000	−1	800	−1
Meiktila	14,399	7	23,000	6	28,000	10	25,000	12	19,000	14
Yamethin	18,889	2	5,000	2	22,000	8	19,000	9	14,000	10
Thayetmyo			34,000	10	28,000	10	23,000	11	14,000	10

Sources: Col. 1: *Census of Burma, Report*, p. 181; Cols. 2, 3, 4 and 5: Adas, "Agrarian Development in the Plural Society", p. 323.

of those enumerated in the censuses in Lower Burma. No distinction
was made in the census series between temporary or seasonal migrants
and settled or permanent migrants, so it is not possible to retrospectively
assign the seasonal migrants to a district of permanent settlement. This
factor complicates the calculations of population in Upper Burma as
well as the delta, as a considerable seasonal flow of labour was necessary
for the agriculture of the dry zone and the northern wet zone. Such
large numbers of people were involved in this migration (over 186,000
from Mandalay district alone between 1891 and 1931) that it is almost
impossible to calculate the "natural" decline or increase in population
in the districts of Upper or Lower Burma.

Some of the intricacies of the internal migration, particularly within
the delta, have been documented by Adas. The migration flow chart,
Figure 1.1, is intended to add to this information by showing the
seasonal migration within and from Upper Burma. The district box
sizes are proportional to the district populations in the census of 1891,
and the arrows to the delta indicate the percentage of the migrants in
1891. The small arrows plot some of the intricate inter-district flow and
counter-flow of migrants in Upper Burma.

Migration shows most readily in the census tables as imbalances in
the sex ratios of districts, as the majority of migrant workers were adult
males. This can be seen, for example, in the Lower Chindwin district,
where a surplus of 29,597 females was recorded in 1891. The problem
in using these figures in a definitive way is, of course, the lack of
information on whether the imbalance was due to permanent or
temporary migration and the additional problem of whether indeed the
sex ratios were also affected by the moving census dates.

The complexity and volume of the internal migration therefore
makes it difficult to estimate distinct population figures in terms of
overall numbers or changes, particularly in Mandalay, Minbu and
Myingyan districts from 1891 to 1911. However, as most of this internal
migration took place within the defined study area, then in terms of the
total population of the territory, it is not a major problem.

Of far more significance to the analysis and interpretation of the
census in Burma than the internal migration was the Indian immigration.
This exogenous migration was encouraged by the colonial government
and had, by 1931, added more than one million to the population
numbers in Burma. Although, due to the large numbers, it was obviously
essential to extract these immigrants from the Burmese population in
the study, it was not simple.

One reason was that until the 1921 census, the Indian population
was classified by religion and not nationality, although attempts were
made from 1881 to 1911 to record the number of inhabitants of Burma

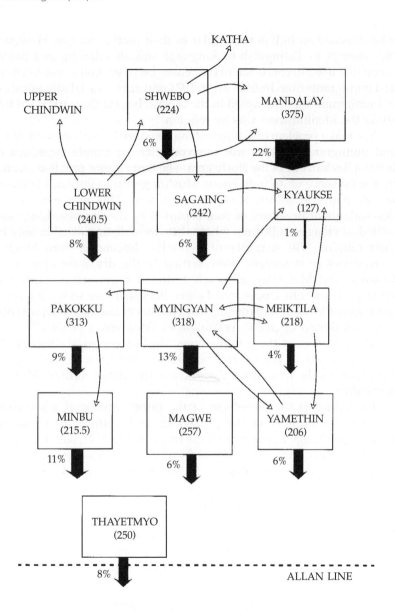

FIGURE 1.1

Migration Flow Chart

Details of district populations in 1891 (in 1,000s), flow of migration within Upper Burma districts and the percentage of migrants born in Upper Burma but enumerated in Lower Burma, by district of origin.

Sources: *Census of Burma 1891.*

who returned an Indian vernacular as their mother tongue. However, this attempt to distinguish by language was also flawed, and Baxter noted that it led to confusion in the census between Arakanese Muslims and immigrants from India.[57] From 1921 onwards, a racial identification of immigrants was attempted in the census, but for the purpose of this study the identification was by religion.

The major problem of distinguishing between the Arakanese Muslims and immigrant Muslims was overcome by the simple expedient of leaving Arakan out of the study area. The more minor problem created by the presence of an indigenous Muslim group in Burma, known as the Zerbadis Muslims, was not overcome. This group were the descendants of prisoners of war, captured by the Burmese kings and settled in villages in Burma, where they were distinguishable only by their religion. The majority of Zerbadis, descended from Moghul mercenaries or Assamese, were settled in the dry zone districts of Kyaukse and Mandalay, although scattered communities existed in other parts of both Upper and Lower Burma. There were also some more recent Muslim settlements, descendants of the forced deportation to Upper Burma of 20,000 Arakanese by Bodawpaya in 1784.[58]

The numbers of these indigenous Muslim groups are thought to be insignificant in the overall population dynamics, so no attempt has been made to extract them from the major Indian Muslim community.

In evaluating the usefulness of the Burma census as a source to calculate the number of the population in the study area and the percentage change in those numbers from 1891 to 1941, so far we have identified three areas of major difficulty — the changes to district boundaries and census areas, the Indian migration, and doubts about the accuracy of the enumeration. Given the lack of alternative data, it was decided that the way forward was to try to overcome these specific difficulties and "smooth" the census data as far as possible. To simplify this, and because the problems in Upper and Lower Burma were not the same, the two territories are discussed separately but with the common aim of overcoming the problems outlined.

Estimates of population in Upper Burma 1891–1941

The priority for Upper Burma was to establish an outer boundary of the study area within which the population would be directly comparable census by census (see Maps B to G). This outer boundary was made up of district boundaries, so those two problems will be discussed together. The enumeration and the different way in which it was accomplished in some areas form part of the boundary discussions, as areas were sometimes excluded from the census. The effects of migration will therefore be considered after the boundaries.

Establishing boundaries and mapping population transfers

The southwestern corner of Upper Burma is formed by Thayetmyo district. Prior to the annexation of the Kingdom of Ava by the British in 1885, Thayetmyo had been divided by the Allan Line, with the southern part belonging to British Burma and the northern part under the jurisdiction of the Burmese kingdom. After the annexation of Upper Burma, the two parts of the district were reunited and the external boundaries remained unaltered from 1887 to 1941.

North from Thayetmyo district, the western boundary of Minbu district formed the outer edge of the study area: no alterations have been found to this boundary between 1891 and 1941. The district of Pakokku lay north of Minbu and provided a long western boundary to the study area, forming a 'finger' into the Upper Chindwin district. The Pakokku hill tracts, which lay to the west of the district, were severed administratively from the main district in 1897–98, were not included in the 1891 census and therefore do not impinge on the boundary of the study area.

The northwestern boundary of the Lower Chindwin district, which formed part of the boundary of the study area, was demarcated in 1888 when the huge Chindwin region was divided into Upper and Lower districts. This part of the district boundary remained constant through the census series, although the accuracy of the population figure for 1891 is questionable, as it was not until 1890–91 that the area known as the Kani Governorship (which formed almost two-thirds of the total area) was brought under the civil administration.

The northernmost and northeast boundaries of the study area were formed by the districts of Shwebo and Katha. Shwebo was constituted in 1895, when the two districts of Ye-u and Shwebo were amalgamated. A slight alteration to the northern boundary of the district, and therefore the study area, was made in August 1891, when a part of the Wuntho state was incorporated into the Katha district. This probably accounts for the discrepancy in the census figures, which show in the 1892 "General Table for the British Provinces and Feudatory States" a figure of 227,804[59] and in the 1901 Upper Burma volume, a figure of 230,779.[60] The larger figure has been accepted as a retrospective adjustment, and is in fact confirmed by the *Burma Gazetteer, Volume B, Shwebo District* (1906).

However the 1891 figure should be regarded with some reservations, due to the post-annexation turmoil in the district, as well as the boundary adjustment. Unrest was admitted to extend to 1890, and the extent may partly be judged by the size of the force (3,520 men) that attacked the town of Taze on 12 June 1886, four years previously.[61]

The Katha district, which forms the northern loop and part of the eastern boundary of the study area, was annexed by the British in 1886 and was originally known as Myadaung. On 15 November 1920, it was amalgamated with Ruby Mines district, which lay to its south between the Shwebo district and the Northern Shan states. To simplify the calculations of population change, the two districts have been treated as one unit throughout the census series.

To the northeast of Katha district lies the area commonly known as the Wuntho Shan state, which forms, in theory, part of the boundary of the study area. It was, however, excluded from the calculations of population change because, although incorporated into Katha district in 1891, Wuntho was not included in the census of that year due to military operations. The population of the Wuntho state was identified in the census figures up to and including 1931, and was therefore easily deducted from the district total. The 1941 population for Katha district, less the Wuntho state, was calculated by assuming that the population change between 1931 and 1941 had been constant over the whole district, and therefore the population in the Wuntho state had grown at the same rate as the rest of the district of Katha; that is, at 1.35 per cent per annum for ten years. The population of the Wuntho state in 1931 was 97,688: when compounded by 1.35 per cent per annum for ten years this gives an estimated figure for 1941 of 111,706. This figure was then deducted from the inclusive figure given for Katha district in 1941 to find the net figure, which was comparable to the previous census.

The other alteration in the Katha district boundaries that affected the study area was a transfer of land comprising most of the Kachin hill tract to the Myitkyina district (which lies outside the study area). This administrative transfer took place between the censuses of 1921 and 1931, and involved (in 1931) a population of 21,762, which was added back to the 1931 census population for the study area. To find the comparable 1941 figure for the Katha district, the 1931 figure of 21,762 was compounded by 1.35 per cent per annum, giving an estimated total of 24,884 for the Kachin hill tracts in 1941. This estimated figure was then added to the 1941 census figure for Katha district, thus keeping the boundary of the study area and the district boundary of Katha constant.

Some adjustment was also necessary to the eastern boundary of the Ruby Mines district. When constituted by the British in 1886, it formed an L-shape round the Shan state of Mongmit. From 2 February 1892, the Mongmit state was incorporated into the Ruby Mines district, but from 31 March 1906, it was administered separately. In order to maintain a constant boundary, the population of the Mongmit state (like the population of the Wuntho state) was excluded from the census series.

Unfortunately, another complication confuses the calculations in the Katha district. The population of the district was reported to be 59,329 in the 1891 census report,[62] but the *Burma Gazetteer, Volume B, Katha District* (1913) gave the population as 90,548 in 1891; and Scott and Hardiman reported the population to be 111,588 in 1891,[63] a variation of more than 50,000. A closer examination reveals that the census figure leaves out the estimated areas of the Kawlin and Katha excluded tracts; by adding these areas back, the census total (excluding the Wuntho state) becomes 81,591. Much of the confusion was due to the Wuntho Rebellion, which started in January 1891 and resulted in the loss of many records, including census returns. To allow for under-enumeration due to the rebellion and underestimation in the excluded areas, the *Burma Gazetteer* figure of 90,548 was chosen as probably the best estimate for 1891.

The districts that formed the remaining eastern border of the study area were Mandalay, Kyaukse, Meiktila and Yamethin. A minor boundary adjustment involving unpopulated land was made to the Mandalay border in 1925,[64] and the only other alteration that has been traced was a transfer of 2.6 square miles of land from Yamethin district to the Southern Shan states on 23 March 1914.[65] No details of population were found, so no adjustment was made.

Meiktila and Yamethin were formed as separate districts in 1886, but in 1894, the former district of Pyinmana was merged into the Yamethin district. Due to the many and intricate boundary changes that took place in the three districts where the populations involved were inadequately recorded, the area has been treated as one large unit throughout the census series.

The Yamethin district forms, with Thayetmyo, the southern boundary of Upper Burma in the study area. In 1914, there were two transfers of territory between Yamethin in Upper Burma and the neighbouring district of Toungoo in Lower Burma. These involved a gain to Yamethin of 36.64 square miles and a loss of 0.99 square miles. No details of population have been traced, and so no adjustment could be made to the calculation of district population figures.

The adjustments described above achieved the first objective of a consistent external boundary to the study area of Upper Burma for the census series 1891 to 1941. Within the border, the individual districts were also adjusted (as far as possible) to boundaries that remained constant throughout the census series: in four cases, by treating two or more districts as one unit.

Myingyan district: study on making adjustments to administrative transfers

The simplest way to illustrate the method used to obtain constant district boundaries is to trace the history of a sample district. Myingyan district was chosen as it represents both successful and, in some cases, unsuccessful attempts to form an area that was comparable census to census.

Prior to 1901 no changes in the district boundaries of Myingyan were discovered, but in the following decade (1901 to 1911), many adjustments were made. These included the transfer of 15 villages from Sagaing district to Myingyan district; the transfer of one village from Myingyan to Pakokku district; and the transfer of two villages from Myingyan to Minbu district.[66]

These adjustments formed part of a series described in the 1911 census: "There have been numerous and intricate transfers between the Minbu, Pakokku, Sagaing and Myingyan Districts. The total of the present areas does not coincide with that of 1901. Attempts at readjustment of the slight differences found have been made, but without success. The present figures are the result of careful calculation and enquiry."[67]

Due to lack of records, the official figures for the 1911 census had to be adopted for all the four districts mentioned above, without adjustment for the "numerous and intricate transfers". The tables in the 1911 census also gave retrospectively adjusted figures for the 1901 and 1891 censuses of the four districts involved, but these figures were not adopted due to doubts about their accuracy. This negative course was not satisfactory but was believed to be less damaging than unjustifiable estimation.

More changes took place in Myingyan district between 1911 and 1921. On 22 June 1916, the administration of Sale township (232,550 acres) was transferred from Myingyan district to Magwe district.[68] The population of Sale in 1913 was listed as 42,617 and, in order to keep the district boundary consistent, the population of this township was added back to the Myingyan district for survival of records of the 1941 census, from the 1931 census figure of 79,919. This was compounded at the rate of increase per annum in the rest of the Magwe district (1.14 per cent), giving an estimated figure for Sale township in 1941 of 89,511, which was then added to the Myingyan district total to re-establish a district figure within a constant boundary. (The same figure was deducted from the Magwe district totals to preserve the balance.)

Two other minor changes occurred in the decade from 1911 to 1921. One was a transfer from Pakokku district to Myingyan district that involved only 105 people; in the other, no population was involved.[69] No adjustment was made for either of these boundary alterations.

The census of 1931 records a further transfer of population that took place between 1921 and 1931 from Myingyan district to Magwe district. This change involved a population stated to have been 2,674 in 1921,[70] and this figure has been added back to the 1931 and the 1941 census figures for Myingyan district, after compounding by a rate of 1.65 per cent per annum from 1921 to 1931, and 1.14 per cent per annum between 1931 and 1941. Both rates of increase were those for Magwe district in the respective decades, and the resultant figures were deducted from the Magwe totals.

Of course, the above description shows only one side of the adjustments. For example, when the population figures for the Sale township were added back to the figures of Myingyan district, the population of Sale township was deducted from the census figure for Magwe district.

Population of Upper Burma in the study area and the effects of migration

Table 1.7 shows the results of the calculations and the adjustments to boundaries that were discussed above with examples. At first sight, the table shows some remarkable inconsistencies: two districts (Mandalay and Thayetmyo) had negative growth from 1891 to 1901 (and also between 1901 and 1911, in the case of Mandalay), while other districts, such as Shwebo/Ye-u, had growth rates of over two per cent in the same decades. Closer examination shows some slight correlation, however. All districts increased their populations overall between 1891 and 1941, though with wide variations in the rates of increase; in Mandalay, for example, the population grew from 374,060 in 1891 to 408,926 in 1941, an overall growth of only 9.3 per cent. By contrast, Shwebo/Ye-u and Magwe districts more than doubled their populations in the same period, exhibiting overall growth rates of 120.4 per cent and 113 per cent respectively.

Another correlation can be seen in the percentage change of population by decade. The table shows that in the decades 1891 to 1901, 1901 to 1911 and 1931 to 1941, nine of the 13 districts experienced population increases of one per cent or more. But in the decades 1911 to 1921 and 1921 to 1931, only three out of 13 districts experienced growth of one per cent or over. This suggests a pattern of growth for two decades, a slowing from 1911 to 1931, and then some renewal of growth, although the former momentum was not regained, as no districts showed a growth rate of 1.5 per cent or over after 1931. The variation in the rates of growth between individual districts raises questions also. The adjustment of boundaries, although imperfect, has produced district

TABLE 1.7

Upper Burma: Numbers of Population by District and Inter-censal Rates of Change per Annum

District	1891 Total Pop.	1901 Total Pop.	1901 % Change	1911 Total Pop.	1911 % Change	1921 Total Pop.	1921 % Change	1931 Total Pop.	1931 % Change	1941 Total Pop.	1941 % Change
Mandalay	374,060	366,507	-0.2	340,770	-0.72	356,621	0.45	371,636	0.41	408,926	0.95
Katha and Ruby Mines*	124,610	138,840	1.08	156,183	1.17	164,799	0.53	178,244	0.78	204,168	1.35
Shwebo and Ye-u	230,779	286,891	2.17	356,363	2.16	391,284	0.93	458,058	1.57	508,681	1.04
Sagaing	247,136	277,769	1.16	312,111	1.16	326,908	0.46	335,965	0.27	387,270	1.42
Lower Chindwin	233,316	276,383	1.69	316,175	1.34	342,880	0.81	372,166	0.81	414,844	1.08
Myingyan and Pagan	351,411	356,052	0.13	441,905	2.16	504,814	1.33	555,625	0.95	632,094	1.28
Pakokku	311,959	356,489	1.33	409,909	1.39	465,771	1.27	499,181	0.69	559,671	1.14
Minbu	215,959	233,377	0.77	263,939	1.23	274,302	0.38	277,876	0.12	302,373	0.84
Magwe	219,190	246,708	1.18	316,909	2.5	360,446	1.28	416,505	1.44	466,889	1.14
Kyaukse	126,622	141,253	1.09	141,426	0.01	142,677	0.08	151,320	0.58	152,506	0.07
Meiktil, Yamethin and Pyinmana	423,661	495,502	1.56	587,241	1.69	613,086	0.43	700,819	1.33	807,214	1.41
Thayetmyo	250,161	239,706	-0.42	248,275	0.35	255,406	0.28	274,177	0.70	297,434	0.81
Wuntho State (Shan)	68,890	80,369	1.54	89,414	1.06	88,926	-0.05	97,688	0.93	111,706	1.34

Notes: * Excluding Wuntho and Monmit states.

Sources: *Census of Burma* (population numbers calculated by district reconstruction).

areas that are more comparable from census to census than the official figures, and it is from these adjusted figures that the inter-censal rates of change have been calculated. They can be considered as more accurate than the official figures, and therefore the inconsistencies in the district experiences, and the rise and fall of inter-censal growth rates need explanation.

Post-annexation disturbance may be a partial explanation for some districts. Kyaukse, Mandalay and Thayetmyo experienced prolonged and heavy fighting after the British invasion (6,000 Burmese guerrillas surrounded Kyaukse town in 1886),[71] but again the picture is inconsistent. Kyaukse district may have been under-enumerated in 1891 due to disturbances, as the 1.09 per cent rise in population by 1901 was the highest inter-censal rise attained by the district during the study period, but Mandalay and Thayetmyo can only be described as suffering from slow depopulation. Some further explanation must be sought. Could migration be a major factor in explaining the inconsistencies in Table 1.7?

As discussed earlier in this chapter, the demographic history of Burma is affected both by the exogenous Indian migrations and the internal seasonal and permanent migration. The Indian immigration was far less significant statistically in Upper Burma than in Lower Burma. Table 1.8 shows the Hindu and Muslim populations in the

TABLE 1.8

Selected Districts of Upper Burma showing the Indian Population as a Percentage of the District Total

District	Hindu					Muslim				
	1891	*1901*	*1911*	*1921*	*1931*	*1891*	*1901*	*1911*	*1921*	*1931*
Mandalay	2.56	3.66	4.71	6.19	7.64	–	–	–	–	5.98
Magwe	–	–	–	2.02	2.47	–	–	–	–	–
Yamethin/ Meiktila	–	–	–	1.41	1.52	–	–	–	–	2.89
Katha	–	–	–	2.42	3.17	–	–	–	–	–
Shwebo/ Ye-u	–	–	–	–	–	–	–	–	–	1.98
Kyaukse	–	–	–	–	–	–	–	–	–	4.82

Sources: *Census of Burma.*

districts in which an Indian population became statistically significant as a percentage of the total district figures that include all races.

The table shows that the only district to be materially affected by a large Indian population was Mandalay, which, far from having exaggerated growth rates, actually suffered a decline in population between 1891 and 1931 (the 1891 figure of 374,060 not being overtaken until the 1941 census). The combined Indian and Muslim populations of Mandalay district in 1931 (at 13.6 per cent of the total, or nearly 53,000) were, therefore, only masking a continuing decline. It should be noted that something of a similar nature happened in 1931 in Kyaukse: after two decades of less than 0.1 per cent growth, the district posted a sharp increase to 0.58 per cent, with Indian Muslim immigrants comprising 4.82 per cent of the population. The other districts identified in the table show relatively healthy rates of growth even when the Indian population is subtracted, again indicating that this immigration cannot be the explanation for the inconsistent inter-censal growth rates in Upper Burma.

If Indian immigrants were not the cause, can the explanations be found in internal migration, due to some districts "losing" excessive population numbers to Lower Burma? This has already been discussed in connection with Table 1.6 and Figure 1.1, but the picture is so confused by the change of census dates and the lack of information as to whether the migrants were seasonal or permanent that definitive conclusions are not possible. Two issues should be noted in particular: that migrants to the dry zone were recorded there in the census whether they were seasonal labourers or permanent migrants; and that the numbers migrating from Upper Burma to Lower Burma showed a steady decline between 1901 and 1931. The first problem means that a seasonal labourer could, for example, be enumerated in Lower Burma when harvesting in one census year, and ten years later might be enumerated in his home district of Upper Burma, vagaries of census, his personal preference and harvest dates permitting. There is no way in which this information can be extracted from the census; thus the district and total population figures for both Upper and Lower Burma are affected. Secondly, the decline in the numbers migrating from Upper to Lower Burma between 1901 and 1931 means that for those districts of Upper Burma suffering from population stasis in the latter decades, out-migration cannot be the major cause. It was a contributing factor, but the figures suggest that other causes must also be looked for.

Before leaving the topic of migration, another reference should be made to Figure 1.1. This flow chart illustrates the extent and complexity of the internal migration within Upper Burma, as well as the seasonal flows from Upper to Lower Burma. It also suggests that out-migration to other districts of Upper Burma cannot account for the slow depopulation of some districts, such as Kyaukse and Mandalay, because these districts were in receipt of seasonal migrants for the rice harvest, and this practice was continued. It seems therefore that neither migration nor post-annexation disturbances can satisfactorily explain the inconsistencies between district growth rates, or the slowing of overall population growth in Upper Burma between 1911 and 1931. It is hoped that later chapters will provide more satisfactory explanations.

Estimates of population in Lower Burma 1891–1941

Having established acceptable district figures of population change in the study area of Upper Burma, an attempt was made to do the same for the districts of Lower Burma using the same methodology. This, unfortunately, was not successful.

The very rapid development of the delta area caused a degree of administrative change, and division and subdivision of districts that made reconstruction impossible. Despite the grave doubts already expressed about the accuracy of the officially recorded changes, especially prior to 1900, there was no practical alternative that could be said to improve on the official figures.[72] This means that the outlines of the study area of Lower Burma, and the boundaries of the individual districts used throughout the calculations all rely on the official, retrospectively adjusted figures.

Two tables, 1.9 and 1.10, can be used to illustrate the above point. Their immediate purpose is comparison only. Table 1.9 shows the population of Lower Burma, by district, from the contemporary census records. Table 1.10 shows the population, by district, but with the retrospective adjustments, made by later census officials, due to boundary changes and the division of districts.

Apportioning the Indian population among changed boundaries

The problem is that the figures in Table 1.10 include the very large Hindu and Muslim populations that were such a feature of many Lower Burma districts; for example, nearly 20 per cent of the Hanthawaddy district in 1921 was Hindu or Muslim. No acceptable figures of population change for the indigenous peoples of Burma could be calculated under such circumstances. Therefore the priority was to establish district population figures that excluded the Hindu and Muslim immigrants, but were within the consistent, retrospectively adjusted boundaries.

TABLE 1.9

Lower Burma: Numbers of Population by District from Contemporary Census Records

District	1872	1881	1891	1901	1911	1921	1931	1941
Sandoway	54,725	64,010	77,134	90,927	102,803	112,029	129,245	139,747
Rangoon district	332,324	* Became Hanthawaddy and Thongwa						
Rangoon town	98,745	134,176	180,324	234,881	293,316	341,962	400,415	500,800
Bassein	322,689	389,419	475,002	391,427	440,988	489,173	571,043	664,724
Myanaung	476,612	* Became Henzada and Tharrawaddy						
Prome	274,872	322,342	360,252	365,804	378,871	371,575	410,651	436,714
Thayetmyo	156,816	169,560	250,161	* Reunited with Upper Burma				
Moulmein town	46,472	53,107	*				*	
Shwegyin	129,485	171,144	198,521	* Split up among Pegu, Thaton and Toungoo				
Toungoo	86,166	128,848	162,132	279,315	351,076	381,883	428,670	*
Hanthawaddy	*	427,720	267,039	484,811	539,109	304,624	408,831	459,422
Tharrawaddy	*	278,255	347,454	395,570	433,320	492,429	508,319	593,909
Thongwa	*	284,063	446,076	484,400	* Became Maubin, Pyapon and Myaungmya			
Henzada	*	318,077	380,927	484,558	532,357	550,920	613,280	693,271
Pegu	*	*	301,420	339,572	429,121	445,620	489,169	582,959
Myaungmya	*	*	*	303,274	334,852	370,551	444,784	488,031
Thaton	*	*	*	343,510	416,975	471,100	532,628	592,638
Maubin	*	*	*	*	305,073	330,106	371,509	428,092
Pyapon	*	*	*	*	256,215	288,994	334,158	385,008
Insein	*	*	*	*	*	293,083	331,452	387,345

Notes: *District not in existence at that date.

Sources: *Census of Burma.*

TABLE 1.10

Lower Burma: Numbers of Population by District and Inter-censal Rates of Change per Annum
(These figures include retrospective adjustments made by the census official.)

District	1872 Total Pop.	1881 Total Pop.	1881 % Change	1891 Total Pop.	1891 % Change	1901 Total Pop.	1901 % Change	1911 Total Pop.	1911 % Change	1921 Total Pop.	1921 % Change	1931 Total Pop.	1931 % Change	1941 Total Pop.	1941 % Change
Sandoway 1825	55,325	65,182	1.82	78,509	1.86	90,927*	1.46	102,803	1.22	112,029	0.85	129,245	1.42	139,747	0.78
Rangoon town	98,745	134,176	3.41	182,080	3.05	245,430	2.98	293,316*	1.78	345,505	1.63	400,415*	1.47	500,800	2.23
Bassein 1852	202,428	268,169*	3.12	320,973*	1.79	391,427*	1.98	440,988*	1.19	489,473	1.04	571,043	1.54	664,724	1.51
Prome	280,288	328,905	1.78	368,977	1.14	365,804*	-0.08	378,871	0.35	371,575	-0.19	410,651	0.99	436,714	0.61
Thayetmyo	156,816	169,560	0.87	250,161	3.88	–	–	–	–	–	–	–	–	–	–
Toungoo 1853	136,816	190,385*	3.67	211,784	1.06	279,315*	2.76	351,076*	2.28	380,797	0.81	428,670*	1.18	474,858	1.02
Hanthawaddy 1852, 1912	115,231	182,607*	5.12	244,057*	2.90	297,015*	1.96	332,569*	1.13	364,624*	0.92	408,831	1.14	459,922	1.17
Tharrawaddy 1852/3, 1878	171,202	272,001*	5.14	339,240*	2.20	395,570	1.53	433,320	0.91	492,429	1.27	508,319	0.31	593,909	1.55
Henzada 1853, 1878	256,753	363,899*	3.88	437,620*	1.84	484,558	1.01	532,357*	0.94	550,920	0.34	613,280	1.07	693,271	1.22
Pegu 1883	100,338	166,120*	5.60	212,116	2.44	299,591*	3.45	382,166*	2.43	446,706*	1.56	489,969*	0.92	582,959	1.73
Myaungmya 1903	56,845	105,369	6.86	181,792	5.45	282,932	4.42	334,852*	1.68	370,551*	1.01	444,784	1.82	488,031	0.92
Thaton 1895	160,429	223,309	3.67	259,108	1.48	333,438*	2.52	405,225*	1.94	472,451*	1.53	532,628*	1.19	592,638	1.06
Maubin (Thongwa) 1903 (1875)	124,442	173,315	3.68	213,738	2.09	278,309	2.63	305,073*	0.91	330,106*	0.78	371,509	1.18	428,092	1.41
Pyapon 1903	39,847	79,226	7.64	145,996	6.11	226,443	4.38	256,215*	1.23	288,994	1.20	334,158	1.45	385,008	1.41
Insein 1912	86,831	138,746*	5.21	184,064*	2.82	227,300*	2.10	265,245	1.54	289,540*	0.87	331,452*	1.35	387,345	1.55

Notes: * Indicates retrospective adjustment.

Sources: *Census of Burma.*

The restricting factor lay within the limitations of the census records. As previously stated, the census commissioners produced retrospectively adjusted population figures for the newly constituted district boundaries; however, no equivalent adjusted figures were produced for the Hindu and Muslim populations. Therefore, although the number of Hindus and Muslims were tabulated for each census, no retrospectively adjusted figures were produced. For example, the Shwegyin district in 1891 contained 5,600 Muslims and Hindus, but by the 1901 census, that district no longer existed because it had become part of the districts of Thaton, Pegu and Toungoo. The Indian populations of these districts in 1901 were 20,033, 23,384 and 9,612 respectively. The difficulty was how to relate and divide the figure for the Indian population of the district of Shwegyin in 1891 to the retrospectively adjusted figures for the district populations of Thaton, Pegu and Toungoo in 1891.

The series of diagrammatic Maps H to M represent an attempt to overcome this difficulty. The maps are based on the 1891 Census of Burma map. By using overlays, it was possible to see (and therefore measure) the change in the district areas from one census to another, and to use this information to reconstruct the transferred areas. The measurement of the districts was made by planimeter, an instrument for measuring plane areas, but it must be emphasised that, despite the technical accuracy of the instrument, the estimations are approximate only. This is due to the diagrammatic nature of the maps and to the inclusion of the area of rivers in the measurements.

The objective was to reconstruct the district boundaries of the 1891, 1901 and 1911 censuses to those boundaries that were in existence in the 1921 census. As an example to illustrate the calculations, a brief look at the figures for the Insein district, newly constituted in 1912, should suffice. Insein district lay just north of Rangoon and had a high Indian population, and is therefore a good example of the necessity for this type of reconstruction.

Land was taken in 1912 from the two districts of Hanthawaddy and Pegu to form Insein; therefore the Indian population of the new district had previously formed part of the populations of Hanthawaddy and Pegu. The technique of reconstruction sought to establish what percentage of a district had been transferred, and then assumed an equal percentage of population had been transferred.

A problem that could not be overcome by reconstruction was the assumption that the Indian population of a district was evenly distributed; that if ten per cent of the land area was transferred, then ten per cent of the Indian population was transferred. While many Muslims worked as traders in the villages, Hindus were often found clustered in the more industrial locations, where they were employed

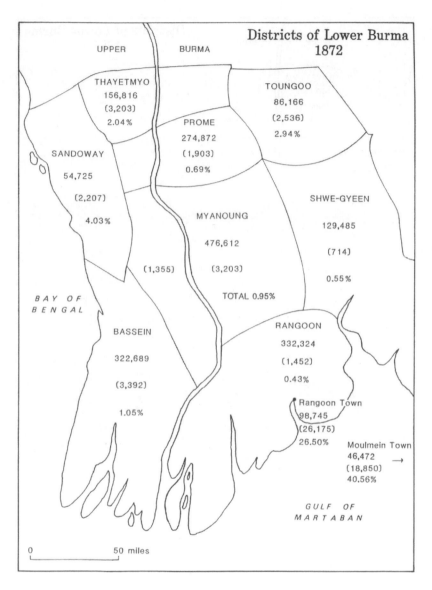

MAP H

in the rice mills, the docks and other places needing coolie labour. The figures for Insein and Hanthawaddy districts in Table 1.10 are the most susceptible to distortion by this bias, due to the density of the population, and also further exacerbated by the changes in the boundaries between Rangoon town and the districts. There was, for example, a transfer of

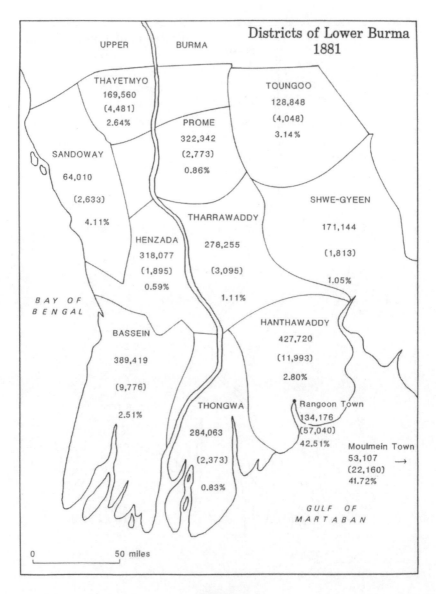

Districts of Lower Burma
1881

UPPER   BURMA

THAYETMYO
169,560
(4,481)
2.64%

PROME
322,342
(2,773)
0.86%

TOUNGOO
128,848
(4,048)
3.14%

SANDOWAY
64,010
(2,633)
4.11%

SHWE-GYEEN
171,144
(1,813)
1.05%

THARRAWADDY
278,255
(3,095)
1.11%

HENZADA
318,077
(1,895)
0.59%

BAY OF
BENGAL

HANTHAWADDY
427,720
(11,993)
2.80%

BASSEIN
389,419
(9,776)
2.51%

THONGWA
284,063
(2,373)
0.83%

Rangoon Town
134,176
(57,040)
42.51%

Moulmein Town
53,107   →
(22,160)
41.72%

GULF OF
MARTABAN

0   50 miles

MAP I

"congested districts" from Hanthawaddy district to Rangoon town between 1901 and 1911, but no details were found.[73]

There was no need to reconstruct the district to obtain the figures of the Indians in the 1911 census — those were given in the 1913 *Burma Gazetteer, Vol. B, Insein District No.6* as 25,500. The next figures to calculate

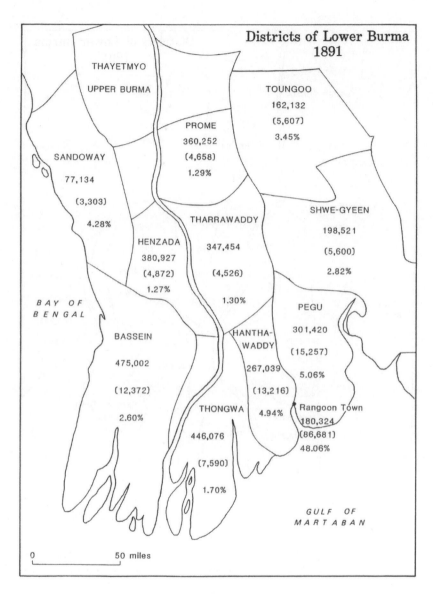

MAP J

were, therefore, the numbers of Hindus and Muslims who, in 1901, were living in the area that later became Insein district.

By measuring the district of Hanthawaddy as it appears on Map L, it was calculated that 38 per cent of that district was transferred to form part of the Insein district in 1912. The total number of Indians in

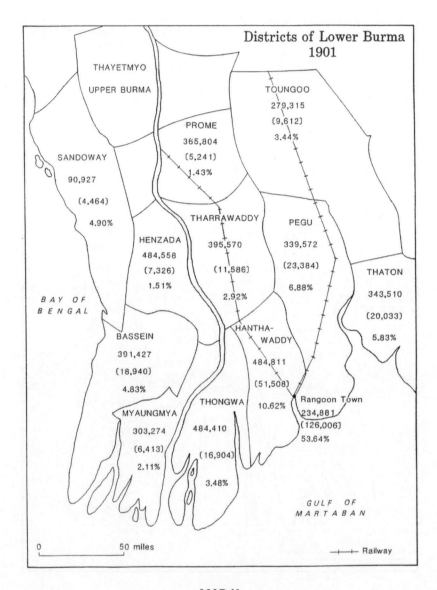

MAP K

Hanthawaddy in 1901 in the 1911 boundaries was 43,782 (having been subject to a separate calculation), of which 38 per cent (or 16,637) were assumed to live in the area transferred to Insein.

The rest of Insein district was composed of land transferred from Pegu district. Using the same technique that had been used for the

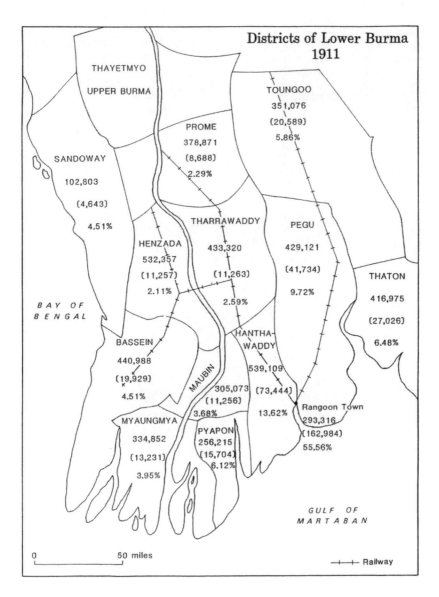

Districts of Lower Burma 1911

THAYETMYO

UPPER BURMA

TOUNGOO
351,076
(20,589)
5.86%

PROME
378,871
(8,688)
2.29%

SANDOWAY
102,803
(4,643)
4.51%

THARRAWADDY
433,320
(11,263)
2.59%

PEGU
429,121
(41,734)
9.72%

HENZADA
532,357
(11,257)
2.11%

THATON
416,975
(27,026)
6.48%

BAY OF
BENGAL

BASSEIN
440,988
(19,929)
4.51%

HANTHA-
WADDY
539,109
(73,444)
13.62%

MAUBIN
305,073
(11,256)
3.68%

Rangoon Town
293,316
(162,984)
55.56%

MYAUNGMYA
334,852
(13,231)
3.95%

PYAPON
256,215
(15,704)
6.12%

GULF OF
MARTABAN

0   50 miles

—┼—┼— Railway

MAP L

Hanthawaddy district, it was estimated that ten per cent of the area of Pegu district had been transferred. It was assumed that ten per cent of the reconstructed 1901 Indian population of 31,110 in the 1911 boundaries of Pegu district was transferred to Insein, or 3,111. Therefore the total Indian population of Insein district in 1901 in the 1911 (and unchanged

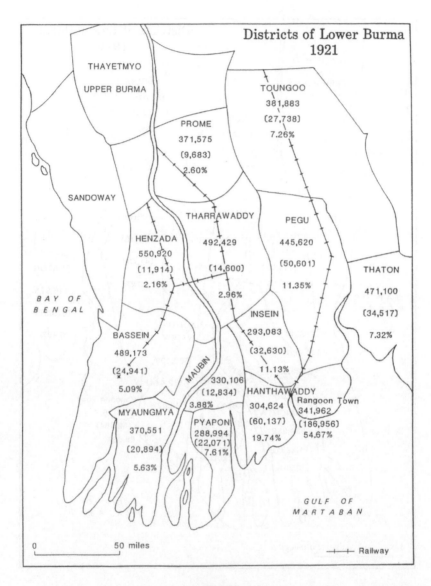

Districts of Lower Burma 1921

THAYETMYO

UPPER BURMA

TOUNGOO
381,883
(27,738)
7.26%

PROME
371,575
(9,683)
2.60%

SANDOWAY

THARRAWADDY
492,429
(14,600)
2.96%

PEGU
445,620
(50,601)
11.35%

HENZADA
550,920
(11,914)
2.16%

THATON
471,100
(34,517)
7.32%

BAY OF
BENGAL

INSEIN
293,083
(32,630)
11.13%

BASSEIN
489,173
(24,941)
5.09%

MAUBIN
330,106
(12,834)
3.88%

HANTHAWADDY
304,624
(60,137)
19.74%

Rangoon Town
341,962
(186,956)
54.67%

MYAUNGMYA
370,551
(20,894)
5.63%

PYAPON
288,994
(22,071)
7.61%

GULF OF
MARTABAN

0   50 miles

+—+— Railway

MAP M

1921) boundaries was estimated at 16,637 (from Hanthawaddy district) plus 3,111 (from Pegu district), making a total of 19,748.

Each of the districts of Pegu, Toungoo, Thaton, Maubin, Insein, Hanthawaddy, Myaungmya, Bassein and Pyapon were reconstructed for some or all of the census periods in this way. Where figures existed in the *Gazetteer* series for the appropriate census years, these figures were accepted as more accurate than reconstruction. The district figures of Indian population by census were therefore drawn from three sources: the reconstructed figures described above; the contemporary census figures where no boundary alterations had taken place; and the *Gazetteer* figures where available.

A complicating factor was the lack of agreement between the *Volume B Gazetteers* and the census maps. This was often due to the lapse of time between the drafting of the census maps and the printing of the *Gazetteers*. Boundary changes that occurred after the date of the last decennial census were incorporated into the accompanying *Gazetteer* series without explanation. For instance, in the 1906 series *Gazetteers*, the Thongwa district does not appear, as it had been replaced in 1903 by the districts of Pyapon and Maubin. (This should not be confused with the township of Thongwa that was described in the 1906 *Gazetteer* series, as it was not the same township of Thongwa recorded in the 1901 census.)

No attempt was made to reconstruct the district boundaries for the 1872 and 1881 censuses, as no census maps exist for these years. Also the need is less, as the number of migrants, except in the towns of Rangoon and Bassein, was low and the census themselves under-enumerated. No adjustment was made for the boundary changes that occurred between Henzada, Bassein and Sandoway districts. The areas affected were largely hill or foothills, and were therefore unlikely to have contained significant Indian populations.

Despite the admitted weaknesses of the reconstruction technique, it is clearly preferable to use it to produce estimations of the Indian district populations (identified by religion) rather than accept total population figures, non-differentiated by race, which would have made calculations of growth rates meaningless. Table 1.11 shows the results of the figures produced by this technique.

After this somewhat laborious and unrewarding work, it was at last possible to fulfil the objective of this section and calculate indigenous population totals for the districts of Lower Burma by subtracting the Indian population (Table 1.11) from the total population (Table 1.10). The resulting Table 1.12, though far from perfect, represents the best attempt that can be made to produce district population figures of the Burmese population of Lower Burma and inter-censal rates of growth.

The annual rates of population growth were, in the earlier years, much higher than those found in the districts of Upper Burma, and reflected the rapid rate of agricultural development. But after this early period, all the districts showed a decline in the rate of growth (after 1911 or 1921) and, with the exception of Thaton and Pegu, each district had at least one decade when growth of less than one per cent per annum

TABLE 1.11

Number of Indians in Districts of Lower Burma (calculated by district reconstruction to 1921 boundaries)

District	1891	1901	1911	1921
Bassein	8,500*	18,940	19,929	24,941
Toungoo	6,650*	9,612	20,589	27,738
Hanthawaddy	7,200*	31,500*	51,000**	60,137
Pegu	13,500*	23,644*	40,000**	50,601
Myaungmya	6,300*	11,047*	13,231	20,894
Thaton	2,200*	20,033	27,026	34,517
Maubin	5,100*	5,677*	11,256	12,834
Pyapon	2,150*	6,423*	15,704	22,071
Insein	9,000*	19,748*	25,500**	32,630

Notes

* Figures calculated by reconstruction to 1921 district boundaries.

** Figures for 1911 from *Burma Gazetteer, Vol. A* for Syriam, Insein and Pegu.

Sources: *Census of Burma; Burma Gazetteer, Vol. A.*

was experienced. The low growth rates between 1911 and 1921 were obviously influenced by the flu pandemic. The high early rates must be treated with a degree of caution, as they would have been influenced by the later improvements in enumeration as well as the flow of immigrants from Upper Burma. Also, of course, it should be remembered that the rates for the years prior to 1891 are not adjusted for the presence of Indian migrants.

Prome, Hanthawaddy, Henzada and Maubin districts experienced lower than average rates of increase: Prome showing a slight decline in population between 1891 and 1901. The experience of Hanthawaddy probably bears little relationship to the other three districts, as nearly 20 per cent of the population of this district was Hindu or Muslim by 1921. This contrasts with Prome, Henzada and Maubin, which were three out of the four districts in Lower Burma in 1921 and 1931 having Indian communities of less than four per cent of their total populations. The other district was Tharrawaddy and the four districts were clustered together in the centre of Lower Burma. There is no evidence to suggest that errors in the calculations of the migrant community have distorted the rates of population growth in these districts.

TABLE 1.12

The Study Area of Lower Burma: Numbers of Population by District and Inter-censal Rates of Change per Annum, Calculated by District Reconstruction to 1921 Boundaries to Subtract the Indian Population (These figures include retrospective adjustments made by the census official.)

District	1872 Total Pop.	1881 Total Pop.	1881 % Change	1891 Total Pop.	1891 % Change	1901 Total Pop.	1901 % Change	1911 Total Pop.	1911 % Change	1921 Total Pop.	1921 % Change	1931 Total Pop.	1931 % Change
Sandoway	53,118	62,549	1.81	75,206	1.84	86,463	1.39	98,160	1.26	106,421	0.80	122,263	1.38
Rangoon town	72,570	77,136	0.68	95,399	2.12	119,424	2.24	130,332	0.87	158,549	1.95	188,280	1.71
Bassein	199,036	258,393	2.89	312,473	1.90	372,487	1.75	421,059	1.22	464,532	0.98	544,002	1.57
Prome	278,385	326,132	1.75	364,319	1.10	360,563	-0.10	370,183	0.26	361,888	-0.22	397,807	0.94
Thayetmyo	153,613	165,079	0.79	–		–		–		–		–	
Toungoo	134,280	186,337	3.64	205,134	0.96	269,703	2.73	330,487	2.03	353,059	0.66	395,167	1.12
Hanthawaddy	115,000	170,614	4.38	236,857	3.28	265,515	1.14	281,569	0.58	304,487	0.78	343,048	1.19
Tharrawaddy	167,999	268,906	5.22	334,714	2.18	383,984	1.37	422,057	0.94	477,829	1.24	493,722	0.32
Henzada	255,398	362,004	3.87	432,748	1.78	477,232	0.97	521,100	0.87	539,006	0.33	600,175	1.07
Pegu	100,338	166,120*	5.60	198,616	1.78	275,947	3.28	342,166	2.15	396,105	1.46	437,871	1.00
Myaungmya	56,845*	105,369*	6.85	175,492	5.10	271,885	4.37	321,621	1.67	349,657	0.83	415,831	1.73
Thaton	160,429*	223,309*	3.67	256,908	1.40	313,405	1.98	378,199	1.87	437,934	1.46	493,969	1.20
Maubin (Thongwa)	124,442*	170,942	3.52	208,638	1.99	272,632	2.67	293,817	0.74	317,272	0.76	356,706	1.17
Pyapon	39,847*	79,226*	7.63	143,846	5.96	220,020	4.24	240,511	0.89	266,923	1.04	304,427	1.31
Insein	86,831*	138,746*	5.20	175,064	2.32	207,552	1.70	239,745	1.44	256,910	0.69	289,885	1.20

Notes: * Population for which no figures of Indians are available.

Sources: *Census of Burma*.

As with Upper Burma, the district population figures and growth rates show interesting inconsistencies that are not readily explained. The decline in the rates of growth after 1911 and 1921 parallels, to some extent, the Upper Burma experience, although none of the districts of Lower Burma suffered from population decrease. Again, it is hoped that later chapters will provide a degree of explanation.

Population numbers for the study area

In the introduction to this first chapter we stated a simple objective: to establish the number of the Burmese population during the period of the British administration. This objective has been far from simple to achieve but, at last, after estimations of the nineteenth-century population, explanations of the establishment of the study area, the adjustments of district boundaries and populations in Upper Burma, and the calculations to remove the migrant Indian populations from the Lower Burma figures, it was accomplished. This was done by totalling all the district populations for Upper and Lower Burma from Tables 1.7 (excluding Wuntho state, which lies outside the study area) and 1.12 for each census year from 1891 to 1931. From these totals, the rate of population change per annum for the inter-censal decades in the study area were calculated, and are shown in Table 1.13.

Two figures are shown in Table 1.13 for the percentage rate of change between 1891 and 1901. The first figure is the actual unadjusted result, and the second figure shows the effect of adding five per cent

TABLE 1.13

The Study Area of Burma: Numbers of Population and Inter-censal Rates of Change per Annum

Census Year	Population Total	% Change per Annum
1891	6,324,278	
1891 + 5%	6,640,492	
1901	7,312,289	1.45/0.96 (+5%)
1911	8,282,212	1.25
1921	8,989,566	0.82
1931	9,974,725	1.04
1941	11,380,088	1.32
1941 + Indians	(11,980,088)	

to the population total for 1891 in the study area to allow for the under-enumeration of that census. Two figures are also shown for 1941: the figure in parentheses is the census figure for the study area including the Indian population, as no differentials by race or religion are available for this census due to the loss of the records. The smaller figure shows the result of deducting an estimated 600,000 Indians from the total for the study area. This is a rough estimation suggested by a total of 648,472 Indians identified in the study area in 1931. The number of migrants resident in Burma declined slightly during the 1930s as a result of the economic depression. This estimated figure (total minus Indian migrants) was used for the calculations of the rates of change per annum between 1931 and 1941.

The figures, not surprisingly, show a decline in the rate of increase per annum after 1911, with a recovery in the 1930s. But the average growth rate from 1891 to 1941 at 1.07 per cent is far from spectacular, and closely mirrors the estimated figure for nineteenth-century population growth. A more rapid growth rate in the twentieth century would be less surprising, given the improved infrastructure and lack of major catastrophe, such as famine (not forgetting the flu pandemic and its losses). If these figures are put into a broader context by comparing them with the growth rates experienced in other Southeast Asian countries and India, a more useful picture emerges (see Table 1.14). From 1921, Burma's inter-censal growth rates are remarkably similar to India's and slightly lower than Indonesia's, but are much lower than their Southeast Asian neighbours.

TABLE 1.14

A Comparison of Inter-censal Growth Rates per Annum in
Twentieth-century India and Southeast Asia

	Burma	India	Indonesia	Malaysia	Philippines	Siam
1901–1911	1.25%	0.56%	1.0%	–	2.0%	1.3%
1911–1921	0.82%	–0.03%	1.0%	1.9% (1918/19)	–	2.2%
1921–1931	1.04%	1.05%	–	2.7% (1929/30)	2.1%	2.9%
1931–1941	1.32%	1.31%	1.5%	1.6% (1936/37)	2.0%	1.8%

Sources: Malaysia, Philippines, Thailand: Hirschman, *Population and Society in Twentieth Century South-East Asia*; India: Dyson, *Indian Historical Demography: Developments and Prospects*; Indonesia: Boomgaard and Gooszen, *Changing Economy in Indonesia*, Vol. 11, p. 82.

Siam, Malaysia, and the Philippines appear to have achieved growth rates of over two per cent in the 1920s, and growth rates well in excess of Burma's in the 1930s; but it should be noted that the figures for these three countries were obtained from untreated census data and therefore may be unreliable.

This comparison emphasises the point already made in this chapter that explanations need to be sought for the slowing in the growth rate of Burma's population in the twentieth century.

2 Birth rates and death rates in colonial Burma

> The components of change in total population are births, deaths, and migrations.[1]
>
> Shryock and Siegal

The influence of migration on population change in Burma was discussed in the first chapter. The objective of this second chapter therefore is to measure the other two components of population change, which are births and deaths. In order to do this, acceptable estimates or calculations of the birth and death rates in Burma for the study period must be found, as information about the number of children born, their survival and their average expectation of life are part of the most basic demographic data. With that knowledge of birth and death rates, plus the information on the numbers and rates of growth of the population, it should be possible to see the structure of Burmese demographic experience between 1891 and 1941.

Because this chapter deals with calculations to provide birth and death rates for Burma, it is inevitably technical in parts. As in the first chapter, an attempt has been made to clarify and simplify the text by dividing it under sub-headings. The sections will look at the setting up of the Sanitary Commission and the introduction of the registration of vital events, followed by an assessment of the accuracy of, and problems in, registration. This will be followed by an introduction to the use of the census to produce birth and death rates, and then a description of how this was applied to the Burmese data, using Model Life Tables. The chapter concludes with a discussion of the estimated rates produced by the calculations.

Before a description of the Sanitary Commission is undertaken, we should define what is meant by birth and death rates. Births and deaths are conventionally measured as the ratios of the numbers of these vital events in a calendar year to the average population in that period. The

Crude Birth Rate (CBR) is usually measured as the ratio of live births per 1,000 of population on the mid-year population, and the Crude Death Rate (CDR) is calculated in the same way using the number of deaths. These are known as "crude rates" when used in this form and not refined in terms of age, sex or, in the case of the death rate, by specific disease, for example. However, for the purposes of this study, crude rates are acceptable, as population structures usually change only very slowly.

The simplest source of the statistics of birth and death in a community are the registers of vital events. These commonly include the registration of marriages and stillbirths, as well as live births and deaths. In Burma, during the period of the study, the responsibility for the collection of statistics of vital events came under the office of the sanitary commissioner. The history of the founding of this office in India and Burma is of some interest.

The sanitary commission in Burma and the introduction of registration

In May 1859, a Royal Commission was appointed to examine the sanitary state of the army in India. The commission reported on 19 May 1863, and one of its recommendations was "the necessity of introducing a systematic registration of deaths". It was as a result of this advice that the registration of births and deaths in India and Burma was undertaken.[2] Both civilian and military registration was attempted.

The Royal Commission also recommended the appointment of a Sanitary Commission in each of the presidencies in British India, and initially, Burma's affairs were overseen by the Sanitary Commission in the Presidency of Bengal. A despatch in 1868 from the Government of India to the new sanitary commissioner in Bengal stated that "the diminution of mortality in the army and the improvement generally of its sanitary state was the primary objective."[3] It was appreciated in the instructions that the improvement would not be "brought about by measures solely directed to the amelioration of the sanitary conditions of the soldier as such, that the interests of the community at large were as much concerned as those of the army."[4] But the primary function of the Sanitary Commission was quite clear — its principal duty was to the army, and the sanitary state of the civil population was important only in that its ill health could indirectly affect that army.

Part of the reason for describing the origins of the Sanitary Commission in Burma is to appreciate precisely the terms of reference under which this body was formed. In later chapters, there are criticisms of the public health authority's concentration of resources and care on the troops, police and European personnel, so it is perhaps salutary to appreciate that their limited responsibilities were decided by a higher authority. There were, of course, enlightened and ethical administrators, but the original terms of their remit defined the health of the European troops as their primary objective.

It was perhaps unfortunate that the system was introduced when Albert Fytche was Chief Commissioner of British Burma. Hall describes Fytche as having far less ability and insight into the Burmese character than Arthur Phayre, the man he succeeded as Chief Commissioner.[5] He certainly had very little interest in, or sympathy for, the Sanitary Commission in Burma. In the Resolution accompanying the health report of 1870, it was stated that the Chief Commissioner "finds it quite impossible, having regard to the calls upon his time, to follow the Sanitary Commissioner through the 119 printed pages of discursive suggestions which form his report for the year 1870." The Resolution goes on to say that the chief commissioner had already stated to the government of India "that no possible advantage is derived by the Province from the appointment of a Sanitary Commissioner as a distinct officer", and that a department of sanitation was a luxury that only highly populated countries with advanced civilisations could afford.[6] This was not the most advantageous atmosphere in which to launch new concepts that would have benefited from central funding.

It was against this background that the collection of vital statistics was started in Burma. The figures were published in the annual reports that the sanitary commissioners were required to return, and by 1864, some major towns in Lower Burma, such as Henzada and Myanaung, were under vital registration. Initially the recording of marriage rates was also attempted, but in 1883 this was quietly dropped.[7]

Despite the initial celerity, however, the extension of registration was slow and patchy. The health report of 1876 was able to comment only on the "tolerable" efficiency of its performance in 17 towns, where registration was "nominally compulsory".[8] In district circles, the registration of births was not yet compulsory, but returns were made from these districts of reported vital events. This led to a situation where, for example, Henzada district was reporting a ratio of births of 8.75 per 1,000 in 1876, which would hardly seem to justify the time spent collating the figures.

By 1897, vital registration had been introduced into eight major towns in Upper Burma, but there were still pockets in Lower Burma, such as parts of the districts of Akyab, Bassein, Toungoo and Thayetmyo, where registration was not enforced. No attempt had been made to introduce the system to the hill areas, such as North Arakan. Even where registration had been established, fluctuations occurred; for example, parts of Toungoo district were exempted in 1898.[9] Yet in the same year, the registration of deaths only was introduced into parts of 11 districts in Upper Burma.[10] The overall picture was of a gradual increase in the registered area within Burma Proper, the districts of Arakan and Kyaukpyu, and parts of the Mergui Peninsula. On 1 January 1907, the last major extension of the system occurred, when the registration of births was started in the non-municipal towns and districts of Upper Burma. The percentage of the population under registration improved greatly between 1901 and 1911. In 1901, the census population was reported to be 10,490,624, but the number under registration was only 5,546,265 (53 per cent); in 1911, the figures were 12,115,217 by census and 9,878,593 (82 per cent) registered.

When the decision was made in 1870 to introduce registration into British Burma, no special agency was appointed to undertake the task, as that would have entailed a large expenditure of public money.[11] Instead, the headmen were made responsible for registering the events and sending a list on the first day of every month to the *myooks* of townships, who would tabulate the information and pass it to their district officer. At district headquarters, a monthly return was to be prepared for each district; this would then be sent to the sanitary commissioner, who was responsible for preparing the return for the province. This return was to be published in the monthly *Gazette*.

By 1875, the difficulties inherent in the system had forced a change, and district returns were ordered to be quarterly, not monthly.[12] The absurdity of the initial requirement had become apparent when some of the returns for July 1870 were not received until June 1871.[13] Many modifications of the system were to follow. One of the most successful was the introduction, in 1883, of the collection of registration counterfoils from headmen by monthly police patrols.[14] This system continued until 1921, though not always smoothly, and in 1891 it was implied that some police patrols had followed the easier path of ordering the headmen to report to the station, instead of the patrols visiting the villages.[15]

Some of the amendments to the system have, in retrospect, a certain macabre humour; for example, it soon became apparent in large towns that there was a need for greater supervision of the burial grounds. In 1879, there were 12 burial grounds in Rangoon for which "no trustworthy particulars could be obtained and where any corpse could be disposed of by paying the gravediggers a trifling fee." In addition to this, all burial grounds were unfenced; so not only could a family dig a grave for an unregistered corpse, but, the authorities belatedly recognised, "this might be done for an enemy" also.[16] Even in 1895, there were still only "recommendations" to municipal committees that certificates of registration should be necessary before burial was permitted,[17] so presumably some illicit and unregistered urban burials continued to occur.

The systems of checking the death registration were constantly amended. By 1897, the official procedure was that vaccinators and the district sanitary or medical officers checked the district figures, and the town figures were checked against the records of the cemetery caretakers.[18] In 1904, the job of compiling the registration returns for each district was transferred from the district officers to the civil surgeons.[19] As these medical officers were supplied with clerks to assist them, it is probably safe to assume that this was an attempt to improve the registration by transferring the responsibility from an overworked, and often disinterested, branch of the service to those with a professional interest in the statistics. In addition to these amendments, there were systems of punishments and fines for defaulting headmen, and warnings given to the police, caretakers and registrars. But what degree of efficiency were these changes and punishments producing in the registration?

The registered birth and mortality rates: an assessment of accuracy

The graph, Figure 2.1, shows the registered birth and mortality rates from 1876 to 1939. From 1876, the birth and death rates rose slowly from

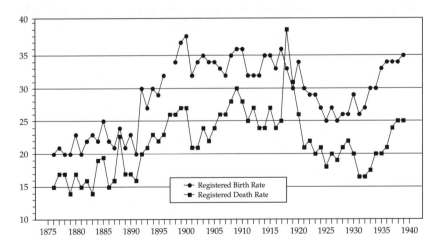

FIGURE 2.1
Burma: Registered Birth Rate and Registered Death Rate
(per 1,000 population)

Sources: *RSAB*.

a very low base until 1900. The underlying upward trend almost certainly reflected the gradual improvement in the registration system rather than increased mortality and birth. The addition of the newly registered areas of Upper Burma is reflected in the lower rates shown after 1901, as the addition of these areas had the effect of depressing the national rates. As these figures are not adjusted in any way, each census year shows an apparent drop in the vital rates. This is due to the larger census population upon which the rates were calculated, without an equivalent increase in the birth and mortality figures because the registration of these was initially poor. From 1911, the registered mortality rate was approximately 24 to 27 per 1,000, until the flu pandemic of 1918 caused the number of deaths to soar. But in the 1920s, the registered death rate slumped to below 20 per 1,000, rose briefly at the end of the decade and then dropped sharply again in 1931. It was not until 1937 that the rates rose to the levels registered between 1906 and 1916.

The central and basic problem, which was commented on year after year in the annual health reports, was that the recorded birth and death rates bore little relationship to the day-to-day experience of the administrators of the scheme. Many of the returns were frankly disbelieved by the sanitary commissioners, whose previous experience in India led them to expect much higher rates from a largely agri-cultural population. The commissioners also made their own calcula-tions of the probable vital rates from the census returns. In 1885, D. Sinclair, the Sanitary Commissioner, estimated the rural birth rate as 40 per 1,000 and the death rate at "somewhere over 30".[20] In 1901, one of his successors (C. C. Little) said that the Sanitary Commission was looking for a birth rate of 42 per 1,000.[21] He had made this esti-mate from calculations of the numbers of women married in Burma compared to India, which were 64 per cent and 88 per cent respectively, and had assumed for the estimation a "normal" Indian birth rate of 48 per 1,000.

Other assessments of the rates followed. In 1905, the birth rate was estimated at 45 per 1,000,[22] and in 1921, calculations from the new census figures produced estimates of "50 per mille or above" for the birth rate, and 40 per 1,000 for the death rate.[23] Clearly there are problems with any calculations made from unadjusted census figures, but this is not a valid reason for discounting the opinions of experienced, contemporary observers, who were also receiving advice from the civil surgeons and district commissioners.

The registered mortality rates in Burma were also tested by comparison with the deaths recorded amongst the convict population in the gaols. This data was used by the sanitary commissioners and can be used now to check the efficiency of the registration. The convict death rate in 1883 was 29.6 per 1,000, which compares to the registered death rate for the province of 13.24.[24] In 1894, the death rate in the gaols was 28.8 per 1,000 and the official death rate was 23.[25] Although the diets in the gaols were poor and infectious diseases spread rapidly in gaol, convict mortality obviously excludes the important infant and child mortality, and presumably some of the deaths from ageing. It would be reasonable therefore, to expect the average convict death rate to be appreciably lower than the rate for the population as a whole. But this was not the case in Burma.

These low provincial rates were an average of the district and urban rates. Much of the harsh comment in the annual health reports was reserved for the huge variations between localities. This was a feature of the registration from 1870, the first year that statistics were returned for most of the province. In that year, a birth rate of between 14 and 64 per 1,000 was returned from the local areas and a death rate of between 14 and 74.[26] Seven years later, a birth rate of 115.82 was returned from Myanaung, and the next year Henzada town returned a death rate of 6.84.[27] These unlikely figures were not confined to the earliest years of the registration. In 1911, the birth rate of Yamethin town was returned as 14.6 per 1,000, and its infant mortality rate as 855.93.[28]

On the few occasions that extreme fluctuations in rates were investigated, they were usually found to be the result of erroneous calculation. If, for example, the recorded number of births in a municipal area was mistakenly calculated as a ratio of the local municipality plus village populations, an absurdly low birth rate would be returned. Or in a district where the death registration was more accurate than the birth registration, the infant mortality rate calculated on these figures would be higher than the true rate. This probably explains the infant mortality rate (IMR) of 772 per 1,000 births returned by Pyawbwe town in 1911; the sanitary commissioner's comment was "one feels justified in suspecting the grossest carelessness in registration of births."[29]

Another way of checking the accuracy of birth registration in Burma is to compare the sex ratio of the recorded births to the standard sex ratio of 104 to105 males born to every 100 females.[30] Deviation from the standard sex ratio in recorded births usually indicates a form of social sexual preference in the society concerned; when the society places a higher value on one sex than the other, it is therefore more likely to register the birth of a child of that sex. In Burma, a male preference is revealed by the registration of births; for example, in the decade between 1902 and 1911, 106 to 108 male infants were registered each year for every 100 female infants registered. In addition to confirming a sexual inequality in Burmese life, these figures also confirm that not all births were registered.

It was abundantly clear to most of the sanitary commissioners that the registration was inadequate. They checked the average rates for Burma against their calculations on census data; they compared the convict death rate to the registered mortality; and they recognised the failure to register the births of some females.[31] The problem that the commissioners faced was that, with no special agency appointed for the task of the registration, the system lacked overall supervision and fundamental control. The commissioners were also aware that too much criticism and pressure could have an adverse effect, by producing the statistics that they required through an act of creativity in the district commissioner's office. In 1894, the sanitary commissioner wrote that "there is some danger of local authorities working up to a preconceived standard".[32]

These problems of inefficiency, inaccuracy and laxity were recorded year after year in the annual reports. In 1879, it was stated that no attempts had been made to ensure that the headmen had a sufficient supply of books.[33] In the 1883 report, it was stated that the 1884 returns for the town of Lemyethna had been calculated on the 1883 figures; this was described as "unpardonable".[34] In 1892, a district commissioner was reported as saying that "it is necessary to say plainly that these rural vital statistics are not, and in no reasonable time likely to be, worth anything."[35]

The problem therefore ran throughout the system. The government had failed to convince the Burmese people of the desirability or necessity of registering vital events, despite using a system of fines, punishments and warnings. The headmen, who received no pay for the task, were understandably reluctant to undertake it or execute the system efficiently. It was stated, in 1871, that "it is hardly to be believed that a Burman will travel a distance of 30 or 40 miles over a difficult country to perform a duty for which he gets no pay and which he looks upon as no use."[36] The headmen were, of course, the easiest target for the administration's criticisms, and were often accused of laziness when submitting inadequate returns.[37] The police, whose job it was to collect the counterfoils until 1923, no doubt also saw it as another and unnecessary chore. On occasions, counterfoils were lost or not collected, and the police disciplined as a result.[38]

Many and varied efforts were made to create and enforce a supervisory agency for the registration, but with indifferent results. In 1882, the annual report stated that "The police sergeant, the head constable, the township officer, the Inspector and Assistant Superintendent of Police, the Sub-divisional Officer and the Deputy Commissioner are all required by standing orders to examine the village registers."[39] Twenty-five years later, it was admitted in the annual report that verification was "probably very perfunctory", as the district officers and civil surgeons did not have the time to do it, nor presumably the will to enforce their subordinates to do it for them.[40]

The form of verification that, in theory, stood most chance of success was when smallpox vaccinators examined the headmen's registers and made house-to-house calls to verify the entries. This idea was resisted by the headmen and the villagers, and before long, by the vaccinators themselves. The Burmese had become familiar with smallpox inoculation before the arrival of the British, and for a long time there was considerable resistance to the new idea of the vaccination of infants and children. The headmen and the vaccinators soon found that attempts at verification of the registers by the vaccinators resulted in fewer births being registered, and in people hiding their infants from the vaccinators when house-to-house calls were made.[41]

Sometimes, periods of intense activity by the sanitary staff brought to light unregistered births and deaths. This happened in Mandalay in 1910 during an outbreak of plague; this had provoked the sanitary officers and the civil surgeon into extensive anti-plague work in the town, and had incidentally uncovered 1,150 unregistered births in that year alone. In the same year, the deputy commissioner of Kyaukse reported the discovery of two bodies buried in a garden. These unregistered deaths were plague victims, buried hastily to avoid the official attention that a notifiable disease attracted, and brought to light only by the increased work of the anti-plague drives.

All these known deficiencies make the use of the registered birth and death figures for the production of crude rates difficult to justify. But there is one other way of interpreting the graph of registration, and that is as an indicator of the administration's efficiency, rather than the health of the Burmese. The fluctuations shown in the graphs of Figure 2.1 represent administrative change and crisis as much, if not more than, mortality crisis.

On some occasions, the magnitude of the mortality crisis overcame the inadequacy of the registration. This is shown on the graph by, for example, the rise in mortality in 1888, when a cholera epidemic was recorded as causing 16,000 deaths. The deaths from the flu pandemic in 1918 took the recorded mortality to nearly 389,000 in that year, and the arrival of plague and its epidemic nature between 1907 and 1911 is also clearly visible on the graph. However, other apparent drops in the mortality and the birth rate are due to change or crises in the administration. It was decided in 1923 that, instead of the statistics being collected by the monthly police patrols, the headmen themselves should be responsible for taking or sending the figures to the civil surgeons. This change was imposed on the Sanitary Commission, and the probable result was predicted in the annual reports with some accuracy. By 1925, the recorded mortality rate had dropped to 18.75 and the birth rate to 25.38, the lowest rates since 1891. The officiating Sanitary Commissioner, G. Jolly, described the results with some exasperation when he wrote: "the inevitable result has been that the whole system of collection of vital statistics has been seriously disorganised."[42]

It was 1929 before the rates again approached even the low levels recorded in 1922, the year before the change in the system, and this "advance" was short lived. In 1930, the Saya San Rebellion broke out. This anti-colonial rising resulted in the deaths and wounding of 288 headmen within a year, and with many districts in turmoil, the registration suffered.[43] It was not until 1938 that the rates came close to the 25 per 1,000 CDR and 33 per 1,000 CBR that had been the approximate rates in the most efficient registration period between 1900 and 1920.

The discussion so far has been limited mainly to a description of the failings of the registration system, but the extent of that failing has not been measured. Three points of comparison were suggested — the convict death rate, which hovered around 29 per 1,000, the sex ratio of births, and the estimates of the sanitary commissioners themselves. The two former have already been discussed, but the differences between the commissioners' calculations and the recorded rates can be seen more clearly in Table 2.1. This is perhaps useful as an aid to judging the extent of under-registration.

This comparison reveals differences of 20 to 40 per cent between the commissioners' estimates and the official registration. The calculations of these health officials are supported by the statement of Sanitary

TABLE 2.1

Birth Rate and Death Rate in Burma (estimated by the sanitary commissioners)

Year	Estimated Rate			Recorded Rate	
	BR	DR		BR	DR
1885	40	30+		25.51	19.89
1901	42			32.07	
1905	42			34.37	
1921	50	30+		29.85	21.45

Sources: Annual health reports.

Commissioner, C. E. Williams, in his annual health report of 1912: "A general review of the recorded birth rates induces the conviction that from 25% to 33% of all births are omitted to be registered in most rural areas, and also in some towns."[44]

Further evidence of the difference between the official rates and the actual rates of vital events appeared in the last decade of the study period. This evidence confirms that approximately one-quarter to one-third of the vital events were not recorded. In 1929, with the aid of a grant from the Rockefeller Foundation, a Health Unit was set up in Hlegu township. The objectives were to conduct a survey of health problems in a defined area, and to try to solve those health problems "with a unit of personnel and equipment on a scale more or less comparable with such services as police protection and general education."[45] A great deal of emphasis was placed on the collection of vital statistics within the Health Unit area. Prior to its inception, the five-year mean of birth and death rates in Hlegu township were 16.89 and 12.72 per 1,000. In 1934, the sanitary commissioner reported "the rather startling fact that the ratios of births and death in the township, for the five years previous to the inception of the unit, were in error to the extent of 122.53% in the case of births, and 76.81% in the case of deaths."[46] It is not surprising that the commissioner was startled, as Hlegu could hardly be described as a remote township. It lies just north of Rangoon, and the commissioner would presumably have been left pondering the probable inaccuracy of the registration of more far-flung townships.

During the ten-year period 1930 to 1939, the average recorded death rate at Hlegu was 21 per 1,000, and the birth rate was 35 per 1,000. Compared to the estimates of the sanitary commissioners, these figures are still low, and it is notable that in the three years 1937, 1938 and 1939, the birth rate rose to nearly 37 per 1,000. I would suggest that this probably indicates improved registration rather than a rising birth rate because the health officials were still detecting a high rate of omissions by 1939.[47] In addition to detected omissions, it is probable that a number of stillbirths and the births and deaths of early neonates were still escaping registration.

On 1 July 1936, what was described as a Rural Uplift Centre was inaugurated at Tatkon in the Yamethin township. It was funded by a grant of Rs. 5 *lakhs* from the Government of India. The responsibilities of the Health Department extended to the whole township, not only to Tatkon and, as with the Hlegu Centre, emphasis was placed on vital registration. The recorded CBR for the years 1937, 1938 and 1939 were 39.71, 46.72, and 48.54 per 1,000. The 1938 figure was 11.44 above the previous five-year mean, or approximately 25 per cent higher. The CDR from 1937 to 1939 was 28.68, 32.65 and 35.04, and again the 1938 figure was 11 above the five-year mean; that is, approximately 33 per cent higher.[48] Surprisingly, the annual reports made little comment on these figures, despite the fact that the statistics from Tatkon were closely in line with the former estimates of the health officials.

The registration data from these two health centres confirmed the former estimates of the sanitary commissioners that between 25 and 33 per cent of vital events were not registered. Indeed, the Hlegu figures implied that nearly 50 per cent of the vital events in that township had formerly not been registered, and this was in an area where at least partial registration had started 70 years previously.

This discussion of the history and the quality of the registration system in Burma leads to the conclusion that between one-quarter and one-third of the vital events were not recorded. It is difficult to make even the most basic demographic deductions from such flawed data, especially as the levels of inaccuracy varied from district to district and town to town. The other possible source of data is the census material: could it be used as an alternative and more accurate source of Crude Birth Rates and Crude Death Rates?

The census of Burma as a source of CBRs and CDRs

The census statistics of Burma, even with under-enumeration, provide more exact data than the registration figures. The problem is to find a technique that could utilise those census statistics. Modern demographers have devised a number of techniques to extract the most accurate information possible from incomplete data, and the most suitable method for the Burma data is one described in the volume usually known as Manual 4, "Methods of Estimating Basic Demographic Measures from Incomplete Data".[49] This describes the techniques for estimating the mortality and birth rates of populations from census survival rates.

The data requirements

The analysis requires a closed population; namely, one that is closed to migration or has detailed records of the gains and losses caused by migration. Other requirements are the details of the distribution of the population by sex and in five-year age groups, and these must be recorded in two or more successive census, five or ten years apart. The data must show evidence of a stable population; that is, with little change in fertility or mortality, and, in addition, each census must refer to the same geographical area. The subsequent paragraphs in this section will examine these requirements in turn and explain how the data from the Burma census was adjusted to these needs.

A closed population

The greatest problem with the Burma census data was the distortion caused by male immigration from the Indian sub-continent. This was a major difficulty, which was bypassed by using only female data. This had an added advantage in that it also eliminated many of the problems caused by internal migration, as much of this was male. It was disappointing to have to discard half the population data, but demographically the most important group was retained and now provided a "closed" population suitable for analysis.

Detailed information on the sex and age distribution

One of the other requirements for the analysis was the detailing of the population by five-year age groups and sex in each census. In the Burma census series from 1891 to 1921, these age groups form part of the Tables of Religion. This means that the population in those tables is listed firstly by religion, then by sex and age groups.

The information was grouped by district so that, for example, in 1921 the reference was to the "Imperial Table VIIB, Age, Sex and Civil Condition by Religion". The population was listed from left to right by sex, and then by unmarried male, female and totals, and then married and widowed males, females and totals. This information was defined vertically under each district, and subdivided into Buddhist, Animist, Hindu, Mohammedan, Christian and All Religions. Unfortunately, in districts where there were only small groups of non-Buddhists, these populations appear in the table as totals only, with no age groups, so it was not possible to include these minorities in the analysis.[50] As approximately 90 to 95 per cent of the women in the study area were Buddhist, this was the safest data to use for the analysis. Unfortunately, this also eliminated the small community of indigenous Muslim women, but their data was not distinguished in every district from the non-indigenous Muslim women, nor were age groupings available for every district. The data-base for analysis had thus shrunk through discarding first the male cohort and then the non-Buddhist women, but the remaining cohort of Buddhist women formed a firm group for which the necessary details were available. They represented the majority of females in Burma and formed, for example, 44 per cent of the total census population in 1901.

A further complication affected the data from the 1921 and 1931 censuses. The division of the population into five-year age groups appeared in the Tables of Race in the 1931 census and not under the

Tables of Religion as earlier. This meant that instead of five-year age groupings existing for female Buddhists in the 1931 census, there were age groupings for Burmese females.

Since the analysis requires two directly comparable cohort groups ten years apart, if the 1931 data was to be used, then a comparable cohort group in five-year age groups had to be found in the 1921 census. This was resolved by using the data for women of "All Religions", less the numbers of Hindu and Muslim women in Burma. This left a cohort consisting of Buddhist, animist and Christian women, plus a few "Others". The very few European Christian women were inevitably included in this cohort, as were the animists, but their numbers were too insignificant to affect the analysis. The reason that Christian women were included in the cohort was that many Karen women were Catholic, and would undoubtedly have been considered as "Burmese" in the 1931 racial category.[51] The main difficulty lay in the subtraction of the Hindu and Muslim females because, as previously explained, the detailed five-year age groups were not available for every district in the 1921 census, and therefore the option of simple subtraction was not possible.

The solution was the method recommended in the UN Manual 4;[52] that is, a reduction in each age group of "All Religions" by the ratio of the number of Hindu and Muslim women to the total number of women of "All Religions". In relation to the Burma census, there was a total of 160,688 Hindu and Muslim women in Burma in 1921 (excluding as far as was possible those born in Burma) and a total female population under "All Religions" of 4,692,400 (both groups included females aged 60-plus), giving a ratio of 0.034 (160,688 divided by 4,692,400). Therefore each five-year age group of "All Religions" was reduced by this figure, thereby providing cohort groups that were comparable to the 1931 census figures. This method makes the assumption that the demographic characteristics (e.g. numbers in each age group) of the migrant population were the same as the indigenous population. In this case, this is a justified assumption, as the Indian females did appear comparable in that respect to the Burmese females (that is each group showed a full age range) but the method could not be used for the male Indian community as most of them were between 15 and 30 years of age.

The 1931 census figures also showed an anomaly. In 1921, 160,688 Hindu and Muslim women had been recorded, but the 1931 records show only 99,131. In the 1931 census, in many districts only Burmans or "Other Indigenous Races" were listed, so it seems probable that the categories of Hindu and Muslim females were incomplete. To smooth this anomaly, the number of "Indian" females in 1921 — 160,688 — was assumed to have grown at the same rate as the rest of the population in the decade 1921 to 1931; that is, by 1.02 per cent per annum, giving a new "Indian" female population figure for 1931 of 177,851. This figure, as a proportion of the total female population, was of course again 0.034, as the number of Hindu and Muslim females and the total female population under "All Religions" had increased at the same rate. Each of the five-year age groups in the females "All Races" table of 1931 was then reduced by this amount.

These adjustments of the 1921 and 1931 census data provided female cohort groups in each census that were suitable for analysis.[53] But unfortunately, further smoothing was found to be necessary on all the census material before it could be used.

The five-year age groups necessary for the analysis appeared only in the 1891 and 1931 censuses. In the 1901 and 1911 censuses, the age groups were in five-year periods only up to the age of 20 years, followed by two 20-year age groups (20 to 40 years and 40 to 60 years), and a 60-plus group. In the 1921 census, the groupings from age 20 to 60 years were divided into ten-year intervals. In 1931, the five-year age groupings were continuous from age zero to five and up to the age of 70. If any analysis was to be done on the material, then continuous five-year age groups were necessary in each census. These were found by sub-dividing the larger age groups in the 1901, 1911 and 1921 censuses into five-year age groups containing the same ratios of the population as they did in the 1891 census.

This was felt to be justified by the correspondence between the ratio of the age groups in the 1891 census to the same groups in the 1931 census. Until the age of 40 years, both these censuses showed almost the same proportions of their populations in each five-year age group. Between the ages of 40 and 60 years there was some disparity, but with the majority of the 1931 population showing a similar structure to that of the 1891 population, it was felt that the sub-division of the intervening census populations by this method was justified.

In 1901, for example, there were 1,100,474 Buddhist females in the study area between the ages of 20 and 40 years. In the 1891 census, 58 per cent of the population in the 20 to 40 year age group were up to 30 years old, and 42 per cent were between the ages of 30 and 40 years. When these percentages were applied to the 1901 figure, 638,275 females were between 20 and 30 years, and 462,199 were between 30 and 40 years. Similarly, of the 20 to 30 year cohort in 1891, 54 per cent of these females were between 20 and 24 years and 46 per cent were between 25 and 29 years.

This method of proportional sub-division of age groups was applied to all the 20-year age groupings in the 1901 and 1911 censuses. The ten-year age groupings in the 1921 census were also proportionally divided by the same ratio as the ten-year age groups in the 1891 census; that is, 54 per cent and 46 per cent between the ages of 20 to 30 years.

It has already been stated that, in order to analyse the 1921 to 1931 data, the number of females of "All Religions", less the numbers of Hindus and Muslim women, was used. As this was done in order to find a comparable cohort group to the 1931 cohort, it was decided to sub-divide the ten-year age groups in the cohort by the same proportion as in the 1931 census; that is, only marginally different from the 1891 groups up to the age of 40 years, but showing more deviation in the 40 and 60 year groups. The major difference lay in the over-50 year groups; in 1891, the 50 to 54 year cohort represented 56 per cent of the population between the age of 50 and 60 years, but in 1931 the same cohort represented 65 per cent of the ten-year age group.

The last problem needing to be resolved before the census data could be used for analysis was that of age misreporting. Age errors, age heaping or age shifting[54] are all terms used to describe the tendency in populations to misreport ages to census officials. In the less bureaucratic populations of the world, where age is often a matter of memory, age-reporting errors are quite common. In addition to simple error, age heaping is caused by a tendency in particular cultures to report ages thought to be lucky or honourable. Age shifting is often seen as exaggeration of age in the elderly. Also very common is the under-reporting of infants.

In Burma, age heaping was very conspicuous in the 40 to 44 year age group of the 1891 census and, to a lesser extent, in the 50 to 54 year age group. This concentration is illustrated more clearly by the accompanying population pyramid (Figure 2.2). From the age of five years to the age of 39 years, each five-year female age group diminished by approximately 35,000. But in the 40 to 44 year age group there were only 7,500 fewer females than in the 35 to 39 year group, and the next age group of 45 to 49 years was 48,000 fewer at 111,496, thus showing a conspicuous age preference for 40 to 44 years. The numbers in the next age group, 50 to 54 years, were 123,778, an increase of 11,000 from the 45 to 49 year age group. The problem was partly solved by the use of the technique of cumulation, which is described below.

Another common error, apparent within the tables of age groups in the Burma census, was the under-reporting of infants up to one year old. This error ran through the whole census series, but was most easily identified in 1921 and 1931, when the under-five-years age groups were subdivided into the first year of life and one to five years. It would be reasonable to expect the infant (zero to one year group) to comprise more than one-fifth of the under-fives, as infant mortality and weaning mortality takes a considerable toll. (The estimates of the

Age group

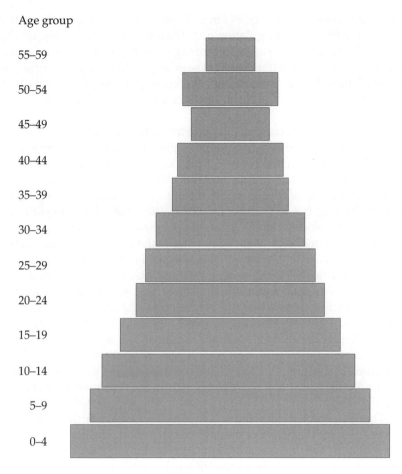

FIGURE 2.2
Population Pyramid Census 1891 Showing Heaping In
Age Groups 40–44 and 50–54

Sources: *Census of Burma 1891.*

extent of infant mortality are found in Chapter Three.) But in 1921, these female infants comprised 20.2 per cent of the under-fives, and in 1931, just under 20 per cent. This is noted for interest only as it does not affect the calculations.

The recommended method of dealing with the age misreporting in census data is cumulation of the age groups from the youngest up to the oldest.[55] This means that when the survival rate of a cohort over a ten-year period is calculated, it is not the survival of the individual cohort between, say, the age of ten to 15 years that is calculated, but the survival of the whole population over the age of ten years. This has the effect of dampening the effect of age misreporting, because the misinformation lies within a larger segment of the age distribution of a population, hence "smoothing" the error. All the census data was cumulated in this way and the result can be seen in Table 2.3.

A stable population occupying the same geographical area
Fortunately, the evidence of a stable population, which is required for the analysis, exists in the census data. As already stated in the discussion of age groups, the 1891 census and the 1931 census showed almost the same proportions of their populations in five-year age groups up to the age of 40 years, but with some deviation after that. This was felt to be evidence of sufficient stability for the purpose of the analysis.

The problem of each census referring to the same geographical area was the most easily overcome. This was achieved by aggregating the data on a district basis and using only those districts that lay within the study area. The total figure for the study area was then used for the analysis. Unfortunately this did not solve all the problems relating to geographical area, as adjustments were necessary for the changes that had taken place in the northeast and southeast boundaries of the study area. These adjustments were calculated in a similar way to those described in Chapter One to provide constant district boundaries to the Wuntho state, Katha and Shwebo districts in the northeast, and Thaton, Pegu, Shwegyin and Amherst districts in the southwest.[56]

One other adjustment that is sometimes necessary with census data is correction for the length of the inter-censal period. The Burma censuses were held in February and March, and, excluding the 1872 and 1881 censuses, the greatest departure from the ten-year interval was the period between the 1921 and 1931 censuses. This interval was three weeks short of ten years. As many more necessary and "heroic" adjustments had already been made to the data, it was decided that the adjustment of the population to a period of three weeks in ten years would be an unnecessary sophistication.

It would be helpful at this point to summarise the adjustments that have been made to the census data in preparing it for analysis. The first and most important was the decision to use only Buddhist female data in order to exclude the Indian migrant community and alleviate the distortion caused by internal migration. The problems caused by the switch from Tables of Religion to Tables of Race in 1931 were overcome by the use of the data for "All Religions" in 1921 and for "All Races" in 1931, less the numbers of Hindus and Muslims born outside Burma for both census years. The other major difficulty, caused by the lack of

TABLE 2.2

Census of Burma 1901: Buddhist Female Data by Age Group (unadjusted)

Age Group	Population	Age Group	Population
0–5	530,476	20–40	1,100,474
5–10	461,808	40–60	546,941
10–15	388,648	60+	247,360
15–20	350,167		

five-year age groups in the 1901, 1911 and 1921 censuses, was overcome by dividing the large cohort groups into the same proportions as existed in the 1891 census. In addition, the data was cumulated to dampen the effect of age misreporting; and finally the figures were adjusted for the changes in the boundary of the study area.

The method of analysis

Probably the simplest way to explain the method used in the analysis to establish CBRs and CDRs is to use one of the census years as an example. The data from 1901 was chosen because this census was neither complicated by underestimation (in the way that the 1891 figures were) nor involved in the change from religious to racial data. Before any adjustment, the 1901 Buddhist female data from the 27 districts of the study area were in the form shown in Table 2.2.

The first step was to divide the population into five-year age groups in the same proportions as in the 1891 census. The numbers were then cumulated from the top; that is, from the youngest to the oldest. Data from the under-tens and the over-60s are not used in the analysis. Table 2.3 shows the data used for analysis.

The analysis requires the use of model life tables, and it was decided to use the West Model series from the Office of Population Research, Princeton University.[57] This choice was influenced by the fact that the West Model tables contain no persistent or consistent deviation from a median world experience of mortality, whereas the North, South and East Model tables express regional deviations. Another advantage of the West family tables is that they include the experience of countries as diverse as Taiwan, Australia, South Africa, Canada and those of western Europe. Since it was not known whether the Burmese data contained a regional variation, the best estimations of mortality would

TABLE 2.3

Census of Burma 1901: Buddhist Female Data in Five-year Age Groups
(adjusted and accumulated)

Age Group	Population	Age Group	Population
10+	2,386,232	35+	750,309
15+	1,997,584	40+	546,941
20+	1,647,415	45+	359,778
25+	1,302,746	50+	229,715
30+	1,009,140	55+	84,995

be produced by the use of these more neutral life tables, rather than a table with a persistent deviation, which might have introduced a distortion.

Establishing the model life table level

The object of the immediate exercise was to find the West Model Life Table level that most closely expressed the experience of the Burmese people. This was done by selecting tables with various levels of mortality, in this case levels 1 to 9, within which the Burmese level was estimated to lie. The technique required that the cumulated female population of 1901 be projected to 1911; that is, the different survival rates of the various levels of life tables were used to project how many of the population of 1901 would survive to 1911 at these differing levels of mortality. These estimates of survival were then compared to the actual survival rates shown by the 1911 census figures. The proximation between the estimate and the actual survival should lie within one or two levels of the West Model Life Table and not across a very broad range of levels. This depends on well-adjusted data and fairly accurate estimations of the probable levels of mortality.

The estimation process is shown in Table 2.4. Columns 2 to 6 show the ten-year survival rates in West Model Life Tables at levels 1 to 9.[58] The 1901 female Buddhist population from the study area is shown in Column 7, divided into five-year age groups. The estimates of the population surviving in 1911 are found by multiplying the census figures in Column 7 by each of the survival rate levels 1 to 9 in the same age group. For example, the number of the female population in the ten to 14 year age group in 1901 was 388,648. When this is multiplied by the ten to 14 year survival rate in level 1, the result 333,305 can be found in Column 9 in the 20 to 24 year age group (namely, the ten to 14 year

TABLE 2.4

Example of the Use of Model Life Tables on Data from 1901 Census
(Buddhist Females) to Find the Survival Levels in 1911

1	2	3	4	5	6	7
	Ten-year Survival Rates in West Model Life Tables					*1901 Census (adjusted)*
Age Group	*Level 1*	*Level 3*	*Level 5*	*Level 7*	*Level 9*	*5-yr Age Intervals*
0–4	0.737	0.7847	0.8232	0.8552	0.8826	530,476
5–9	0.8736	0.8946	0.9121	0.9271	0.9401	461,808
10–14	0.8576	0.8808	0.9001	0.9167	0.9312	388,648
15–19	0.8286	0.856	0.8789	0.8986	0.9158	350,169
20–24	0.805	0.8358	0.8616	0.8838	0.9032	344,669
25–29	0.7841	0.8178	0.8461	0.8704	0.8917	293,606
30–34	0.766	0.8018	0.8319	0.8578	0.8805	258,831
35–39	0.7518	0.7884	0.8193	0.8459	0.8692	203,368
40–44	0.7267	0.7649	0.7972	0.8251	0.8496	187,163
45–49	0.675	0.7177	0.7539	0.7853	0.813	130,063
50–54	0.592	0.6415	0.684	0.7216	0.7541	144,720
55–59	0.482	0.5384	0.5875	0.6308	0.6696	84,995
60+	0.3617	0.4202	0.4721	0.5185	0.5605	247,360

8	9	10	11	12	13
	Projected Figures from Ten-year Survival Rates in West Model Life Tables				
Age Group	*Level 1*	*Level 3*	*Level 5*	*Level 7*	*Level 9*
0–4					
5–9					
10–14	390,961	416,265	436,688	453,663	468,198
15–19	403,435	413,133	421,215	428,142	434,146
20–24	333,305	342,321	349,822	356,274	361,909
25–29	290,150	299,745	307,764	314,662	320,685
30–34	277,459	288,074	296,967	304,618	311,305
35–39	230,216	240,111	248,420	255,555	261,808
40–44	198,265	207,531	215,322	222,025	227,901
45–49	152,892	160,335	166,619	172,029	176,767
50–54	136,011	143,161	149,206	154,428	159,014
55–59	87,793	93,346	98,054	102,138	105,741
60+					

continued

TABLE 2.4

continued

14	15	16	17	18	19	20
	Projected Figures from Ten-year Survival Rates in West Model Life Tables					*Cumulated 1911 Census*
Age Group	*Level 1*	*Level 3*	*Level 5*	*Level 7*	*Level 9*	
0+						
5+						
10+	2,500,486	2,604,022	2,690,077	2,763,535	2,827,474	2,705,009
15+	2,109,526	2,187,758	2,253,389	2,309,872	2,359,276	2,232,301
20+	1,706,090	1,774,624	1,832,174	1,881,729	1,925,130	1,835,884
25+	1,372,786	1,432,303	1,482,352	1,525,456	1,563,221	1,458,603
30+	1,082,635	1,132,559	1,174,589	1,210,794	1,242,537	1,137,215
35+	805,177	844,484	877,622	906,176	931,232	853,892
40+	574,960	604,373	629,202	650,621	669,423	631,282
45+	376,696	396,843	413,880	428,596	441,522	415,257
50+	223,804	236,507	247,261	256,567	264,755	265,138
55+	87,793	93,346	98,054	102,138	105,741	98,101
60+						

age group ten years later). Therefore, if the survival rate of Buddhist females of that age in 1901 corresponded to the level of mortality found in the West Model Life Tables level 1, then 333,305 of the original 388,648 would have survived to make a 20 to 24 year age group in the census of 1911. These calculations are repeated for each age group across the range of the survival rates 1 to 9, and the results are shown in Columns 9 to 13.

The next stage on the table shows the results of cumulation. The projected figures from Columns 9 to 13 are shown in columns 15 to 19, after cumulation. The last column, number 20, shows the cumulated female Buddhist population of the study area from the 1911 census. The projected figures in Columns 15 to 19 are then compared with the actual population in Column 20 to find the model life table level with the closest proximation to the actual Burmese experience. The table shows that the levels closest to the Burmese experience lie between 3 and 7 with one exception. This is the 50-plus age group, where the cumulation has been less effective in smoothing the age misreporting in the 40-plus

TABLE 2.5
Summary of Median Life Table Levels

Inter-censal Period	Median Life Table Level
1891–1901	8.88
1901–1911	5.15
1911–1921	3.54
1921–1931	3.46

and 50-plus age groups. But otherwise the result shows a consistency that justifies the extensive preparatory smoothing of the data.

One more calculation was needed to find the exact level of mortality that would produce the projected population that precisely matched the census population of 1911. This level was found by interpolation. For example, at age group 20-plus, the proximation to the actual 1911 population figure lay between levels 5 and 7, and was in fact very close to level 5. The calculation to find the intermediate level was: $([1,835,884 - 1,832,174] \div [1,881,729 - 1,832,174]) \times 2 + 5 = 5.15$.

A calculation was made for each age group from ten-plus to 55-plus and the median level of 5.15 was then selected as providing the most accurate estimate of the level of mortality for Buddhist females between 1901 and 1911. These calculations were then repeated for the other inter-censal periods, and the results are shown in Table 2.5.

It is obvious from these figures that either the level of mortality between 1891 and 1901 was lower than that of subsequent years or that there was a problem with the data. If, as discussed in the first chapter, the 1891 census suffered a greater degree of under-enumeration than subsequent census, then the survival calculations would be distorted. The result would be a falsely high survival rate, which would explain the margin between the estimated level up to 1901 and after 1901. Unfortunately there is no way in which the 1891 census figures could be adjusted for under-enumeration without prejudging the estimated survival rate. A calculation of survival rates following an adjustment by an additional ten per cent for under-enumeration in 1891 produced a median estimate of level 2.58. I would suggest that probably the true level for that inter-censal period lies between the two estimates of 8.88 and 2.58 and that the survival level was approximately 5-plus, and therefore very close to the 1901 to 1911 level. A more definitive interpretation would rely too much on subjective decisions and circularity, and could not be justified.

TABLE 2.6

Example of the Use of West Model Life Tables to Calculate the Mortality Rate
Corresponding to Survival Levels

1	2	3	4	5	6	7	8
Age Group	Mortality Rate Level 5	Mortality Rate Level 6	Mortality Rate Level 5.15	1901 Pop. 1,000s	1911 Pop. 1,000s	Mean Pop. 1,000s	Av. Annual Deaths 1,000s
0–4	112.28	99.84	110.42	530.4	564.1	547.2	60.42
5–9	10.33	9.37	10.19	461.8	546.2	504.0	5.13
10–14	8.00	7.26	7.89	388.6	472.7	430.6	3.39
15–19	10.51	9.56	10.37	350.1	396.4	373.2	3.87
20–24	13.20	12.03	13.02	344.6	377.2	360.9	4.69
25–29	14.84	13.53	14.64	293.6	321.3	307.4	4.50
30–34	16.82	15.33	16.60	258.8	283.3	271.0	4.49
35–39	18.49	16.88	18.25	203.3	222.6	212.0	3.88
40–44	19.88	18.21	19.63	187.1	216.0	201.5	3.95
45–49	21.51	19.82	21.32	130.0	150.1	140.0	2.98
50–54	28.05	25.92	27.73	144.7	167.0	155.8	4.32
55–59	36.04	33.43	35.65	84.9	98.1	91.5	3.26
60+	86.69	84.27	86.33	188.1	252.4	220.2	19.00
					Totals	3816.2	123.88

Sources: Cols. 2 and 3: West Model Life Tables [$n^m(x)$]; Cols. 5 and 6: *Census of Burma*, adjusted.

Estimating the crude death and birth rates

The calculations of the life table levels also provided the key to the estimations of inter-censal CBRs and CDRs. Again the methods used were those described in Manual 4,[59] and the data used was the average inter-censal populations for each age group and the West Model Life Table mortality rates for each age group corresponding to each inter-censal survival level. An example of the calculation to find the CDR between 1901 and 1911 is shown in Table 2.6. The mortality rate corresponding to level 5.15 (Column 4) was calculated from the level 5 and 6 data (Columns 2 and 3), and the average inter-censal population (Column 7) was calculated from the census data (Columns 5 and 6).

TABLE 2.7
Summary of Average Crude Death Rates

Inter-censal Period	Average CDR
1901–1911	32.5
1911–1921	37.4
1921–1931	37.6

The average annual deaths for each age group (Column 8) was found by multiplying Column 4 by Column 7. The average CDR was then found by dividing the average inter-censal population by the average yearly number of all deaths. In this example: 123.88 ÷ 3,816.2 = 32.5.

This figure was taken as the most accurate estimate for the average inter-censal CDR from 1901 to 1911 for Buddhist females. These calculations were repeated for the 1911 to 1921 and 1921 to 1931 inter-censal periods, and the results are shown in Table 2.7.

The second step was the calculation to find the CBRs for the same inter-censal periods. This in theory was very simple; the estimated CBR is calculated as the sum of the CDR plus the rate of natural increase (calculated in Chapter One, see Table 1.13). But here a problem arose, as the rate of increase calculated in the previous chapter was for the total indigenous population and not for the female Buddhist population alone. It had not been possible to calculate the rate of increase for males and females separately, due to the limitations in the census data and the problem of Indian immigration. There was no reason to expect unusual differences in the mortality experiences of the sexes, however, so it was decided to use the rates from Chapter One. Obviously this use of general rather than sex-specific data must slightly smudge the accuracy of the result, but not to the point where confidence is lost in the results.

The estimates produced here cannot compare in accuracy with figures from modern, bureaucratic countries. They attempt to improve on the rates from the poor vital registration statistics, and I think that an accuracy level of probably plus or minus one or two is achieved. The calculation for the CBR is shown in Table 2.8.

It should be noted that using the population growth rate for both males and females in this calculation may have raised the estimated birth rate marginally. But this is probably more than compensated by the probability of downward bias in the mortality rate. The estimate of childhood mortality[60] (i.e. the mortality up to ten years old) was extrapolated from the West Model Life Tables, and if that pattern of

TABLE 2.8
Calculation of Crude Birth Rates

Inter-censal Period	CDR	Natural Increase	CBR
1901–1911	32.5	+12.5	= 45.0
1911–1921	37.4	+08.2	= 45.6
1921–1931	37.6	+10.4	= 47.9

mortality is not valid for Burma, then the birth and death rates may be biased. It may be that the mortality level of very young Burmese children was higher than that shown by West Model Life Tables, and if that were so, then the birth and death rates would be under-estimated. But these are marginal differences only, and for the present time, given the existing data, I think that these are the best estimates possible of the Buddhist female CDR and CBR for Burma between 1901 and 1931.

Limitations/shortcomings of the available data

Several attempts were made to estimate the inter-censal survival rate of Buddhist males in the study area. The analysis was not successful, as it produced a wide range of survival levels amongst the age groups in each census. The only inter-censal period producing a narrower range was that between 1901 and 1911, and the median life table level for that period was 2.68. The median level for the inter-censal period 1911 to 1921 was 6.28, but the other periods produced survival levels ranging from 1 to over 11. Little confidence can be felt in median levels calculated from such widely scattered results, and the attempt to produce a CBR and CDR for Buddhist males was abandoned. These poor results had been anticipated and were one of the main reasons for the use of female data only, as that was less influenced by the distortions of internal migration.

Attempts were also made to analyse individual districts using female data, but again the results were too erratic to inspire confidence. This may have been due to seasonal agricultural movement across district borders involving female labour, whereas the movement across the study area boundaries to cut wood or search for minerals was more commonly male. Therefore the total female Buddhist data for the study area was accurate enough for analysis, but on an individual district level, there were too many distortions.

More disappointing than these failures was the lack of any detail in the 1941 census, making analysis of the 1931 to 1941 inter-censal period impossible. The 1930s were a period of change in medical thought, when the most detailed health reports were produced and when the health officials showed the beginnings of an interest in the welfare of the rural community in Burma. But it is possible to state that there is nothing in the health reports to suggest that there was any substantial change in the CBR and CDR in that decade from the rates prevailing in the 1920s. The effect of the Saya San Rebellion on the registration has already been discussed. In addition, there is plenty of evidence in the health reports that the registration was still affected by chronic shortcomings. In 1930, a report from Myaungmya district mentioned a headman who, in six years of office, had never submitted the counterfoils of registration to either the police or his township officer![61] This type of incident was only one example of a more constant complaint about the inefficiencies of the registration.

During the 1930s, the registered BR, DR and IMR were frequently compared to the rates recorded in the provinces of India, and it was noted that although the BR and DR in Burma were comparatively low, the IMR was one of the highest.[62] The health officials were not attempting to stress the high number of infant deaths in Burma but the inefficiencies in the registration system. By contrast, when for example Yamethin township was recording a DR of 34-plus and a BR of 48-plus, this was attributed to "good registration".[63] Although there is only negative evidence, the lack of firm statements in the health reports about a decline in mortality should be accepted as an indicator of a sustained rate of mortality. It is inconceivable that the health department would not report such an achievement as a decline in mortality if they believed it had occurred.

Figure 2.3 compares the registered birth and death rates with the CBRs and CDRs estimated from the model life tables. This gives a better illustration than mere figures of the disparity between the official and estimated rates. Although it must be emphasised again that the techniques used to produce these estimates depend on the stability of the population figures used for analysis, there is nothing in the data to suggest that these levels of mortality are inaccurate.

To summarise the available evidence therefore: the official registration figures continued to be under-recorded, and the health officials were still of the opinion that rates, such as those recorded at Yamethin township, were closer to the correct level. In addition, the evidence from the rural health centres at Tatkon and Hlegu supported the view of a sustained mortality in the 1930s, similar to that experienced in the 1920s. But this cannot be attributed to the major epidemic diseases of

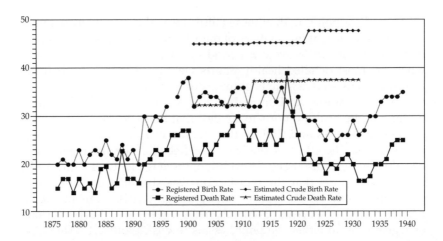

FIGURE 2.3

Burma: Registered Birth and Death Rates with Crude Birth Rates
and Crude Death Rates Estimated from West Model Life Tables
(per 1,000 population)

Sources: Registered rates: *RSAB*; crude rates: Model Life Tables.

smallpox, cholera and plague, as they had been steadily declining as
causes of mortality since 1912. This obviously poses the question, what
were the determinants of this high death rate? This is investigated in
Chapter Six.

3 Infant mortality

In colonial Burma, parents frequently had to come to terms with the bereavement caused by the death of an infant child. For every 100 children born alive, 25 to 35 would not survive to their first birthday. The rate of loss was commented on from the early days of the British administration in Lower Burma; in 1862 the deputy commissioner of Bassein wrote that "The rate of death among the native Burmese is decidedly higher with the infantile portion than the adult community".[1] This chapter will examine the rate of infant deaths as well as their causes.

The first section of the chapter explains the terms used to define infant mortality and then assesses the effectiveness of the registration in recording infant deaths. An estimate of the infant mortality follows, with a discussion of nutrition, disease and the British response to the persistently high mortality.

Infant mortality and how it is calculated

Infant mortality is the mortality of live-born children who have not reached their first birthday. It is usually measured as the number of infant deaths in a given year divided by the number of live births in that same year, and this is commonly known as the Infant Mortality Rate, or IMR, quoted as deaths per 1,000 births. This definition does not include stillbirths, miscarriages or abortions.

Infant mortality consists of two components — neonatal mortality (which occurs in the first month) and post-neonatal mortality (occurring from the age of one to 12 months). This is an important aid to analysis, as a high percentage of mortality occurs in the first, vulnerable hours after birth. Periodisation is further refined by the term "perinatal mortality", which includes the mortality in the first week of life, plus stillbirths and all foetal mortality occurring after the twenty-eighth week of pregnancy. Prior to 1920, the only age details available for infant death in colonial Burma were deaths under one year. From 1920, the deaths were detailed by age, as occurring in the first week, up to one month, from one month to six months, and from six to 12 months. The problem with the use of these figures is that an estimated 30-plus per cent of the infant deaths were not recorded.

Another way of analysing infant mortality is to divide it into "endogenous" and "exogenous" mortality. This is a way of distinguishing between causes that precede the birth or come from the birth itself (endogenous), and those causes that are external (exogenous), such as infection, inadequate nutrition and poor hygiene.[2]

The infant mortality rate is, however, an imprecise measurement in demographic terms. This is because deaths measured in a given year will include many infants whose birth was registered the previous year. For example, a child born in June 1893 may die at the age of nine months in March 1894, and be recorded as part of the infant mortality rate measured on the number of births in 1894. Equally a child born in December 1894 would be recorded in the 1895 IMR figures if it died before its first birthday. Catastrophes, such as famine or pandemic, can cause gross distortion, and if abrupt differences occur in the number of births from year to year, then this also can be misrepresented by the IMR.[3] But for historical data, which is often imprecise, averaged periods of several years of IMRs are acceptable.

The IMR is more vulnerable to distortion than most other demographic rates because two registered rates are needed for its calculation. If the births are under-registered, then the infant deaths will be divided by a figure that is too low, resulting in an artificially high IMR. Conversely, if the infant deaths are inadequately recorded, then the IMR will be artificially low. In colonial Burma, both these potential errors were known to occur. Health officials believed that deaths were more likely to be registered than births, on the grounds that deaths involved a ceremony and were therefore more noticed and noticeable. But, "On the other hand, deaths of infants often escape registration".[4]

The method of measuring infant death rates for some of the colonial period in Burma was to divide the yearly number of infant deaths by an estimate of the population aged under one year. The estimate was in practice the last census figure for that age group and was therefore inaccurate, as it could be (at most) nine years out of date, and, as discussed in Chapter Two, infants were under-enumerated in the census. In later years, the method of calculation was to divide the deaths under one year by the number of births in that year (the method described earlier), although the tables still claimed to show a figure calculated on the ratio per 1,000 living. For the sake of easy comparison, the figures on the accompanying graph, Figure 3.1, are all calculated as infant deaths per 1,000 births for the same year; that is, as an IMR.

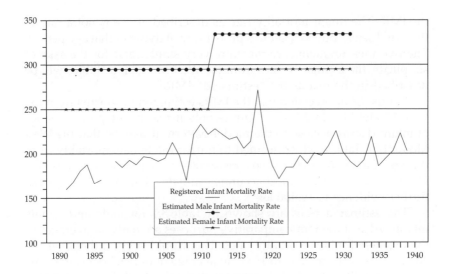

FIGURE 3.1

Burma: Registered Infant Mortality Rate, Calculated as Births Over
Deaths for Each Year, Estimated Rates from West Model Life Tables
Appropriate for Each Inter-censal Period

These official figures suffer, of course, from the same registration
defects that were described in some detail in Chapter Two. However,
it can be seen that during the period of most efficient registration, the
recorded IMR rose to a peak of 233 per 1,000 in 1910, but declined in
the early 1920s, when registration was disrupted. By 1929, it had risen
to 225 per 1,000, only to fall sharply during the period of the Saya San
Rebellion.

It was obviously necessary to find more accurate estimates of the
IMR during the colonial period. It is not possible to use calculations of
survival rates for infants. Therefore only indirect estimation is possible,
and this is done quite simply by reading from the appropriate column
of the West Model Life Table at the level estimated in Chapter Two for
each inter-censal period. The life tables show the numbers in a model
population dying in each age interval, and from these we can deduce
the numbers per 1,000 of infants expected to die before their first
birthday in each mortality level of the life tables. Estimates of infant
mortality for each inter-censal period can therefore be obtained from
the tables.

Although these "rates" taken from the life tables are the number per
1,000 dying in that age interval, they are very close to the definition of

the IMR. The infant mortality rate as described above is not a rate in the usual sense, but is closer to a probability of dying in that age period. The two measurements are therefore very similar and for the sake of simplicity, the estimated rates from the West Model Life Tables will be described in the text as the "estimated" IMR.

It must be appreciated that the IMRs estimated for Burma from the West Model Life Tables are accurate only if that country's experience of infant deaths is close to the model pattern. It may be that the West Model Life Tables, which seemed to mirror the female mortality from the age of ten to 60, may not so consistently model the infant mortality. However, these are the most accurate estimates that can be made until further evidence is available.

The estimated rates are shown in Table 3.1 for male and female infants. Also shown for comparative purposes are ten-year averages of the registered infant mortality rates. This would suggest that over the 40-year period from 1891 to 1931, an average of only 68 per cent of the infant mortality was officially registered; that is, the difference between the registered rate of 200 deaths per 1,000 and the estimated rate of approximately 300 per 1,000. To put it another way, for every ten children born alive in British Burma, at least one arrived and then died before its first birthday without entering the registration system.

The significance of the infant mortality rate

There are obvious reasons why the extent of infant mortality is important, the most significant being the cost in human terms. There is also an

TABLE 3.1
A Comparison of the Estimated IMR and the Registered IMR

	Estimated Rates from West Model Life Tables		Registered Rates (ten-year averages)	
	Female	Male		
1891–1901	250	295	1891–1900	178.0
1901–1911	250	295	1901–1910	200.5
1911–1921	295	335	1911–1920	220.0
1921–1931	295	335	1921–1930	196.6
			1931–1939	199.8

Sources: Coale and Demeny, *Regional Model Life Tables and Stable Populations*, pp. 42–45; Annual health reports.

economic factor — each infant death can be regarded as a lost investment. In addition, infant mortality is a very potent determinant of
demographic growth and therefore needs to be carefully explored in
that context. But there is a more subtle reason why infant mortality is
important, and that is it has been accepted for more than 100 years that
the level of the IMR is a measure of the health and prosperity of a
community as a whole.

An 1861 paper by Dr W. T. Gairdner, which was among the
*Transactions of the National Association for the Promotion of Social Science
in Great Britain and Northern Ireland*, observed that the sanitary state of
very young children was a most delicate test of the real health and wellbeing of the parents, that is, of their social and moral condition at the
productive period of their life.[5] In 1976, a standard demographic textbook
makes the same point: "It [the conventional infant mortality rate] has
been widely used as an indicator of the health conditions of a community
and, hence, of its level of living".[6]

The British health officials in Burma were well aware of this factor,
and their sensitivity to potential criticism runs through the records. A
bald summary of the situation was made in 1909 by C. E. Williams, the
sanitary commissioner, when he commented that the high infant
mortality in Thayetmyo town was "intimately associated with the social
and sanitary conditions under which the towns-people live",[7] and in
1939, a statement very close to the 1976 definition appeared in the
health records: "The death rate among infants under one year is
considered as a useful index to the social circumstance of a country."[8]

A convenient way to examine the significance of Burma's infant
mortality is to compare the figures with those of neighbouring countries.
As infant mortality is such an important part of total mortality, it is not
surprising to find that, again, Burma's experience appears to differ
somewhat from her neighbours. In the Straits Settlements (S.S) and
Federated Malay States (F.M.S), the IMR had declined by the 1930s from
well over 200 to 168.3 (1936 S.S.) and 142.0 (1936 F.M.S.).[9] In the city of
Bangkok, the average IMR from 1932 to 1934 was 168.0.[10] In India, the
probability of dying in the first year of life declined after 1920
"from the highest values of 301 per 1,000 live births (1911–20) for
males and 284 for females (1901–11), to 190 and 175, respectively, in
1941–50".[11]

It makes little difference whether these neighbouring rates are
contrasted with either the registered IMR for Burma or the estimated
IMR, as neither rate indicates a decline in the infant mortality. The
average official rate for 1931 to 1939 is almost identical with the rate for
1901 to 1910, as both are within 0.7 of 200 per 1,000. The estimated IMR
paints an even worse picture of an increasing rate rather than the

decline seen in neighbouring countries. The following sections on infant malnutrition, disease and the British administration's response will argue that a combination of cultural traditions, infections, particularly malaria, and lack of commitment by the responsible authorities effectively condemned these infants.

Infant nutrition

The first public health report for British Burma, written in 1867, commented on the "excessive mortality amongst Burmese children"[12] and attributed this chiefly to indigestible food. This theme of poor infant nutrition was constantly pursued in the reports up to the 1930s, although not all sanitary commissioners were prepared to admit "excessive" infant mortality within the jurisdiction of Burma.

In 1899, the first link was made in the annual health reports between poverty and high infant mortality. This judgement by C. C. Little, the sanitary commissioner, anticipated twentieth-century opinion, while blaming Burmese ignorance, by recognising the sensitivity of infants to "unhealthy surroundings and morbific conditions generally".[13] Two years later, however, in the health report of 1901, Little is found defending the IMR of Burma as not exceptionally high compared to the other provinces of India.[14]

The somewhat confused nature of this reasoning continued in the official records. A reluctance to admit that the IMR in Burma was high vies with an anxiety to explain that the reason why infants were dying was the ignorance of the mother and her provision of harmful foods to the child. The deputy commissioner of Bassein in 1862 commented "bitterly on the want of care of parents for their offspring and the general indifference to sanitation."[15] In 1904, the high IMR was attributed to "improper feeding, neglect, insanitary surroundings and improper clothing".[16] By 1905, it is blamed on the lack of available cow's milk, the cesspits and flies.[17] The governor of Burma, Sir Herbert White, added his weight to the argument: "Evidence in other countries points rather to the conclusion that improper feeding is the main cause of infantile mortality."[18] Even more sweeping criticism is found in the 1915 Henzada issue of the *Burma Gazetteer*: "The reasons for this extremely high mortality rate amongst the children are the employment of ignorant midwives, improper feeding, and the insanitary conditions in which the children are born and reared. Burmese mothers must rank amongst the worst mothers in the world."[19]

By 1913, empirical enquiry had replaced such sweeping criticism in some of the reports, and local charitable societies for the prevention of infant mortality were being developed with support from the government. The Mandalay Society for the Prevention of Infant Mortality conducted an enquiry into the 2,124 infant deaths in Mandalay in 1912, and reported that 24.9 per cent could be attributed to malnutrition and 22.5 per cent to prematurity.[20] In 1915, the health officers of Mandalay and Rangoon provided statistics that analysed the infant deaths in those towns due to a grouping of causes, which included malnutrition (the others in the group were premature birth, debility and atrophy). They attributed 41.39 per cent of the deaths in Rangoon and 23.9 per cent of those in Mandalay to these four causes.[21] For 1916, an updated set of figures is available for Mandalay only, in which 20.2 per cent of infant deaths is said to be caused by this group, excluding atrophy.[22]

The 1920 health report gives causes of infant death for Mandalay, Bassein and Rangoon, although for varying periods. Unfortunately the terminology has changed, becoming "deficient vitality (premature birth, debility etc.)", but as the only figure given for Rangoon is the 1915 figure of 41.39 per cent, it can be assumed that the classification is constant. The figure for Bassein of 39.74 per cent is presumably an average as it covers 1910, 1911 and 1914. The figure for Mandalay, covering 1913 to 1916, is 28.48 per cent.[23]

There are a number of obvious difficulties concerning the use of these figures. Firstly, the registered IMR is, by my estimates, severely under-counted. Secondly, the deaths are attributed to these causes after the infants' demise, either from a description given by the parents or from the appearance of the body. It is possible that a few of the children were treated by the health oficer or seen by a charitable society midwife, but for the majority, a cursory examination after death would be the nearest approach to diagnosis. Thirdly, the figures are urban only, but no significant variation between urban and rural infant diet is suggested in the records. These are reasons for caution, but are not sufficient for discarding the only figures available, which put prematurity and "nutrition related" deaths at 20 to 40 per cent of the total.

Although references to infant diet continue in the annual health reports, in the 1920s and 1930s they are mainly confined to brief comments on ignorance, debility and malnutrition,[24] as the main emphasis in the 1930s switched to the study of infectious disease.

Criticism of infant diet in Burma is probably the most consistent theme running through the British health official's explanations of infant mortality. Even when allowance has been made for the prejudice implied in much of this comment, the consistency of the criticism and the results of the few investigations made suggest that the infant diet of this period should be examined.

Maternal diet and its effects on in-utero nutrition

Infant nutrition is not solely a matter of the child's diet but is, perhaps, equally concerned with maternal diet. There are two obvious stages of infant nutrition, the *in-utero* and the post-natal. At both these stages the child may be dependent on the quantity and quality of its mother's diet, making the chronic under- or malnutrition of the mother a threat to the child's health.

The foetus *in-utero* is totally dependent on the mother nutritionally, but post-natally, the human infant is commonly fed on breast milk supplemented with other foods as available. This means that there are three particular aspects of nutrition to consider for the Burmese infant. Is there evidence to suggest that malnutrition, at any or all of these stages, contributed to the high rate of infant mortality? I suggest that evidence (which augments the official British comments) supports the hypothesis that many, if not the majority, of infant deaths in Burma were diet-related.

Malnourishment could start in foetal life, but to find evidence of such a private, domestic matter as the diet of pregnant Burmese women in the period of the study is not easy. A few references to a poor state of health in pregnant and parturient women do exist. In 1915, when discussing the high stillbirth rate for Mandalay town (26.5 per cent), the sanitary commissioner considered this a reflection of "a very serious state of health of the pregnant or parturient mother".[25] From Akyab, there is a comment by the health officer in 1931, that, "With so many sickly, poorly nourished mothers, ... puny, weakly babies are inevitable".[26]

The health report of 1939 contains more concrete evidence in the form of an extract from the report of a lady assistant district health officer from the Sanitary Department. In the course of investigating the high IMR of a Burmese town, this health officer visited mothers and infants at their homes and reported the following.

> From the infants I inspected during my home visits, I have formed a very strong conviction that most of the deaths which occur within the first three months are primarily due to malnutrition. Most mothers even those of the middle class that can afford luxurious diet, try to starve themselves during pregnancy. This I may say is due to the Burmese custom and prejudices that they still follow even now. They believe that if during this period they live strictly on rice diet with some dried fish and other dried products, they are bound to be free from ailments that people who take plenty of fresh and rich foodstuff would suffer from. In some very poor cases pregnant mothers would restrict themselves to such an extent that they would eat nothing but rice and a few grains of salt as they cannot afford to have dried fish.

Is there any wonder then that a child born of such a mother is so poorly nourished? On examination some mothers were found to be devoid of subcutaneous fat, some have angular stomatitis and gastro-intestinal disturbance, etc. The infants are also devoid of subcutaneous fat, their bones are very soft, and on the whole they are very undersize.

Report on the State of Public Health in Burma, 1939, p. 42

The suggestion that dietary deprivation amongst pregnant women was widespread in Burma receives support from more modern sources. In 1959, C. V. Foll, the Chief Medical Officer of the Burmah Oil Company, described the cultural beliefs prescribing the diet of pregnant women in Burma. He reports that "the main concern of antenatal diet is concentration on those foods which are believed will bring about a not-too-heavy baby with a small head."[27] Also the diet is restricted by the avoidance of those hot or harsh foods (like chillies or honey) or green vegetables, which are believed harmful to the child *in-utero*.[28]

These restrictions are confirmed by an undated paper (probably from the 1970s) written by Dr Ma Ma Tin, which reports on an investigation of feeding patterns in the Mandalay region. In the section concerning dietary beliefs during pregnancy, Dr Ma Ma Tin confirmed the exclusion of green vegetables, fruits, hot foods and first-class proteins (such as beef and fish) from the diet, as they could be harmful to the baby. The reduction in the quantity of the food taken by the mother, with the object of reducing the pressure on the uterus and to keep the baby small, is also discussed in the paper.[29]

Additional supportive evidence comes from a paper by Dr Cho Nwe Oo, discussing the results of a survey carried out in Hlegu township in 1974. Dr Cho Nwe Oo found the protein and calcium intake of pregnant women deficient, and concluded that the low average birth weight (2.75 kg) of babies in Burma was "not a genetic characteristic but is due in part to maternal malnutrition".[30] The conclusion of this paper is that one of the two most detrimental factors "affecting child health are [*sic*] dietary inadequacy during pregnancy with consequent low birth weight and increased perinatal mortality."[31]

Other important surveys have been carried out since the Second World War, and these have included a World Health Organization (WHO) nutrition project during which 2,127 expectant and lactating mothers were examined between 1955 and 1957. Dr S. Postmus, a senior WHO officer, in the text of one of his reports, drew on the detailed knowledge of the superintendent of the Children's Clinic in Mandalay for details of the diet of pregnant women in Burma. The superintendent had 25 years of experience in the clinic prior to 1955, which means that his observations fall well within the period of the study and are therefore particularly valuable in confirming the other data. He observed that "many expectant mothers are afraid that a rich diet will result in a big baby and, consequently, in a difficult and painful delivery; they prefer to go hungry, eating very sparingly for fear of the consequences."[32] The superintendent confirmed that, during pregnancy, vegetables, fruit, eggs, milk and sugar are avoided.

The dietary survey also confirmed the pre-war findings of Dr U Maung Gale, who, in 1939, established that the eating of highly milled rice was widespread in Burma. The WHO found that home-pounded rice was eaten in Myitkyina district, but that only highly milled rice was eaten in Payagyi district, "rural" Rangoon, Maymyo and Lashio. The result of eating highly milled rice was a diet deficient in thiamine, which could, given the stress of pregnancy, produce beri beri.

These post-1940 reports of the beliefs and practices that affected the diet of pregnant women in Burma strengthen the pre-war evidence that malnutrition during pregnancy affected the viability of the new-born child. It was to these infants' disadvantage that their mothers' diet was restricted by custom as well as by the vagaries of harvests and food shortages. A diet that reduced the protein, mineral and vitamin intake, and was also designed, understandably, to restrict the size of the baby for parturition purposes, thereby placed the child at great risk especially in the first, most hazardous, month, when the principal causes of death are low birth weight and neonatal tetanus.[33]

Postmus found that average birth weights in Burma were low. He reported an average male weight at birth of 2.763kg from 2,012 boys born, and an average female weight of 2.719kg. But within these averages there were 26.4 per cent of boys and 30.9 per cent of girls born with a weight lower than 2.5kg, the official definition of prematurity.[34] Other studies in Burma have shown high numbers of infants born below 2.5kg. In 1957, Foll recorded 19 per cent of males and 25 per cent of females born below this weight,[35] and a major collaborative project with WHO in 1981 reported 22.4 per cent of all deliveries under this weight.[36] This weight, of course, is a "world" standard, and it could be argued that it is not necessarily applicable to Burma. But it would appear that the relationship between malnutrition and small stature is perpetual, that small babies and children grow up to be small adults. These female adults then desire a small rather than a large baby; their diet also dictates a small infant, and therefore "racial characteristics" may really be ancestral malnutrition.[37] "Adult nutritional status is therefore an outcome of past and present nutrition."[38]

Statistical evidence of malnourishment *in-utero* would appear in high numbers of infant deaths in the first month of life. Only very

TABLE 3.2
Urban Age-Specific Infant Mortality Rates Prior to 1920
(Figures shown as percentage of total registered IMR for Burma)

Town	Year	Deaths at 1 Week	Deaths at 1–4 Weeks	Deaths at 1–3 Months
Thayetmyo	1909	26.0	24.0	
Mandalay	1915	26.8	11.6	26.9
	1916	35.6	11.8	16.9
	1917	30.0	14.0	
	1918	28.0	16.0	
Bassein	1918	"Similar" to Moulmein	13.0	
Moulmein	1918	20.0	13.0	

Sources: *Report on the Sanitary Administration of Burma.*

scanty information is available for Burma before 1920. From that year, details of ages of death under one year were published annually in the public health records.

Information prior to 1920 consists of a few urban details only, shown in Table 3.2. The difficulty with these figures and those post-1920 figures shown in Table 3.3 is that the dividing line between the age groups should be regarded with some suspicion. The difference between a baby dying at seven days or eight days old for example, may be a matter of opinion and, after that, a matter of memory.

In addition to this difficulty, it should be remembered that one-third of the infant deaths were very likely not registered. The probability is high that the majority of these young lives were lost within a few days of birth, thus lessening the significance to the community of both their arrival and departure. This would probably help to explain the difference between the urban figures, on which the charitable societies or the health officials occasionally made special enquiry, and the lower provincial figures (Table 3.3), which were recorded only by the local headmen.

The urban, pre-1920 figures suggest that between 20 and 35 per cent of infant deaths occurred within the first week. Most of these would be endogenous; that is, from malformation, debility or obstetrical trauma,[39] and I suggest that the majority were related to malnutrition.

TABLE 3.3

Comparison of Officially Registered Infant Deaths

Year	Total deaths (<1 year)	0–1 week				0–1 month		1–6 months		7–12 months	
		Males	Females	Total	Total as % of Total (<1 yr)	Total	Total as % of Total (<1 yr)	Total	Total as % of Total (<1 yr)	Total	Total as % of Total (<1 yr)
1920	61,935	6,497	5,243	11,740	18.9	23,717	38.3	25,814	41.7	12,404	20.0
1921	55,826	6,069	4,691	10,760	19.2	20,311	36.4	23,213	41.6	11,802	21.1
1922	59,255	5,420	4,231	9,651	16.2	19,081	32.2	27,642	46.6	12,539	21.2
1923	58,799	5,256	4,065	9,321	15.8	18,566	31.6	28,569	48.6	11,664	19.8
1924	58,683	4,708	3,766	8,474	14.4	17,413	29.7	28,699	48.9	12,571	21.4
1925	51,906	4,114	3,304	7,418	14.2	15,118	29.1	25,998	50.1	10,790	20.8
1926	60,130	4,592	3,664	8,256	13.7	16,887	28.1	30,285	50.4	12,958	21.5
1927	53,754	4,022	3,205	7,227	13.4	15,063	28.0	27,640	51.4	11,051	20.6
1928	58,643	4,305	3,436	7,741	13.2*	15,749	26.9	31,419	53.6	11,475	19.6
1929	64,629	4,370	3,333	7,703	11.9	15,070	23.3	36,155	55.9	13,404	20.7
1930	63,198	4,721	3,716	8,437	13.3	15,950	25.2	34,880	55.2	12,368	19.6
1931	61,276	4,741	3,783	8,524	13.9	15,651	25.5	34,474	56.3	11,151	18.2
1932	61,972	5,043	4,031	9,074	14.6	17,007	27.4	33,422	53.9	11,543	18.6
1933	69,397	5,151	4,019	9,170	13.2	17,060	24.6	39,023	56.2	13,314	19.2
1934	80,238	5,405	4,324	9,729	12.1	18,031	22.5	46,989	58.6	15,218	19.0
1935	74,375	5,660	4,479	10,139	13.6	18,135	24.4	43,210	58.1	13,030	17.5
1936	81,022	5,652	4,505	10,157	12.5	19,052	23.5	46,950	57.9	15,020	18.5
1937	84,889	6,142	4,662	10,804	12.7	19,698	23.2	49,351	58.1	15,840	18.7
1938	93,170	6,216	4,679	10,895	11.6	20,097	21.6	57,946	62.2	15,127	16.2
1939	87,194	6,017	4,653	10,670	12.2	19,585	22.5	53,019	60.8	14,590	16.7

Sources: Annual health reports.

These figures contrast strongly with the official registration figures in Table 3.3, which show a declining percentage of mortality in the first week and in the first month, during the period 1920 to 1939. But significantly, the total mortality between birth and six months remains constant at 80 per cent; it is the distribution that has altered. It is possible that these figures indeed imply a gradual swing from neonatal mortality to a mortality between one and six months, but the constancy of the 80 per cent and the degree of under-registration make it difficult to form firm conclusions on this point.

Maternal diet and breast-feeding

The second stage of the Burmese infant's nutrition, breast-feeding, was universal and prolonged. Early commentators such as Sir Arthur Phayre and K. N. MacDonald remarked on the duration of breast-feeding, which Phayre described as two to three years,[40] and MacDonald observed as not uncommon until three to four years old.[41]

Although the British administrators took for granted the necessity of breast-feeding, they would appear to have found the duration of the practice offensive. Phayre suggested that it was a cause of the excessive infant mortality,[42] and in the annual health report of 1894, the officiating sanitary commissioner G. T. Thomas described breast-feeding for two years as an "insanitary habit which requires correction".[43]

Foll, writing in 1958 and 1959, confirmed the extended duration of breast-feeding in Burma, and said that exceptionally this may be prolonged beyond three years of age.[44] Over a decade later, the writers of the collection of papers *Beliefs and Practices about Foods and Feeding*, which describe local dietary practices in Burma, also confirmed that the practice of prolonged breast-feeding persisted in Burma after 1940, and quoted durations of between six months and three years, with an average period of two years.[45]

Firm evidence therefore exists about the prolonged breast-feeding practised in Burma,[46] but does this negate or enforce the hypothesis of the importance of malnutrition in the high IMR? I would suggest that the dietary beliefs and practices of Burmese women, thought by them to protect the child, affected the efficiency of their lactation and contributed to the nutritional impoverishment of their infants.

The strongest evidence for this dietary restriction appears in the health report for 1928. The assistant district health officer of Bassein, Dr Saw Kyaw Zit wrote: "It is very usual for women in Burma, in their anxiety to have healthy children, to restrict their diet to rice and salt only during lactation. I think this voluntary semi-starvation practised by the over-anxious mother contributes much to the unhealthy condition of the suckling mother and consequent high infant mortality."[47]

I would suggest that this statement by Dr Saw Kyaw Zit should be taken as strong evidence of a widespread practice. In his position as a Burmese doctor, with intimate knowledge of his family and patients, his assessment must be of greater value than the often more cursory understanding of a European doctor.

Post-1940 evidence supports this hypothesis. Foll stated that the lactating mother must avoid "hot" or "harsh" foods, as they will affect the baby.[48] The collection of papers describing local dietary practices in Burma contains several references to proscribed foods during lactation. Dr Ma Ma Tin, reporting on her survey of 170 mothers in the Mandalay region, found that the diet restrictions included avoidance of peas, legumes, gourd and tamarind leaves, flour and wheat, tomatoes, brinjals and chillies. The diet thought most propitious to produce more milk were soups with a little quantity of fish or prawns, with garlic or pepper, or soups made from mutton bone or oxtail.[49]

From the northern Shan states, Dr Sao Yan Naing reported that the (non-Chinese) mothers omit animal proteins from their diet and "usually survive solely on rice, oil and salt". Dr Sao Yan Naing quoted the belief that meat causes "putrefactive stools in the young and vegetables cause colic and pulses produce diarrhoea".[50] Dr Aung Kyin reported briefly from Magwe district in central Burma, that "almost all the mothers soon after childbirth lived on rice, oil of vegetable origin and salt."[51]

A hint that these practices are not confined to Burma is contained in the Food and Agricultural Organisation 1956 *Report of the Nutrition Committee for South and East Asia, Fourth Session*: "It is a common practice in certain countries to restrict the diet of the mother drastically for a few weeks before and after delivery".[52]

One customary practice for which no evidence has been found for the period of this study, is the habit of expressing and discarding the colostrum. Foll claimed that this action was customary but is now (1959) unusual,[53] but Dr Ma Ma Tin claimed that it was still customary in the Mandalay region. "Colostrum is expressed and discarded. It is not given to the baby because it causes diarrhoea."[54] Both these researchers say that the baby was fed on water sweetened with honey or sugar until the mother's milk "came in". A detailed report of a survey carried out between March and April 1974 in Yankin village, near Hlegu town, showed that of 42 children examined, only 50 per cent had been "put to the breast" during the first three days of life. Nineteen per cent were given water only for that period and 16.6 per cent were given sugar solution. The remaining 15-plus per cent were given rice water, milk formula or honey.[55] It is noteworthy that as late as 1974 in Hlegu township, just north of Rangoon, 50 per cent of babies were not "put to the breast" in the first three days of life.

With no direct historical evidence, this interesting customary practice cannot be definitely said to have occurred in the period of the study. But it would seem highly probable that the traditional practice was to discard the colostrum with its high protein content and immunity value for the infant.

The above discussion about diet during pregnancy and lactation has ranged beyond the study period and area in an attempt to offer substantiation to fragmentary historical data. To summarise the argument so far: the hypothesis is that the inadequate nutrition of the pregnant woman in colonial Burma contributed to the high IMR by effecting low birth weights. There is now the additional hypothesis that the lactating mother in Burma also experienced malnourishment through a deficiency of protein- and vitamin-rich foods. Did this malnourishment during lactation also increase infant mortality?

There are two main issues to the question. Does malnutrition of the mother affect the breast-feeding child by the diminution of the quantity or the quality of her milk? It is, of course, impossible to make a direct historical assessment of the quantity or quality of breast milk in colonial Burma, but it is possible to look at modern analyses of Burmese lactation, and to consider whether factors affecting modern lactation could also have affected breast milk during the period of the study.

A study of the lactation of Burmese mothers, carried out by Khin-Maung-Naing and associates, and reported in 1980, concludes that maternal under-nutrition affected the potential milk output during lactation.[56] A cohort of 90 mothers was divided into four groups by their nutritional status, and the variation of their mean potential milk output was measured. The range was from 934ml per day for the highest status group to 767ml per day for the lowest.[57] The researchers reported little difference in the composition of the breast milk.[58]

Another study by Tin Tin Oo and Khin Maung Naing on the lactation of Burmese women in low socio-economic groups, reported their milk output as "lower than the 850ml per day assumed by the FAO/WHO Expert Committee on Calorie Requirements."[59] The potential volume from the mothers in this study was 822ml per day, but the consumption by the infants was only 687 ml. Foll, writing in 1958, had also suggested that low intake of breast milk by the infant was a factor in the high infant mortality rate.[60]

This effect of socio-economic grouping on milk output confirms the earlier findings of the WHO survey in Burma. Of 1,500 lactating women examined between 1955 and 1957, 40 per cent reported having insufficient milk for suckling. The figure for the poorer families was nearly 54 per cent of the women examined, whereas the figure for middle-class women was 35 per cent.[61] Perhaps of even more significance than socio-economic grouping was the number of children in the family, as 40 per cent of all multiparous women reported insufficient milk.[62]

Evidence therefore exists that poor nutritional status and/or multiparity in the modern Burmese woman lowers the quantity of her breast milk output. The historical data suggests that in addition to periodic food shortages due to climatic conditions, the lactating woman in Burma was malnourished due to traditional practices. It is not unreasonable to deduce that this malnourishment would have reduced her lactation capability.

This is probably the right point in the discussion to add a note of caution. The role of nutrition in lactation and birth weight is not simple. Field studies, which appeared to establish association between low birth weight and mild maternal malnutrition, were not controlled for other interacting factors, but the dietary supplementation of women has been found to have a positive effect in increasing the birth weight of babies.[63] The birth weight is probably also a determining factor in the quantity of the mother's breast milk; that is, the production of a larger, stronger baby results also in a larger lactation capacity. But the supplementation of the lactating mothers' diet with vitamins and minerals has demonstrably improved the quality of the breast milk.[64] This was confirmed by Postmus, who supplemented the mothers' diets with milk powder, vitamin tablets and vitamin injections, and obtained marked improvement in the condition of the Burmese mother and her infant.[65]

These opinions do not dispute the overall importance of nutrition in pregnancy and lactation, but show that some caution is necessary in attributing an apparently obvious relationship in what is a complex subject. For example, Jane Pryer and Nigel Crook suggest that the nutrition of the pregnant woman affects not only the birth weight but also therefore her lactation capacity.[66]

The second issue for consideration was the question of whether the malnutrition of the mother affected the infant through the diminished quality of her breast milk. Again analysis of direct historical evidence is not possible, but modern data may be helpful.

Dr Cho Nwe Oo's study of nutrition in 1974 reported low intakes of riboflavin, thiamine and calcium in both the lactating and the pregnant women surveyed. This low intake was attributed to the avoidance of pulses and leafy green vegetables in the diet, and had a potentially adverse effect on the child. Dr Cho Nwe Oo related the low thiamine content (111.2µg per day per 800ml) of breast milk to the low thiamine intake of the mothers.[67] Postmus found only 60.0µg of thiamine per

800ml of milk from poor mothers and 68.0µg in the milk of the middle-class mothers.[68] Many of the women in both groups showed clinical signs of thiamine deficiency. A very positive statement comes from Dr Daw Sein May Chit that a low content of thiamine is found in the breast milk of lactating mothers "who restrict their diet to rice alone".[69]

It would seem reasonable to assume that similar dietary restrictions in colonial Burma would have a similar effect; namely, that the thiamine content of the mother's breast milk would be diminished.

The thiamine content of breast milk may be influenced by the method of rice husking used locally, as well as by abstention from other foodstuffs. The introduction and extension of industrially milled rice under British rule certainly produced adult beri beri, especially when combined with prolonged storage of the rice.[70] The difference in the quantity of thiamine retained by hand-milling rather than machine is not negligible, as there may be as much as 2.4µg per gram in home-pounded rice compared to 1.0µg in milled rice. In addition, there is considerable loss of protein due to machine milling.[71] The post-war incidence of beri beri in pregnant and lactating women is well documented. Postmus found clinical beri beri in nearly 40 per cent of the primiparous women and nearly 50 per cent of the multiparous women examined.

It would be reasonable to assume, therefore, that the quality of the breast milk produced by the lactating woman in colonial Burma was diminished by her diet. The traditional practices, which excluded vitamin- and mineral-rich foods from the diet, were almost certainly exacerbated in Burma by the use of industrially milled rice. This emphasis on thiamine is due to its proven link with the disease infantile beri beri, which produces high mortality in infants between the ages of one and six months.[72]

Infantile beri beri

In 1957, the FAO *Report of the Nutrition Committee for South and East Asia, Fourth Session* stated that the incidence of infantile beri beri in the 1950s was unknown, but speculated that it was causing a high mortality. Due to the nature of the disease, often acute and quickly fatal, it was seldom seen by trained medical staff and therefore went undiagnosed.[73] A 1928 comment in an article on epidemic dropsy confirms that, although the adult disease was well documented, the infant disease was not: "With regard to infantile beri beri this has not been reported from India or Burma so far as we are aware".[74]

Investigations of the disease in modern Burma conclude that "infantile beri-beri is an extremely important cause of infantile mortality yet reliable figures and real incidence of the disease are not yet known."[75] Kywe-Thein and associates carried out a study of 200 infant beri beri cases admitted to Rangoon Hospital in 1965 and "found that the thiamine levels of the milk of mothers of beri-beri infants were significantly low in both total and free thiamine." Of the 200 infants admitted, 198 were fed totally on breast milk and yet, of the 78 mothers evaluated, only three showed clinical signs of thiamine deficiency.[76] It is evident from this report that women who show no clinical signs of beri beri can still create a potentially fatal thiamine deficiency in their breast-fed infants.

The age of onset of infantile beri beri is usually between the first and fourth month of life, though in the Rangoon study, seven per cent were less than one month old. Thirty-nine per cent of the cases occurred in the second month of life.[77]

A study in Thailand in 1960 found a characteristic history of breast-feeding, the onset of a mild infection and then sudden death in an apparently otherwise healthy child. The majority of these beri beri cases, on whom an autopsy was performed, were three months old.[78] This study and the Rangoon report both link the onset of infantile beri beri to the additional stress caused by even a minor infection.

Perhaps the most significant part of the Rangoon study for the purpose of historical comparison, is the reason given by the mothers for the initial seeking of medical treatment. These were convulsions and dyspnoea (or laboured breathing),[79] both of which were frequently quoted as causes of infant death in the annual health reports in pre-war Burma.

In 1957, Dr Postmus produced figures of infant deaths that he attributed to beri beri. The 532 multiparous mothers in the study (between 1955 and 1957) reported the deaths of 470 children, of whom 89 (19 per cent) died as neonates and 213 (45.3 per cent) died between the ages of one and six months. This, he stated, was "an avowed symptom for infantile beri beri".[80] Later, Postmus was able to refine the ages of the infant deaths in a larger group: he found that 67.8 per cent of those whose mothers were classified as "poor" died between the ages of two and five months. A slightly smaller percentage, 65.7 per cent, of the offspring of "middle-class" mothers died in that age group. He noted that "Many mothers volunteered the suggestion that their milk must have been poisonous because many of their seemingly healthy babies had died suddenly."[81]

It would be satisfying here to be able to point to Table 3.3 as evidence of the importance of infantile beri beri in Burma between 1920 and 1939. The table indeed shows an increase of 20 per cent over this period in the numbers of infant deaths between the critical ages of one and six months but, as stated previously, it shows no change in the overall mortality between birth and six months. It would seem unlikely that the British health programmes and infant welfare societies had really reduced neonatal mortality by nearly 20 per cent, whilst at the same time this reduction was neatly counterbalanced by an equivalent increase in beri beri deaths in the one to six months age group. If the evidence is taken at face value, it could certainly be said to confirm the hypothesis that infantile beri beri took an increasing toll in colonial Burma. Certainly this is supported by the evidence of dietary change with the increased use of white, highly milled rice in the population. But while up to one-third of the infant mortality remains, by my calculations, unregistered, only tentative conclusions can be drawn.

It can be suggested therefore, that infantile beri beri was probably an important cause of death in colonial Burma, but no firm statistical evidence exists. It probably became increasingly important as the consumption of milled rice spread, but whether that factor is likely to have accounted for 20 per cent of the registered infant deaths can only be considered possible, but not proven.

Supplementary foods for infants

It now remains to examine the third aspect of infant nutrition — supplementary feeding. This was a more visible aspect of infant diet than those which affected maternal nutrition, and as such was widely commented on by the British medical staff.

This comment was almost uniformly hostile, derogatory and sometimes bigoted. The supplementary feeding of Burmese infants was usually boiled rice, to which was gradually added plantain and then, sometimes, small amounts of proteins, usually fish, by the age of one year. Despite the bland nature of boiled rice, its use as an infant food received no praise from the British. These criticisms of the feeding of Burmese infants date from the first official Public Health Report in 1867. The surgeon of Toungoo, Dr Lees, attributed the sparse population "not to any want of prolificity amongst the Burmese but excessive mortality in their children", which he ascribed chiefly to their "indigestible food" as well as their scanty clothing.[82] Again in 1868, but from the surgeon at Moulmein, there are criticisms of the terrible mismanagement of Burmese children by their mothers, their want of clothing and "early cramming with rice, improper food".[83]

Several sources quote the feeding of small balls of rice to young babies, sometimes supplemented by wild plantains. The health report of 1870 also states that fish curry was used in addition to plantain, plus a few whiffs of the cheroot for the infant. The author of the 1870 report, J. McNeale Donnelly, considered that under this treatment "natural selection soon winnows the weakly children from the robust."[84] In the report of 1901, the sanitary commissioner, C. C. Little, suggested that the feeding of infants with balls of rice contributed to a mortality, which he claimed, was not exceptionally high.[85]

Other notable commentators on the diet of Burmese infants include Phayre, who attributed the level of mortality to giving infants "acid wild fruits", as well as prolonged breast-feeding and a deficiency of clothing at night.[86] Colonel William Laurie, who was an advocate of the wrap-them-in-flannel school of thought,[87] also criticised the "evil" want of clothing and "the pernicious practice" of giving week-old children boiled, chewed rice.[88]

A slightly less derogatory description appeared in the *Indian Medical Gazette* in July 1920, written by N.K. Kunhikannan, a sub-assistant surgeon who spent 14 years in Burma. He described the method of feeding as "the mother chews boiled rice, and, when it has been reduced to a semi solid mass, spits it into the mouth of her infant, who swallows the bolus without difficulty."[89]

It was this preparatory chewing of the boiled rice by the mother or other relative which offended many medical staff and aroused them to invective. The district health officer for Sandoway reported in 1931 in the following manner:

> Swelling of the abdomen with flatulence, wasting, vomiting, anorexia, purging, a lump on the right side of the abdomen, the child wails and cries continuously, loss of sleep and finally death from inanition — a complete picture of what an otherwise healthy child would suffer from if improperly fed. A few questions elicited the following facts about infant feeding. At four months the child is given chewed rice to eat, at six months plantain is added. The quantity is progressively increased, till at twelve months the child is brought on to scraps of fish, and anything else the parents may eat. The disgusting habit of chewing rice is undoubtably responsible for much of the infantile mortality. Granny gives a hand in keeping baby quiet. She takes a bolus of boiled rice in her grubby fingers, and pops it into a septic mouth. There the rice is intimately mixed with saliva, film from unbrushed teeth and possibly pus from pyorrhoea. This is then fed to the baby. Violent gastro-enteritis is the only possible result. Further septic feeding continues until the baby is killed.

> *Report on the Public Health Administration of Burma*, 1930, p. 13

No mention is made here of the high rate of malaria then recognised in Sandoway, nor is allowance made for the poverty which makes the human vehicle probably the most feasible way of pulping food for babies.

No precise information is available prior to 1939 on the quantities of the supplementary foods given to Burmese babies, so only tentative comment can be made. It is possible that the diet, as reported by the health officials, was deficient in protein, especially if the introduction of fish was delayed until the infant was a year old.

The FAO's *Third Report of the Nutrition Committee for South and East Asia* (1953) described widespread protein deficiency amongst infants in the region.[90] Burma sent no representative to the meeting and the country was not specified in the report. But again, more information is available from the collection of papers (probably of the 1970s) describing local dietary practices in Burma, which was referred to previously. Dr Daw Ohn Kyi reported from the Mon state that very young children were given boiled rice and salt only, as spiced adult foods were considered unsuitable.[91] From Mandalay, Dr Ma Ma Tin reported on a survey of 170 children between the ages of six months and two years, and found the commonest age for the commencement of mixed feeding to be nine months. Of the 170 mothers in the survey, 150 used rice, oil and salt only as supplementary food. Dr Ma Ma Tin stated that the animal proteins such as eggs, meat and fish were withheld from the child until it was two to three years old, from a combination of cultural dietary beliefs and poverty.[92] Dr Sao Yan Naing's and Dr Daw Tin E's reports from the northern Shan states and the Kachin state confirm that for infants up to one year, the normal supplementary food is boiled rice. In both these areas, meat is withheld from infants as it is thought to produce worm infestation.[93] Dr Po Po, writing in 1965, confirmed that for the majority of infants in Burma, supplementary feeding would consist of "rice, salt and oil". This was because vegetables were thought to cause indigestion; pulses, peas and beans caused colic or diarrhoea; and eggs (in addition to being expensive) would ensure "that the child will be late in talking".[94] The source of the superstition about eggs is not explained by Dr Po Po, but the reluctance to feed meat is attributed to Buddhist values rather than fear of parasites. These papers and reports strengthen the hypothesis that protein malnutrition would have existed amongst infants in colonial Burma.

The question of what calorific value a Burmese infant would have received from traditional weaning foods during the study period is almost impossible to answer. Again, the only possibilities can be derived from modern studies. Tin Tin Oo and Khin Maung Naing, in their article "Breast Feeding and Weaning Practices for Infants and Young Children in Rangoon", showed that traditional Burmese weaning foods such as rice, or rice and oil, contributed only 100 to 200 calories a day, or only 17 to 30 per cent of the infant's total daily calorie requirement. This was "inadequate for the nutritional needs of the child as judged by FAO/WHO requirements of calories for age or calories for weight."[95] This would seem to confirm that breast milk plus "rice alone or rice with oil twice a day appears to be inadequate for nutritional needs".[96] An earlier 1956 study of protein under-nutrition in Rangoon children also confirmed that the protein content of infant diet was inadequate.[97] It would therefore seem safe to assume that the calorific and nutritional values of the traditional supplementary foods were inadequate during the study period also.

Before leaving the subject of feeding the infant with boiled, chewed rice, one other aspect of this diet should be considered. In Southeast Asia, there may well be a "widespread belief in the strength-giving, nutritional and mystical qualities of rice".[98] Certainly for the Burmese people rice has great importance, and it could be that by chewing and offering the rice to her infant, the mother is both bonding and offering her infant the best food that she can. Kunhikannan noted, in 1920, the symbolic strength given to the infant with its first rice; that there was a belief "universal amongst Burmans that unless an infant soon after birth is given some boiled rice it will never have the strength to bear the pain of the bite of an ant."[99]

The vulnerability of the Burmese infant to malnutrition would appear to have followed the child in its journey through the *in-utero* stage and up to its first birthday. This can therefore be considered as the most important underlying cause of high infant mortality. As Dr Daw Sein May Chit said, "the debilitating effects [of malnutrition] render more deadly the common infectious diseases of childhood"[100] and "there is a close and pernicious connection between infectious diseases and malnutrition."[101]

The first health report for Burma covered the year 1867. It would appear that, in the 72 years leading up to 1939, much was written in criticism of infant nutrition, but too little was done to improve it. It is notable that in 1930, when the district health officer for Sandoway was describing with disgust the Burmese methods of supplementary feeding, the Infant Welfare Society in that town had not functioned during that year.[102] The indignant health officer would perhaps have been of more help to infants in Sandoway if he had put his energy into resurrecting a society that offered practical help and advice to Burmese mothers.

Infant disease

In the nineteenth and early twentieth centuries, diseases tended to be classified by their symptoms rather than by a specific pathogen. Thus fevers were described as "remittent" or "intermittent", which described the pattern of the symptoms instead of identifying the underlying or causal organism. This obviously creates problems for the historian of disease who wishes to identify causes of death.

"Convulsions" was one of the half-dozen blanket terms used in this period to cover a variety of infant diseases in Burma. It appears as a "cause" of infant death from the first health report in 1867. In 1881, 254 deaths in Prome were attributed to convulsions, although it is not clear whether all of these were infant, or whether some of the deaths represented adult, mortality.[103] The earliest infant statistics come from the civil surgeon at Thayetmyo, who, in 1909, said that of 91 infant deaths investigated, 61 had a history of convulsions.[104] Reports from Mandalay and Rangoon in 1915 describe neonatal tetanus and convulsions as jointly causing nearly 19 per cent and 25 per cent of infant deaths respectively,[105] and in 1916, the percentage in Mandalay had risen to nearly 40 per cent.[106]

Other extracts that appear in the annual health reports attribute 27 per cent of infant deaths in Rangoon in 1924 to convulsions only, and in 1928, convulsions is listed as one of the seven major causes of infant death in Rangoon. Even in 1934, the health report names convulsions as one of the four main causes of infant death, and in Pakokku town for 1939, 25 per cent of the infant mortality is attributed to convulsions.

Evidence therefore exists of the importance of "convulsions" in the high IMR for Burma, but detailed analysis is lacking. The inaccurate nature of classifying diseases as "convulsions" was recognised in the health report of 1931, when the sanitary commissioner said that it might mean anything "from cerebro-spinal meningitis or tetanus to simple diarrhoea, fever or unsuitable feeding".[107] The commissioner's exasperation was understandable, when one of his own health officers had returned, out of a total of 103 infant deaths, 94 attributed to convulsions.

There is little doubt that high fevers may cause convulsions, which could then have been listed as the cause of death, but deaths from diarrhoea, dysentery and the respiratory diseases should have been recorded under those separate headings in the registration tables, not under convulsions.[108] There is now no way of judging how many of those deaths were wrongly recorded as convulsions, but it is probably reasonable to suggest that the majority of these "convulsions" deaths were due to infantile beri beri or neonatal tetanus.

Neonatal tetanus

It was suggested previously, with reference to Table 3.3, that the division in the registration of infant deaths into "under one week" of age or "under one month" may well be inaccurate. This is significant in attempts to assess causes of death retrospectively. The recognised incubation period for neonatal tetanus is six to 14 days, and although its incidence in Burma was noted by some district health officers, its true impact in lives lost was unknown. Most tetanus deaths occur in the second week of life, as the infection is normally introduced through the open wound of the severed umbilical cord.[109] Certainly the overall losses during the eight to 30 day period in Burma were high. But the accurate age of death figures, which can be diagnostic, are not available for colonial Burma.

Age-specific data for the onset of neonatal tetanus in Burmese infants exists only from studies in the 1960s and 1970s. Ko Ko U and Khin May Khi's 1970 study in Rangoon showed that in 31 per cent of cases, symptoms of neonatal tetanus appeared within five days of birth, and in 60 per cent of cases within five to ten days of birth.[110] A Mandalay study (by Shwe Oh in 1971–73) used slightly different age groups, but produced a very similar overall result: 91.6 per cent of cases showed the onset of symptoms of tetanus between the second and tenth day of life. Furthermore, death occurred within one week of the onset of symptoms in 78 per cent of all fatalities (this data was available for the Mandalay study only).[111] This would place most of those deaths within the second week.

Scattered evidence of tetanus as an important cause of infant death does, however, exist for the period of the study, together with suggestions of how the bacillus was introduced to the child in Burma. The Burmese were largely an agricultural people who shared their spatial area with their buffalo and other domestic animals. The tetanus spore is widespread in the faeces of both man and his domestic animals, "and in the environment surrounding habitations of animals or man".[112] Despite the growth in the population in the period of study, the ratio of urban and domestic population remained constant, and as domestic animals were frequently found in the towns as well as the countryside, some parity of incidence of the disease can be expected.

Contamination of the cut umbilical cord easily occurs from dust, from the instrument employed to sever the cord or from the mother's faeces. (Ko Ko U and Khin May Khi's study found that in 248 home deliveries, 92 mothers were not washed at all, 71 had a partial wash and 87 had a washdown.)[113] The umbilical cord affords an ideal port of entry for the tetanus spore.

A rough guide to the possible incidence of tetanus in Burma can be gained by looking at similar agricultural or "economically dis-advantaged"[114] countries where the disease occurs largely today. In a series of studies carried out between 1960 and 1982 (detailed in Table 3.4), it was found that between 30 and 64 per cent of neonatal deaths were caused by tetanus, and in the Khanna study of Indian villages, tetanus was described as "the leading cause of neonatal deaths".[115]

All these modern reports discuss factors and living conditions that were also common to colonial Burma, such as an agricultural community,

TABLE 3.4
The Incidence of Neonatal Tetanus in Selected Countries Between
1960 and 1982

Country of Study	Neonatal Tetanus Incidence
Bangladesh (1)	30% neonate deaths
Bangladesh (2)	30–40% neonate deaths
New Guinea	80 deaths per 1,000 live births
Thailand	38% infant deaths
Uganda	64% neonate deaths

Sources: Bangladesh (1): Islam et al., "Infant Mortality in Rural Bangladesh",
p. 295; Bangladesh (2): Rahman, "The Effect of Traditional Birth Attendants",
p. 163; Thailand: Stahlie, "The Role of Tetanus Neonatorum in Infant Mortality
in Thailand", p. 17; New Guinea: Schofield, Tucker and Westbrook, "Neonatal
Tetanus in New Guinea", p. 788; Uganda: Bwibo, "The Role of Neonatal Infection
in Neonatal and Childhood Mortality", p. 89.

poverty and a traditional system of midwifery. The instruments used
in the those countries to cut the umbilical cord include knives, trowels,
sickles, scissors, razor blades, split bamboo, reed and bark. The cord
stump was then dressed, again using traditional materials such as ash,
cow dung cake, ghee, oil, burnt earth, powdered pepper, herbs, turmeric
or soot. The higher ranges of mortality would appear to occur in
communities such as New Guinea, where the cord is left untied. In one
Bangladesh study, the overall neonatal tetanus mortality was 27 per
1,000 live births; but for those infants where the cord was left untied,
the mortality rose to 111 per 1,000 live births.[116]

The purpose of the preceding discussion is not to pre-empt the
conclusions of history and say this must be what happened in colonial
Burma, but rather to attempt to evaluate and understand skimpy
historical data.

The first reference to neonatal tetanus appears in the Public Health
Report of 1868, when six per cent of total infant mortality is attributed
to the disease.[117] Most of the statistical evidence comes from the
indefatigable Dr Mullan, health officer for Mandalay. In a report of
1913, he attributed 23 per cent of all infant deaths in Mandalay to
tetanus, and showed that out of a total IMR of 417 per 1,000, 174 per
1,000 occurred in the first month.[118] Dr Mullan also provided figures for
1914,[119] 1915[120] and 1916[121] when he attributed 29.8 per cent (or 133

deaths), nearly 25 per cent (134) and nearly 34 per cent (135) respectively of all infant deaths to tetanus and convulsions. The only evidence for Rangoon is the figure of 18.6 per cent for infant deaths from tetanus and convulsions in 1915.[122] The obvious difficulty with these figures is that they are not specific to tetanus only.

The 1913 figures for Mandalay are the only statistics that are specifically for tetanus, except the very early figures from 1868, which are perhaps more useful in indicating that tetanus was recognised at that period than in recording its incidence. If Dr Mullan's figure for 1913 of 23 per cent of registered infant deaths were due to tetanus out of a total IMR of 417, this gives the number of those deaths as 96 per 1,000. This would mean that more than half (55 per cent) of neonatal deaths that year in Mandalay were due to tetanus. As this is only one year, it is important not to lay too much emphasis on it, but it is worth noting that it lies within the upper range of "similar" countries' experience.

This suggestion of a high prevalence of tetanus in Burma is supported by data from 1867 onwards. In Toungoo, tetanus was "stated to have caused 24 deaths", though the report (1867) continues by saying that tetanus "does not appear so prevalent here as along the sea coast."[123] The health report of 1913 identifies tetanus as a frequent cause of mortality in new-born infants,[124] as does the 1920 report, when considering the high infant mortality in Mandalay.[125]

Unfortunately, medical opinion in Burma, when struggling to come to terms with the causes of a high IMR, did not always receive support in its diagnosis from the senior administration. The Resolution accompanying the 1920 report states firmly that "Tetanus is not a disease which ordinarily causes infant mortality".[126] It is easy to imagine the exasperation an under-funded Public Health Service must have felt when reading that comment.

The link between tetanus incidence and septic cord severing was recognised by the British medical staff as early as 1894. The health report of that year mentioned that the practice of cutting the umbilical cord "with a piece of dirty bamboo still persists in some places" and that "At Akyab the Civil Surgeon ascribes the prevalence of infant lockjaw to this relic of barbarism."[127]

Either the incidence at Akyab must have been very high, or the civil surgeons of the town must have had a particular interest in obstetrics, because in 1931, there is further comment: "Tetanus neonatorum was responsible for 18 deaths under one month. It is entirely a preventable disease and is due to dirty midwifery."[128] In 1920, the health report again mentions tetanus, which is "said to be a common cause of infant mortality in Mandalay and for which the dirty methods practised by native midwives are responsible",[129] although interestingly (and confusingly) the report states that this is the chief reason for the high mortality in the first week.

No historical evidence so far has been found to describe the materials commonly used for umbilical cord dressings in colonial Burma. In 1959, Foll confirmed the use of bamboo or a knife to cut the cord, and said a dressing of saffron paste is then used.[130] Studies of neonatal tetanus in Rangoon (1964) and Mandalay (1971–73) have revealed a wide range of instruments and dressings used for the umbilical cord. Scissors, blades, razors, kitchen knives, bamboo, thread and saws were recorded as cutting instruments in Mandalay,[131] revealing that the instrument used is one that is close to hand. A wide range of dressings was also used on the cord, and these included ash and saffron paste, as well as indigenous medical powders and modern antiseptics.[132] This evidence suggests that saffron paste was probably the traditional dressing for the cord in Burma.

The continuing tetanus incidence in Burma must be regarded primarily as an example of failure by the colonial authority. The disease was recognised in 1867 as causing high mortality in Burmese infants, was linked causally to specific practices with the umbilical cord in 1894, but in 1931, was still causing high losses in those same areas. What was needed was improved midwifery practice especially in the rural areas. The problem was recognised, but little progress was made in the provision of an aseptic midwifery service, except in those towns where an infant welfare society was created.

The depressing picture thus presented of low birth weights, malnutrition, infantile beri beri and neonatal tetanus is not the end of the story of the perils to which Burmese infants succumbed. Dysentery, diarrhoea and respiratory diseases also caused heavy losses during the first year of life.

Dysentery, diarrhoea and respiratory diseases

The earliest official health reports, those of 1867 and 1868, though rich sources of information, often do not distinguish between child mortality and infant mortality; that is whether death occurred over or under one year. For example, the reports refer to tetanus as one of the many children's diseases causing mortality, although this is nearly always a neonatal disease. The following references were made to respiratory disease in those reports, some of which again may refer to infants. In 1867, the surgeon at Moulmein reported that the most frequent source of mortality amongst children was croup or inflammation of the lungs with fever.[133] In the same year from Sandoway, the report lists a severe form of bronchitis.[134] The 1868 report, again for Moulmein, attributes children's deaths to lung diseases, bowel complaints and measles.[135]

The health report of 1910 contained suggestions from the civil surgeons as to the causes of the high IMR. The report from Mandalay included bronchitis and pneumonia, the report from Bassein mentions "disease of the alimentary tract",[136] and from Prome and Paungde, the high rates were attributed to a list including dysentery, diarrhoea, respiratory diseases and intestinal diseases.[137]

It was the Society for Prevention of Infant Mortality that produced the 1913 figures for Mandalay. They attributed 23 per cent of infant mortality to respiratory disease and 5.9 per cent to bowel complaints.[138] Through the efforts of the society and Dr Mullan, the health officer to the municipality, more information is available for Mandalay than any other town in Burma. The available statistics on infant deaths due to bowel complaints or respiratory diseases are shown in Table 3.5. These figures have two limitations — they are urban only and are attributed by description to the registrar and not by medical diagnosis, but they still provide a guide to possible levels of infection.

These figures suggest that the incidence of respiratory disease was higher in the dry zone of Burma than in the delta area, but few further conclusions can be drawn. The rate of respiratory disease in Mandalay may have been linked to the high malarial rate in that district, but again the lack of diagnosis makes the data unreliable. Occasional notes appear in the records linking a high disease incidence with a single causal

TABLE 3.5

Percentage of Registered IMR Attributed to Respiratory and Bowel Disease in Some Urban Areas

Town	Year	Dysentery/Diarrhoea/ Digestive	Respiratory Disease
Bassein	1910/11/14	28.3 (av.)	11.14
Mandalay	1913	5.95	23.0
	1914	—	19.5
	1915	4.4	25.7
	1916	7.7	29.1
Rangoon	1915	8.33	21.16
	1924	7.3	17.4

Sources: Annual health reports.

factor, such as the outbreak of dysentery in Shwebo in 1924, which caused a large number of infant deaths.[139] The dysentery was blamed on the acute scarcity of water that occurred during the dry season.

The blanket nature of the terminology "diarrhoea" and "respiratory disease" probably concealed the links in the infant death pattern between malnutrition, virus and secondary infection. For example, very little evidence exists as to the prevalence of measles in Burmese infants, the only reference being in the 1868 Moulmein report, which also included child mortality. But incidents of epidemic measles were reported, with fatalities, and from 1921, the disease was listed separately in urban areas.[140] The health report of that year recognised that "Very little information is on record as to the prevalence and the case mortality of measles in this country, and probably only a few of many outbreaks in rural areas are reported to the sanitary authority."[141]

The reason for this apparent digression into a discussion of measles is that the disease affords an excellent example of a viral infection that may attack six- to 12-month-old infants. Evidence exists of adult mortality from this disease in Burma, but it does not appear to have been considered by the sanitary authorities in relation to infant mortality. The reason for this could well be that it is an example of a viral infection which can become rapidly fatal when complicated by secondary infection, either pneumonic or diarrhoeal.[142] Measles deaths could therefore be included in those urban infant deaths listed above that were attributed to respiratory or bowel disease.

Many modern studies explore the links between infection, secondary infection and malnutrition.[143] Research in Trinidad in 1960 found a "widespread pneumonia in infants dying soon after the onset of symptoms of tetanus."[144] In 1984, G. T. Strickland in *Hunter's Tropical Medicine* reported that malnutrition is a predisposing factor in *Escherichia coli* infection,[145] which in infants has a summer peak of incidence. Infection by *E. coli* also leads to deterioration of the nutritional state, with dehydration the main cause of death.[146]

Venereal diseases and congenital syphilis
Some British health officials in Burma recognised these links between malnutrition, sanitary conditions and infectious disease. But there were still some medical officers who, despite acknowledging the need for improved sanitation, preferred simplistic solutions. Captain Kelsall, civil surgeon for Thayetmyo town, attributed the high IMR at Thayetmyo in 1909 largely to syphilis, despite admitting that there was no verification of this theory from the town hospital statistics.[147] In 1910, Kelsall, still concerned about venereal disease ("congenital syphilis is largely the cause of deaths in Thayetmyo"), had found a more external and

Darwinian cause. "A further factor tending to increase the mortality (of infants) is the extraordinary amount of mixed breeding in Thayetmyo whereby the high vitality of the Burman is lowered by the large admixture of the physically weaker Madrass."[148]

Syphilis undoubtedly existed in Burma and should therefore be considered as a possible cause of infant mortality. Comments attributing adult mortality to venereal diseases appear in the health reports from 1868 onwards. The reports are all vague and generalised, and although comment was made on the prevalence of syphilis, especially in the sea-ports and riverine towns of Burma, the reports disclose that the true incidence and prevalence was not known.[149]

Congenital syphilis must have contributed to the high IMR in Burma. The difficulty is to differentiate between the apparent prejudices of the medical officers and the lack of statistical substance in their reports. Captain Kelsall was not alone in his opinions; the sanitary commissioner in 1924 suggested that venereal disease was one of the major causes of the high IMR in Burma.[150] The health officer of Akyab attributed the large number of stillbirths in 1931 to the "widespread prevalence of venereal disease".[151] In 1937 and 1938, similar references appear concerning the towns of Chauk and Taungdwingyi respectively.[152] Venereal disease amongst the parents was also blamed for playing "not an unimportant part in the deaths amongst infants" in Yamethin district.[153]

Congenital syphilis (or more accurately pre-natal syphilis) when untreated, is estimated to cause stillbirth in 25 per cent of foetuses, and a mortality of 25 to 30 per cent amongst infected infants born alive.[154] The "snuffles" in infants, which is "almost diagnostic",[155] plus the fact that "Neonatal death is usually due to liver failure, severe pneumonia, or pulmonary haemorrhage",[156] may indicate that infant syphilis deaths were registered as respiratory diseases.

Pre-natal syphilis must have taken infant lives in Burma but, due to lack of diagnosis during the colonial period, an estimate of the extent of the mortality is impossible. Only one statistic appears in the health records, and that assigns one death to congenital syphilis out of a total infant mortality in Mandalay of 1,907 in 1916.[157] It is perhaps reasonable to suggest that the increased incidence of venereal diseases following the British annexation, especially of Upper Burma, might have raised the infant mortality rate,[158] but the extent is unproven.

Smallpox and malaria

There were two other major diseases in Burma that are part of this story of infant mortality. The Public Health Department could eventually regard the history of one of them, smallpox, as a partial success for their administration; the history of the second disease, malaria, can only be regarded as representing mistaken priorities.

The smallpox vaccination programme, started in 1866, was a constant source of worry to the registrars of births and deaths. Vaccination was resisted in some parts of Burma where traditional inoculation was preferred, and registration of the child's birth was avoided in order that the attention of the vaccinator should not be alerted.[159]

Infant deaths from smallpox, when considered over a 50-year period from 1880 to 1930, declined from approximately 20 per cent of the total registered smallpox mortality to 4.5 per cent. The total registered adult mortality also showed a tendency to decline, but as the disease pattern went in three- to six-year epidemic waves, the decline was not constant in either infant or adult mortality.

The highest figure recorded for infant smallpox deaths was 1,088 in the epidemic of 1884. Registration then was, of course, confined to Lower or British Burma only. But by 1930, the figure was only 41 registered infant deaths for the whole of Burma.

There was probably considerable under-registration of infant smallpox deaths. The sanitary commissioner regularly, and probably correctly, suspected concealment of deaths from notifiable diseases, including smallpox cases.[160] But if smallpox is considered as a proportion of total infant mortality in Burma, even allowing for under-registration, it gradually became a relatively insignificant cause of infant mortality. In 1890 for example, of 10,947 registered infant deaths, 636 or 5.86 per cent were attributed to smallpox. By 1930, out of 63,198 infant deaths registered, only 41 or 0.06 per cent were due to smallpox. Sadly, this decline of smallpox had no effect on the overall IMR, and so we will have to look at malaria.

The history of infant deaths from malaria is hidden in the mortality from "Fevers" and "All Other Causes". Yet I would suggest that malaria was not only, to a considerable degree, responsible for the maintenance of the high infant mortality rate in the twentieth century, but also contributed to the rise in the rate which, I think, occurred after 1911.

It is argued in other chapters that the British efforts to contain or treat malaria in Burma were concentrated on areas where troops, the police or European personnel lived, or areas of industrial development. Although some interest was shown in malaria by the official medical services following the 1910 publication of Ronald Ross's work on India, *The Prevention of Malaria* (in 1902, Ross had received a Nobel Prize in recognition of his work on malaria), the application of this research to protect the average, rural Burman was under-funded and unenthusiastic.

If it is difficult, therefore, to assess adult mortality from malaria, it is impossible to give accurate figures for the number of infants dying from, or due to, the disease. The great majority of these deaths occurred in the rural areas of Burma where, even if the child's birth or death was recorded, certainly no treatment or diagnosis was readily available from medical staff. Analysis of the size of the problem can only be attempted through hints in the health records and the use of some of the available knowledge of the epidemiology of the disease.

Fortunately, opinion on the effects of endemic malaria on the IMR would appear to have been constant from the late 1920s to the 1980s. Some of the data written about India would appear to be applicable to Burma, especially where it concerns primary research on the effects of endemic or epidemic malaria. Samuel Christophers, John Sinton and Gordon Covell were all members of the Indian Medical Service with a particular interest in malaria. A report written by them in 1928 included discussion of the greatly increased numbers of stillbirths found in areas of epidemic malaria of the autumnal type.[161] Sinton, in his work *What Malaria Costs India* (1939), states that non-immune women, when entering a highly malarious area, are likely to have a much-increased rate of abortion and stillbirth.[162] He also suggested that in epidemic areas infantile convulsions are found, and that there is a close relationship between malaria and increased numbers of deaths from respiratory and diarrhoeal diseases.[163] Interestingly, he saw most early infant deaths as due to the indirect effects of malaria, for example premature birth or malnutrition due to the mother's illness, and firmly concluded that "malaria appears to have a very definite influence in raising the infantile mortality rate."[164]

Sinton had drawn widely on this work on the pioneering investigations of men like Christophers and C. A. Bentley. It was Bentley who wrote, in 1925, the famous *Malaria and Agriculture in Bengal*,[165] when he was the special deputy sanitary commissioner there. But Sinton's conclusions also differ little from those of G. J. Ebrahim, who was editor of the *Journal Of Tropical Paediatrics*, in 1984. Ebrahim's comments on the effects of malaria in infancy are positive, agreed with those of Sinton (made 45 years previously) and bore close parallels with some of the causes of the high Burmese IMR that have already been discussed. He stated that in endemic areas, the infant's first encounter with malaria is in its foetal life when during pregnancy malarial immunity in the mother becomes attenuated, resulting in increased parasitaemia. For the mother, this higher infestation could mean anaemia and possibly premature labour.[166]

Perhaps even more pertinent to colonial Burma is Ebrahim's report that placental infection can be common, resulting in retardation of intra-uterine growth. He estimated that this could cause a potential weight loss of 165g to 250g. This factor alone, when combined with Burmese cultural dietary practices during pregnancy, must contribute greatly to neonatal mortality due to low birth weight. Ebrahim considered that despite the maternally derived immunity acquired by breast-fed babies, "heavy malarial infection is not unknown in infants and usually presents as severe anaemia."[167] His summary was close to Sinton's; "In endemic areas malaria may be an important cause of abortion, late foetal and neonatal deaths."[168]

The picture that emerges from these reports is that of increased stillbirths in epidemic areas, and a high IMR in endemic areas due to the morbidity of the mother affecting the birth weight (and thus the chances of the infant's post-natal survival). Added to this is the possibility of malarial infection in infancy as a predisposing cause of death.

A 1980 thesis on epidemic malaria in colonial Ceylon by E. Meyer describes a very similar situation. Meyer said that those most affected in an epidemic were infants, new-borns, women and those of low castes.[169] He noted that in the 1928 epidemic, there was a reduction in births, that is, an increase in abortion and neonatal mortality.[170]

Is there historical evidence to suggest that this pattern of events occurred in colonial Burma; and further, does this evidence suggest that infant deaths from malaria increased during the British presence? I believe that there is enough statistical and qualitative information to confirm the first point, and sufficient qualitative evidence to make the latter distinctly possible.

The official health reports contain very few references prior to 1910 that would implicate malaria as a cause of infant mortality. The report of 1883 contains a quotation from the health officer of Rangoon, who talked of "little children" ill with fever, and "distressing scenes" of whole families infected with a fever that he believed to be malaria. No specific reference is made to infants and no further reports linking infant death and malarial fevers have been found until those from the early twentieth century.

Omission from the reports does not mean that infants were not dying of malaria or related diseases, but it probably means that they were doing so unobserved in the rural areas. By 1909, however, the awakening interest in infant mortality coincided with the rising world medical awareness of malaria. The first investigation into infant mortality that mentioned fever was Captain Kelsall's 1909 enquiry into the Thayetmyo death rate.[171] He mentioned fevers as a cause of infant deaths; as did the report from Paungde town in 1910, which described them as occurring in January, July and August.[172]

It was in these health reports for 1909 and 1910 that the difference between the IMR in Upper and Lower Burma is first discussed. The commissioner, C. E. Williams, noticed that the IMR for Upper Burma was higher than that for Lower Burma, the rates differing by 45 per 1,000 in 1907, by 21 per 1,000 in 1908, and 23 per 1,000 in 1909.[173] In 1910, the difference between the rates was 39 per 1,000; and the commissioner stated that the increase in the provincial rate from 222 per 1,000 in 1909 to 233 per 1,000 in 1910 had come from the rural areas.[174] This discussion about the differing rates between Upper and Lower Burma continued in the health reports because, unfortunately, the officials could not be sure whether they were observing varying degrees of registration efficiency or disease patterns.

From 1914 onwards, Mandalay was to be identified in the health reports with the two other Upper Burma districts of Kyaukse and Shwebo as having excessive infant deaths in their rural districts. Each year in the official reports, the commissioners discussed which urban and rural districts had particularly high or low IMRs. It should be understood that no separate rural tables of infant deaths were published, so the only way of obtaining rural figures, as against district figures that included the towns, was when the rural rate of a district was so high that it warranted special mention in the health reports. The consistency with which these districts were named is therefore highly significant, as is their consistently high rate compared to the average

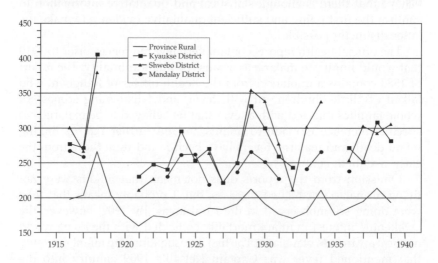

FIGURE 3.2

Registered Infant Mortality Rate for All Rural Districts and Rural Rate for
Kyaukse, Shwebo and Mandalay Districts

rural rate for the province. The IMRs for these rural areas are plotted on the graph (Figure 3.2) for those years in which they were quoted in the official reports.

The graph shows that the IMR peaked in those three districts in approximately five-year cycles. It is possible that irregular rainfall patterns are implicated in the cycles — in May 1934 there was a deficit of rain, and in May 1938, an excess of rain, both of which years showed a surge in the IMR in those districts. But although irregular rainfall may be sometimes implicated in malaria incidence, there are not enough detailed district-by-district rainfall figures to establish this.

It would appear unlikely that these figures reflect solely registration errors. It may be more rational to look for a common disease pattern, especially as all three districts had areas of ancient irrigation and had their agricultural irrigation systems considerably extended under the British. This type of change upsets the balance of the relationship between man and vector in diseases such as malaria, and, by providing more breeding grounds for the mosquito, can radically alter the pattern of contact. In 1917, the prevalence of malaria in Mandalay and Kyaukse was extensively discussed in the health report. The implication in the report is that endemic malaria in these districts had been aggravated to possible epidemic proportions by the extension of irrigation.[175]

As malaria is discussed elsewhere in this book, it is important here to concentrate only on those issues affecting infants. One of the issues discussed in the reports of 1916 and 1917 was the deficit of children under ten years in Kyaukse, Mandalay and Shwebo, and this surely must be partly due to stillbirths and infant mortality. The report of the Society for the Prevention of Infant Mortality in Mandalay, which attributed causes to infant deaths in 1913, did not mention malaria. The society did, however, attribute 22 per cent of the deaths to prematurity. Table 3.6 lists the figures given in the 1916 health report for the numbers

TABLE 3.6
Upper Burma: Number of Children per 100 Married Females
of Child-bearing Age

Malarial Districts		Districts Less Affected by Malaria	
Kyaukse	183	Magwe	245
Mandalay	188	Sagaing	244
Shwebo	218	Meiktila	244

Sources: *Report on the Sanitary Authority of Burma*, 1916.

of children per 100 married females of child-bearing age. The first column represents malarial districts and the second column, other districts in Upper Burma considered to be less affected by this disease.[176]

There were other districts that also figured prominently in the health reports and were consistently identified as "highly malarious". Those districts, for example Minbu, Yamethin and the Lower Chindwin, were recognised as having excessive rural infant mortality (but were not quite so regularly named in the reports as having had the highest IMR, as the malarial districts named in Table 3.6).[177]

The evidence is therefore cumulative that those rural areas that were regularly identified in the reports as highly malarious, and sometimes with spleen indexes (that is, a splenic enlargement noticeable on palpation of the abdomen in children of up to ten years of age) of up to 100 per cent, were those rural districts that had the highest IMR.

The problem with this argument is, of course, that it contains elements of circularity. The health officials felt bound to explain why those districts often returned high IMRs. Therefore the losses are attributed to malaria, which was known to be a problem in the irrigated districts of the dry zone. The researcher then finds evidence in the reports that the high IMR was due to malaria. But even given the scepticism with which all Burma health statistics should be approached, the consistency and weight of the evidence would appear to confirm the importance of the disease.

Some concrete evidence exists in the form of reported spleen indexes. A malaria survey was carried out in Mandalay district in 1917, and this reported an "endemic index being over 50% and in many places 90% and 100%".[178] An enquiry in the southeast of Kyaukse district "revealed a very high splenic index among the child population".[179] In addition to this, there is a broad spectrum of evidence from the *Gazetteers* and the annual health reports about the impact of malaria on infant mortality. In 1901, J. G. Scott and J. P. Hardiman described a fever called "Lnget-pya" in Kyaukse district, which occurred in November, December and January, and reported: "The Burmans die annually in large numbers from this fever, and the infant mortality is especially great at this time of year."[180] The comment in the health records was persistent; for example, in 1926 from Kyaukse district, "a highly malarious one and a high infant mortality is therefore to be expected",[181] and in 1930: "Malaria accounts for many infants' deaths in this district."[182]

As already stated, malaria was known to be implicated in the high IMR of other districts besides Kyaukse, Mandalay and Shwebo. The districts of Yamethin, Thayetmyo, the Lower Chindwin, Sagaing, Akyab, Amherst, Katha, Tharrawaddy and Kyaukpyu were all named in either the health reports, the Volume A *Gazetteers* or malarial reports as suffering infant losses due to malaria. The deaths were sometimes attributed to malaria "weakening the constitution of the mother", or as "chronic malaria causing premature delivery", but more frequently to a statement that malaria partly accounts for the high IMR.[183]

The reports arising from malarial investigations confirm the link between infant deaths and incidence of the disease. Major N. P. O'Gorman Lalor stated in his report of 1912 that malaria was the chief cause of the lowered birth rate, increased infant mortality and ill health in Kyaukpyu district. Furthermore, the source of the endemicity was attributed to the importation of "malaria stricken coolies" to work on the oil refineries, the roads and the Kyaukpyu embankment.[184] He claimed that Kyaukpyu municipality was previously a healthy area, and its population decline dated from the 1880s, when the embankment was raised and coolies imported, thus providing additional breeding areas for anophelines and a source of potential infection in and from the coolies. O'Gorman Lalor also conducted a malarial enquiry into the incidence at Wuntho town in Katha district in 1913, where he reported that he had examined 25 infants aged 12 months or under, of whom 13, or 52 per cent, had splenic enlargement.[185] One of these infected infants was less than three months old.

Evidence therefore exists that in colonial Burma tiny infants were directly affected by malaria, in addition to the less quantifiable but strongly probable theory that they were also exposed to infection *in-utero* and put at risk by their mothers' debility. Ma Htay Nwe has written a very clear description in a modern (1980) report on Lashio township of the malarial symptoms present in very young infants. The difficulties of correct diagnosis are made very apparent — the infants commonly presented symptoms such as jaundice, respiratory distress, fever, vomiting, diarrhoea and, in cases of severe malaria, pulmonary complications.[186] Just as O'Gorman Lalor found malaria infection in babies under three months, so too did Ma Htay Nwe, who reported that it was not uncommon to see very tiny infants with very enlarged spleens, "as large as 3 to 4 fingers in babies as young as 3 to 4 months."[187]

Some tentative guidance to the possible importance of malaria in the IMR may be drawn from a comparison of the rates of infant death in the two health centres established in the 1930s, though, of course, the comparison is not controlled in any way for other diseases. The Rural Health Unit at Hlegu recorded an IMR of 154 in 1935, while the Rural Uplift Centre at Tatkon had an IMR of 235. Three years later, in 1938, Hlegu posted a rate of 162.6, which contrasts with the rate of 300 in Tatkon. (The graph of rural rates, Figure 3.2, shows that 1938 was a peak incidence year in the three districts in Upper Burma.) Both the centres were still finding large numbers of omissions of both births and deaths, probably implying that the rates are under-recorded. Yamethin district, within which the Tatkon centre is found, was admitted to have water supply problems in some areas during the hot months. But malaria was seen as the main killer. In the opinion of the sanitary commissioner in 1938: "A vast majority of deaths among infants in the malarious regions ought really to be attributed to malaria."[188]

Sadly, this belated recognition in the late 1930s of the importance of malaria in infant mortality was too little, too late.

The British response

Some aspects of the health officials' response to the high IMR have already been discussed in this chapter but the practical actions, such as the development of a midwifery service, have only been touched on. This short section will comment on the response of the British administration, and try to assess its effectiveness.

Quite often response was effected through a combination of charitable and official money. Hospitals, hospital wards and maternity shelters were built from subscriptions raised from the public, but they were often maintained largely by government or local authority funding. An example of this was the Dufferin Hospital in Rangoon, which was opened in 1897 "under the aegis of the Countess of Dufferin Fund".[189] The hospital was run until 1923 under a combination of the Dufferin Fund and government support, and until 1934, by a newly formed trust and government support. It became the main teaching institution for midwifery and gynaecology in Burma, although the Mandalay and Moulmein hospitals also developed teaching facilities for midwives.

Most of the midwives, after their 18 months' training, were employed by the municipal authorities.[190] They were usually employed as "Results System Midwives", an arrangement whereby they received a small basic salary from their employers, which was augmented by an additional payment for each confinement attended. The only record found so far of the rates for this "piece work" was that earned by midwives employed by the voluntary society in Mandalay. Each of the two nurses employed had to attend a minimum of eight confinements, and for every confinement above this minimum they were paid two rupees.[191] Unfortunately, the report does not state whether this minimum figure was per month or per year. During 1917, only 231 confinements were attended in total by the two midwives and the lady visitor, so presumably the minimum of eight confinements was an annual figure.

The effect of this system was to confine the midwives to the towns. A midwife living in the rural area would spend an unreasonable amount of time travelling between villages to confinements, even in the dry weather. The result was that by 1934, there were unemployed trained midwives in Burma who were waiting for vacancies to arise in municipal areas. The health authorities' suggestion was that these midwives should go into private practice in the rural areas, some possibly on a part-time basis.[192] It is a little difficult to conceive how they could have made a living, as the major problem of travelling long distances without any means of transport remained.

Voluntary societies or infant welfare societies, such as the one at Mandalay, also employed midwives within the urban areas. The first Society for the Prevention of Infant Mortality in Burma was inaugurated on 15 September 1906 and was a Burmese initiative, not a British one. It was started by Burmese men of "known influence" and Burmese ladies of "recognised position" as a central committee from which, eventually, local organisations developed in most of the major towns in Burma.[193] The original objective of the society was to make trained midwifery assistance available to women in Burma, and as the need became apparent, attempts were also made to provide a health visiting service. It was appreciated that aseptic birth conditions were not enough, that the mother required advice and treatment — both ante- and post-natal, and that some medical supervision of the child during its first year was advisable.

The local societies were of charitable origin but many, once formed, were "grant aided" by local councils. The societies at Rangoon and Maymyo were amongst the most successful. By 1929, the Rangoon society had 1,223 confinement cases in its care, all of which took place in maternity "shelters".[194] There were four shelters under the management of a matron superintendent in Rangoon, and the society employed on average seven to nine midwives. But voluntary subscriptions had long ceased to be adequate, and by 1929, the society in Rangoon was largely funded by the government. The Maymyo society, established in 1926, was from the beginning well organised and active. It established a system of home visits, distributed food, clothing, advisory pamphlets and medicines, and arranged public health lectures. The society also established a Maternity and Child Welfare Centre, and employed a trained health visitor.[195] Many of the local societies acted as supervisory bodies to the Results System Midwives employed by the local councils; others, such as the Sagaing society, supervised the maternity ward of the local hospital.[196]

The original central committee, which started the first Society for the Prevention of Infant Mortality, became the Child Welfare Endowment Fund in 1921, and its objective was the co-ordination of the local societies. By 1923, this fund was being administered by the Burma branch of the Indian Red Cross Society, which had itself been revived in 1922. The

Red Cross was to become an important contributor to infant welfare in Burma, as most of the local societies became affiliated to it. In addition, the Red Cross funded the training in Delhi of ten health visitors for Burma, and in 1935, it largely underwrote the initial costs of a training centre for health visitors in Burma.[197]

There was, however, a major problem with all this charitable activity. Successful voluntary committees often rely on the enthusiasm of a very few members, and if those members leave or move on, then the enthusiasm leaves with them. This pattern was frequently seen in the district branches of the Society for the Prevention of Infant Mortality. For example, in 1920 the societies in Pyapon, Sandoway and Taungdwingyi undertook no activities, and the society in Toungoo ceased to exist. In 1922, it was stated that at "Syriam and other places in the Hanthawaddy District, the stimulus necessary for carrying on the work failed with the departure of Mrs. Ward Perkins."[198] In some urban areas of great need, the necessary stimulus was unfortunately lacking. In 1939, the registered IMR of Myingyan town was 394.5, but the town had no infant welfare society.[199] Kyaukse town also lacked an active local society until the 1930s.

Finance was often a problem: in 1931, a slump in local subscriptions was attributed to the economic depression.[200] Three local societies — Mandalay, Prome and Pegu — sacked midwives that year as an economy measure.[201] The training centre for health visitors, originally planned for 1929, was delayed due to "financial stringency", before being rescued by the Red Cross in 1935.[202]

How extensive was this network of voluntary societies and domiciliary midwives? By 1939, there were 270 midwives employed by local authorities, and they attended 29,351 confinements in that year. Fifty-two local societies employed a total of 25 health visitors and an additional 34 midwives, who attended 5,540 confinements. To put the figures in some perspective, the percentage of registered births attended by trained midwives in urban areas was 35.98 per cent, and in rural areas only 3.86 per cent.[203] This meant that, out of the total of 427,738 births registered that year, only 34,891 or 8.16 per cent of mothers received trained assistance. Far more financial commitment on the part of the government would have been necessary to raise the number of trained attendances whilst approximately nine-tenths of the population remained in the rural areas.

With the advantage of hindsight, it is easy to see that the only possible answer for the rural areas would have been the formal training of the traditional birth attendants — a practice that is widely followed now. This was attempted on an experimental basis at Maymyo in 1929, but the project was abandoned the following year.[204] Two years later, in 1932, traditional birth attendants were barred from practising in the town under the first application of the Burma Nurses and Midwives Act, 1922, and Maymyo was said to be proving itself as a pioneer in child welfare work.[205]

A possible bar to progress in the maternity field was the reluctance of the administration to appoint women doctors. In 1913, a petition from Burmese and European ladies was presented to the lieutenant governor in Burma. This requested that 21 of the existing 25 vacancies for doctors in the government service be offered to the suitable and qualified lady doctors who were already in the province, and who could be usefully employed in the towns where there was no female medical aid.[206] A few women doctors worked in Burma, but these were mostly employed in the private or charitable sector. An experimental appointment in Akyab had shown that the employment of a female doctor increased the number of confinement and gynaecological cases at the Civil Hospital.[207] Many women prefer to be attended by a doctor of their own sex, and it would seem that the reluctance to appoint women doctors resulted in patients being deterred from seeking help, as well as lowering the total number of doctors practising in the province.

One highly popular initiative was the introduction of "Baby Shows". The first show was held in Rangoon in February 1916 and by 1927, baby shows were being held in 16 towns in Burma.[208] Exhibitions, or "Baby Weeks", also became a feature of the programmes of enthusiastic voluntary societies. Both the shows and baby weeks were opportunities for the voluntary societies and the health officials to present hygiene exhibitions, advise on infant feeding and distribute official publications about infant welfare.

These publications covered a wide range of hygiene and disease problems, and there were 95 booklets available by 1929. The Hygiene Publicity Bureau published these books — some in English, some in Burmese — and by 1929, there were ten available dealing with aspects of infant and maternal care, such as *Hints on Sickness of Babies* and *Care of Infants*.[209] If the administration's priorities can be judged by the number of these publications distributed, then infant welfare came well down the list. The only booklets that had a distribution of 30,000 or more were about plague and smallpox (more than 70,000 copies of one booklet about smallpox had been distributed), but the widest distribution of booklets concerning infant welfare was 13,000.

Did these efforts by the administration and the voluntary societies have a measurable result? Was there a decline in the IMR as a result of these efforts by midwives, committees and the Publicity Bureau? There is no doubt that in some of the small areas of urban Burma, where trained midwives worked and records were kept, a measurable decline in infant mortality did occur. Not many figures are available, but a note for Mandalay in 1915 gives a rate of 265 infants per 1,000 dying before their first birthday, having been attended at birth by a trained midwife, against a registered IMR for the city as a whole of 444.8.[210] In 1920 in Mandalay, 159 infants per 1,000 died before their first birthday after delivery by a trained midwife, as against a registered IMR of 360 for the whole city.[211]

In the country as a whole, however, the registered IMR by the close of the 1930s was still well over 200 per 1,000, and the estimates of the IMR for the 1920s certainly do not indicate a mortality decline. It has already been calculated that by 1939 only 8.15 per cent of the registered births were attended by trained personnel. If the figure is calculated to include the estimated 25 to 30 per cent of unregistered births, then the attendance figure drops to approximately six per cent. If it is surmised that a trained birth attendant approximately halved the probability of an infant dying before its first birthday, but that only six per cent of births were delivered in this way, then the total effect of these efforts must have been negligible. No doubt the efforts of the administration and the voluntary sector were saving lives, but measured against the problem, the efforts were puny. Given more time, it seems probable that in the urban areas there would have been a measurable decline in infant mortality, but the Second World War ended any hopes of immediate improvement.

4 The family and childhood in colonial Burma

"Family" is a word that is interpreted differently by different academic disciplines. To a demographer, a family is a kinship unit residing in one dwelling,[1] but a sociologist or anthropologist would define a family in terms of kinship relationships and not residence. The word is used in the title of this chapter in a fairly elastic way, and was chosen to cover the examination of a number of aspects of Burmese life that could be practically grouped under the concept of "family". These include the aspects of the demographic structure that govern family life, such as the age of marriage, childbirth, birth control practices and the level of fertility. The size of the family unit, the proportions of male and female children in the total population and the diseases and mortality of these children can also be discussed in this framework.

The chapter is divided into two main sections; the demographic aspects of the family are discussed first, while the second section examines the morbidity and mortality of children in colonial Burma, their nutrition and patterns of disease.

The Burmese family

In modern Burma the "nuclear family", that is a married couple and their children, is the normal and most desired household unit.[2] Within this unit the husband is, in many senses, the dominant figure; as a man he is on the highest spiritual level, one that no woman may attain.[3] But family relationships are full of subtleties, and the wife is "viewed as the pivotal person in the family".[4] This is exemplified by the Burmese term for family, which translated means the "mother-child group", because the mother is considered to be the primary influence on her children.[5] The Burmese woman also has economic strength within the family; she is the manager of the family budget and often contributes to the family finances through her own retail trading. Her financial independence is

TABLE 4.1
Household Size in Burma

Census Year	Number in Household	Census Year	Number in Household
1891	5.34	1921	4.84
1901	5.01	1931	4.67
1911	4.90	1941	4.75

Sources: *Census of Burma*.

strengthened by her equal property and inheritance rights. These rights are matters of traditional and customary law "and have been so for centuries".[6]

The family in colonial Burma was similar in many ways to the modern family unit. The available data has been exploited to provide an image of the colonial family as far as possible. The simplest evidence, that of household size, can be read directly from the census records as shown in Table 4.1. This reveals a steady and continuous decline in household size in Burma until 1931, but a slight rise in 1941. These 1941 census figures are provisional only, and the apparent rise must therefore be treated with some caution.

One explanation for this shrinking household size may be a change in customary practice. Father Sangermano, writing in 1833, stated that a bridegroom was expected to live with his new parents-in-law for the first three years of the marriage.[7] This arrangement provided the household with a pair of young "hands", an important asset in a largely agricultural society. Mi Mi Khaing, writing in *The World of Burmese Women* in 1984, said that the custom has now "fallen into disuse in its entirety".[8] This decline in matrilocal residence could certainly account for the change in household size, but there may also be other factors that are not yet apparent.

One of the most useful and basic demographic measurements is a calculation of the proportion of the population that lies in each age group, especially the proportions of children and women of marriageable age. Table 4.2 shows that the percentage of population in each age group was relatively constant from 1891 to 1931, typical of a stable population. The constancy of these percentages confirms that the mortality levels did not fall, despite the steady decrease in the proportion of deaths from cholera, plague, and smallpox. In fact, the table suggests the opposite: the proportion of children, especially boys, declined after

TABLE 4.2
Percentage of the Population by Age Groups in Burma

Census year	0–15 Years		15–20 Years		20–40 Years	
year	Male	Female	Male	Female	Male	Female
1891	39.6	37.5	9.2	10.2	29.6	28.9
1901	39.4	38.7	8.8	9.8	30.5	30.8
1911	39.9	38.9	9.1	9.7	29.8	29.6
1921	37.8	37.3	10.0	10.9	29.5	29.0
1931	37.9	38.0	9.2	10.0	30.5	31.5

Sources: *Census of Burma.*

1911, and implies instead some increase in mortality. Some of this mortality between 1911 and 1921 can be attributed to the flu pandemic in 1918, which would have disproportionately affected the most vulnerable age groups of the very young and the very old. But the proportion of children, especially males, was still low in the 1931 census, indicating that other factors were implicated in the short term.

The sex and age ratios shown in Table 4.2 were calculated from data for the study area only, and those from 1891 to 1921 show figures for Buddhists in the study area; the figures for 1931, on the other hand, were calculated from data for Burmese males and females. This was due to the change in the presentation of census data in 1931, when the five-year age groups were shown in the Tables of Race, whereas formerly they were shown in the Tables of Religion.

The significance of the 20- to 40-year-old age group is that these are the main reproductive years for Burmese women; but another useful demographic measurement, known as the "child/woman ratio", uses the theoretically possible child-bearing ages of 15 to 44 years. This ratio can be used as a rough indicator of fertility and was calculated for each census year by taking the number of children aged from zero to nine years and dividing it by the number of women between the ages of 15 and 44 years. From 1891 to 1921, this was calculated using Buddhist data, and for 1931 it was calculated using Burmese data. The results are shown in Table 4.3. The child/woman ratio shows a fall in the number of 0–9 year olds compared to the number of women in the child-bearing age. The ratio declines from 1.2 in 1901 to 1.1 in 1921, with very little recovery in 1931.

TABLE 4.3

The Child/Woman Ratio in Burma, 1891–1931

Census Year	Ratio	Census Year	Ratio
1891	1.18	1921	1.10
1901	1.20	1931	1.11
1911	1.19		

Sources: *Census of Burma.*

It was mentioned above that the main reproductive years for Burmese women were from 20 to 40 years, although the child/woman ratio is commonly calculated on the 15- to 44-year age group. In Burma, the age of marriage for women is approximately 20 years and, as there is very little fertility outside marriage, this marks the onset of the reproductive years. The Singulate Mean Age of Marriage (SMAM) was calculated from the census data and is shown in Table 4.4. From 1891 to 1921, this was calculated on the data for all Buddhists in the Province of Burma, and for 1931 from the data for all Burmese in Burma (governed by the availability of the data in the census records).

The age of marriage is important as a determinant of total fertility levels in the Burmese context. A mean age of 20 years is late for marriage compared to South Asia, but may be in line with other Southeast Asian countries. Peter Smith and Ng Shui-meng calculated a female SMAM

TABLE 4.4

Singulate Mean Age at Marriage in Burma

Census year	Age in Years	
	Male	Female
1891	23.8	20.5
1901	23.8	20.2
1911	23.7	20.3
1921	24.0	20.8
1931	22.9	21.0

Sources: *Census of Burma.*

of 20.9 years from the 1903 census data in the Philippines, and as their estimates of the crude birth rate (CBR) in the Philippines (at 40 to 45 per 1,000) was also close to Burma's, the demographic structure of the two countries in 1900 may have been very similar. Table 4.4 shows that the age of marriage in Burma changed very little between 1891 and 1931, indicating that its effect on fertility was also constant.

Sir Herbert Thirkell White, a former commissioner of Upper Burma, discussed in his reminiscences of 1913 the age at which Burmese women married. He suggested that "as often as not a Burmese maiden does not marry till she is eighteen or nineteen, or even older", although marriages at 14 or 15 years were not uncommon.[9] A research project in 1981 suggested that 87.5 per cent of those married in Burma had done so between the ages of 15 and 24 years.[10] The SMAM calculated at just over 20 years would seem an acceptable figure to lie between Thirkell White's unqualified observations and the more reliable modern data. There is no way of ascertaining the mean age of menarche in colonial Burma, but again modern data may be used as a guide. A 1970 study of 1,031 girls in Rangoon found that the mean age of menarche was 12.4 years.[11] The age may be affected by malnourishment, but even if the age of menarche in colonial Burma was 13 to 14 years, then more than six years of possible fertility were not exploited due to the later age of marriage.

A picture of the indigenous family in colonial Burma is starting to emerge from the data but what is still needed is a description of the number of children in the Burmese family. The General Fertility Rate (GFR) is calculated on the number of births in one year divided by the female population in that same year. But to have any meaning in the Burmese situation, calculating the GFR would require far more accurate birth registration than the records provide. In Chapter Two it was estimated that only 70 to 75 per cent of total births were registered, thus making a calculation of the General Fertility Rate meaningless.

There is, however, one way in which the average number of children per family can be estimated, and that is from Model Stable Population Tables. The stability of the Burmese population between 1891 and 1931, which was discussed in Chapter Two, has been further confirmed by the constant age ratios, and it seems sensible therefore to exploit the additional knowledge that can be gained from the model tables. To estimate the number of children born in a family, or the Gross Reproduction Rate (GRR), from the tables, two parameters are needed. These are the levels of mortality (Life Table levels of approximately 5.1 in 1891 to 1911, and 3.0 to 3.5 in 1911 and 1921), and the annual rates of population increase (approximately one per cent), which were calculated in Chapters Two and One respectively.

By using the above data, the number of children born to the average Burmese family was read from the West Model Stable Population Tables. These are, six to six-plus children per family between 1891 and 1911, and seven to eight children per family between 1911 and 1931.[12] These figures are approximate and are only useful if viewed in the context of a very "broad brush" approach. They can only serve as a guide to the number of children born to the average Burmese family in colonial Burma. It is also important to remember that between one in three and one in four of these children died before their first birthday, and that further childhood mortality would occur, especially in the crucial weaning period.

Some more specific evidence is available to substantiate these estimates from the beginning of the colonial period and from post-war data. In 1856, Dr Stewart, who was appointed to the Pegu Light Infantry, conducted an enquiry into the number of children born to 100 women in the town of Myan-Oung in Burma. The women were aged between 30 and 83 years, and the average number of births per woman was 5.68. Of these children, 257 had died under ten years of age.[13] Unfortunately there are no further details regarding the ratio of women in the reproductive age group, but obviously some of these women had not completed their reproductive life, which would tend to lower the average births per woman. Also there is a recognised tendency amongst women to under-report births, due either to forgetfulness or deliberate suppression. It is not unusual for a mature woman to forget a stillbirth or a child that died as an early neonate, and Susan Scrimshaw reported the probable suppression of a first or second birth when that child was a girl who subsequently died.[14] The 5.68 births reported by Stewart was therefore probably an underestimate due to incomplete family size and under-reporting. The true figure may well have been nearer to the six or seven births per woman estimated from the model tables.

More modern data comes from Daw Tin Tin Nyunt, who calculated GRRs from Burma's post-war census. The data from the rural areas and the Union of Burma resulted in GRRs for 1954 and 1973 of between 2.6 and 3.1 female births, thus giving a total number of births per woman of 5.3 and 6.4 respectively.[15] The urban data produced a lower rate of between 2.3 and 2.9 female births; however, this may be affected by family planning methods.[16] This information should be considered in conjunction with the lowered infant mortality, which had dropped to under 200 per 1,000 by 1954 and to under 50 per 1,000 by 1974, which would tend to lower the fertility rate by increasing the birth interval. With that consideration, the modern data is probably comparable with the estimate for the colonial period.

The data described has produced considerable information about the Burmese family. The average woman married at just over 20 years of age; she probably had six to seven children born to her; and the household size was four to five people. In addition, the data has revealed that, during the colonial period, nearly 40 per cent of the population was under 15 years of age. But what this data does not reveal is the attitude of Burmese parents to marriage or to their children.

Burmese attitudes towards marriage and children

Marriage in Burma was not universal. The percentage of Buddhist females who were married between the age of 20 and 30 years formed only 70 to 75 per cent of the total female Buddhist population in that age group (the figure was calculated on Buddhist data for the Province of Burma between 1891 and 1921). This meant that 25 to 30 per cent of the females in those prime reproductive years were not in an established sexual union. As there was very little fertility outside marriage, this obviously must have acted as a depressant of general fertility, as did the later age of marriage.

How did the Burmese regard their children? Did they see them as having "value", a concept that is sometimes applied to pre-industrial societies but is difficult to assess in the society of colonial Burma? John C. Caldwell's theory of a high, uncontrolled fertility as part of a necessary cultural superstructure maintaining the means of production may not necessarily apply to Southeast Asian cultures.[17] The society that he described is one in which wealth and power flow upwards to a venerated patriarch and where, therefore, an increase in family size brings an increase in wealth and power to the head of the family unit. But although respect for age is clearly characteristic of Burmese society, Caldwell's concept of a patriarchal society, in which the woman and her daughter-in-law have no power outside the home, does not fit the more independent role of the Burmese woman. Also Caldwell's society is one in which a system of arranged marriages is necessary to keep the marital bond weak by comparison with the child/parent bond, and thus retain the power of decision-making over reproduction in the hands of an older generation who are not biologically involved.[18]

It has already been suggested that Burmese society tended to be matrilocal, especially in the earlier part of the colonial period, but it is also clear, from the later age of marriage and the non-universality of marriage, that there was no pressure on the daughter to marry. June and Manning Nash have suggested that in modern Burmese society an unmarried member of the household is economically valuable to the family unit, and it may well be that in this sense the Burmese did see their children as having value, but not within the rigid and patriarchal structure that Caldwell described.[19]

It is also clear that, except for the decrease in the custom of the son-in-law taking residence in the bride's home, other concepts about children did not alter radically during the colonial era. It has already been argued that the Burmese population was stable and therefore, by definition, the fertility and mortality rates were unchanged in the long term. This does not, of course, exclude temporary fluctuations in the rates as a short-term response, but no evidence has emerged of changes in fertility restriction practices during the colonial period. Nor is there real evidence of any change in the fertility from pre-colonial times. Anthony Reid and Norman Owen have speculated that there may have been an increase in fertility in nineteenth-century Southeast Asia as a result of changes in agricultural practice from swidden to settled farming, and also as a result of the spread of the major religions.[20] However, these changes had already taken place in the developed parts of the study area in Burma. It is possible that the development of the delta as a rice-growing area from 1850, may have influenced fertility through improved security and nutritional status, but this is only speculation.[21]

It is also possible that the Burmese adjusted their fertility at times of crisis by delaying marriage or through sexual abstinence. For example, it would be logical to expect that fertility declined naturally during the great famine at the beginning of the nineteenth century, but was there also a positive attempt by the Burmese to limit conception during the crisis? For the present, these possibilities must remain conjecture, but, given the information that is emerging about the adjustment and control of fertility in European and Asian history in response to economic pressures, the emergence of some form of population adjustment history in Southeast Asia would not be surprising.[22]

Burma's pattern of fertility during non-crisis periods would seem to lie somewhere between the uncontrolled fertility that Caldwell described, and the restricted family size that Sarah Hanley and Kozo Yamamura portrayed in Tokugawa, Japan. Some of the fertility control mechanisms in Burma have already been described — these were the late age of marriage and the high numbers of unmarried women. But there are other factors that may have influenced Burmese fertility, such as prolonged breast-feeding. Many cultures practice post-partum sexual abstinence and also abortion and/or infanticide: it is possible therefore that they were customary in colonial Burma.

Fertility control and family size

The universal and prolonged breast-feeding that was customary in colonial Burma has already been discussed as an aspect of infant nutrition. In this chapter, it is the significance of lactation as a birth control method that is important. Firstly, it must be stated that the physiological relationship between anovulation and breast-feeding is not yet fully understood, although its demographic importance in lengthening the intervals between births "is now universally acknowledged".[23] The effectiveness of breast-feeding in prolonging amenorrhoea would appear to depend on the frequency and duration of suckling, including the continuation of night suckling. The introduction of supplementary feeding can increase the chance of ovulation, if it is associated with a decline in suckling.[24]

The effect on fertility of breast-feeding for two years in a South Asian population was discussed in the Khanna study, conducted in 1971 by John Wyon and John Gordon. The detailed information about the reproductive cycles of the participant women studied was gathered during monthly visits to their homes. The average interval between live births was slightly more than 30 months, and the children were breast-fed for an average of 24 months. Ovulation did not occur until ten months after childbirth, and the interval between the first menses and conception was a further ten months. The prolonged breast-feeding was found to lengthen the birth intervals in this population by nearly 50 per cent.[25] The birth rate of the participant women, at 38 per 1,000, was lower than the estimated birth rate for colonial Burma, but the infant mortality rate (IMR) in the Khanna study, at under 200 per 1,000, was also considerably lower. A high IMR, especially when many deaths occur in the perinatal period, raises the birth rate through a shortened post-partum amenorrhoea and, consequently, shortened birth intervals.

Can a post-war study in South Asia provide a guide to the pattern of ovulation and conception in colonial Burma? The Khanna study probably does provide a practical model for other societies in Asia, given certain reservations. The main reservation is, of course, the level of the IMR, but, given the situation where the child in colonial Burma survived its infancy, the study would probably provide a good model, especially as the duration of breast-feeding is very similar. There is, however, no guide to the possible length of the menstruating interval if the Burmese child died in infancy.

Post-partum sexual abstinence can affect the length of the menstruating interval in some societies, but no historical evidence has yet been found on this subject for Burmese society. Tin Tin Nyunt reported a modern post-partum abstinence of about six weeks in her study of 1978, which is low compared to some societies. (In the Khanna study, a post-partum abstinence of four months was reported, which, however, had little significance as the lactation suppressed ovulation for ten months.[26])

There is a possibility that other socio-cultural factors may have delayed conception in Burma. The poor diet that was eaten by lactating women could have prolonged the post-partum amenorrhoea. Michel Carael reported on a 1978 study of women in Zaire, which examined the relationship between birth intervals and nutrition. The study found that one group of rural women had a post-partum amenorrhoea of 18.7 months, whereas the three other groups surveyed had intervals of between 9.3 and 10.7 months. Carael suggested that this prolonged amenorrhoea was related to a "moderate, chronic malnutrition, characterised by unbalanced supplies in protein and lipid". No conclusions about the situation in colonial Burma can be drawn from this study, but Carael's suggestion of a "possible self-regulating fertility mechanism through chronic malnutrition" is, at the very least, interesting, and also relates to other hypotheses of population control in Southeast Asia.[27]

Robert Whyte suggested in his work *Rural Nutrition in Monsoon Asia* (1974) that most Asian societies have in-built, traditional systems for limiting population growth. This, he said, was done by "applying during the critical phases of life the selective power of reduced nutrition on the mother and child".[28] This is an interesting idea because it suggests that the apparently opposing aspects of food taboos (namely, the protection of the mother and child from "harmful" foods, which often leads to deficiencies and under-nutrition) are not, in fact, contradictory, but are designed to protect the community from an excessive burden of dependants. The validity of this idea may be somewhat strained when applied to the Buddhist Burmese society, where merit is earned by the donation of food to others. But despite this, the effect of the food taboos in Burmese society must have been a higher mortality in the very young, and these taboos were therefore a contributory factor in slowing population growth.

Scrimshaw, in an article in 1978, assessed the socio-cultural factors in infant mortality, including the withholding of protein-rich foods from infants.[29] She suggested that the sex, spacing and birth order of the child may determine its allocation of family resources in time, food and medicines, and that the conscious or unconscious actions of the parents may affect the viability of the infant. This means, in effect, that parents may decide whether a child should live or die, and that one of the controlling mechanisms is nutrition.

The discussion so far has touched on three ways in which nutrition may possibly affect population control. It has been suggested that nutritional deficiencies may prolong post-partum amenorrhoea, that food taboos might reduce the number of (vulnerable) dependants in a society, and that the parental control of infant nutrition could consciously or unconsciously act as a form of infanticide. This is not a suggestion that these forms of population control necessarily operated in Burmese society, but is a suggestion that nutrition may be implicated in traditional methods of fertility restriction. It was argued in Chapter Three that the under- or malnutrition of the mother and child were important factors in infant mortality, and, given that hypothesis, it should also be considered that these dietary preferences might also have had a cultural role in the history of population control.

There is no suggestion, however, in the evidence so far examined, of the practice of blatant infanticide in Burmese society. Arthur Phayre commented in 1862 that there was "no suspicion of the prevalence of infanticide or the exposure of children".[30]

It is difficult to discover whether abortion was practised in colonial Burma because abortion, like infanticide, is usually hidden within the indigenous community. No evidence has been found of the use of induced abortion in colonial Burma, but most societies have practised some form of abortion and the Nashes described it as frequently performed in Upper Burma in 1963 to prevent a forced marriage of young people.[31] Without direct historical evidence, however, it must remain an unquantified probability in colonial Burma.

There is one more subject to be discussed in this section of the chapter, and that is childbirth — an event of great demographic importance and family significance. Childbirth is also a time of risk for both the mother and her infant. It is not known how many or what percentage of parturient women died in colonial Burma. During the last 20 years of registration, 1921–41, figures of deaths in childbirth were recorded in the major towns, but like most of the registration data, it was admitted by the health authorities to be very inaccurate. In 1939, the number of maternal deaths recorded was 531, against a figure for live births in the same towns of 49,836. The maternal mortality rate is normally calculated as the number of deaths from pregnancy, labour or the lying-in period divided by the number of live births, and expressed per 10,000.[32] In 1939, therefore, the rate for the towns of Burma was less than 1.1 per 10,000 which is close to the modern rate for developed countries, whereas "in historical populations values as high as two or three deaths per 100 births have been observed."[33] The low rate in Burmese towns therefore offers only the information that the deaths were not accurately recorded.

The annual health report of 1868 expressed concern about the rate of maternal deaths, and stated that 149 of 762 female deaths, or one-fifth, were maternal.[34] The Burmese midwifery methods were described in this report as crude and barbarous, but in the discussion, it was accepted that Burmese women preferred to give birth in their houses rather than hospitals and that only women were accepted as midwives. A post-war description of traditional Burmese midwifery appears in an article by C. V. Foll, chief medical officer for Burmah Oil. In 1959, he wrote that childbirth management in Burma involved "considerable interference from the local midwife, the woman's mother and her relations."[35] He also described the local obstetric practice as "vigorous abdominal massage with kneading the fundus of the uterus."[36]

The period after childbirth, the puerperium or lying-in, is attended by tradition in many societies. Father Sangermano described the Burmese practices in the early part of the nineteenth century. These involved the "heating" of the post-parturient woman by laying her near a fire for ten to 15 days. He described the woman as naked, badly blistered from the heat and, by the end of the period, "the poor woman is quite scorched and blackened."[37] Roasting after childbirth was a common practice in Southeast Asia,[38] but Sangermano's account appears highly sensationalised. It would seem unlikely that Burmese women, who are physically very modest,[39] would lie naked by the fire or allow themselves to become scorched and blackened. The object of roasting was to speed recovery after childbirth and prevent loss of the body heat. Some 45 years after Sangermano, K.N. MacDonald, in *The Practice of Medicine Among the Burmese* (1879), described how the Burmese doctors would order a large fire to be placed near a woman after childbirth, but only in cold weather. She should also have ginger and pepper in her food.[40] More recently, in 1978, C. Mougne described the practice of "lying by the fire" in her work on northern Thailand, and the custom in those villages was admitted to have another important function — this was "drying out the womb" to space births.[41]

No evidence has been found to suggest that the "roasting" in Burma was seen as a device for fertility control, but as northern Thai society and Burmese society have many cultural similarities, it is probable that this belief was shared. Mougne documented alternative methods of "drying out the womb" such as squatting over infusions of bark or leaves, or plastering the belly with a hot brick smeared with a poultice of bark and leaves.[42] Foll described massaging the abdomen with a hot brick for seven days after childbirth in Upper Burma to help involution of the uterus.[43] He also described another method that was traditionally thought to space births; this involved the uterus being "displaced through the stomach".[44] It is clear that Foll had not witnessed this traditional practice of lifting and twisting the uterus, but he commented that it was said to be effective. No clear historical evidence exists to establish that Burmese women used customary methods after childbirth in an attempt to control their fertility, but these modern descriptions of traditional practices make the probability very high. This is not to suggest that the practices described were effective methods of birth control but that Burmese and Thai women were prepared to endure great discomfort in an attempt to limit their fertility.

Morbidity and mortality of children

This section of the chapter will examine the mortality and disease of children between the ages of one year and 15 years in colonial Burma. There is much less information about this age group and its mortality in the annual health reports than about infants and their mortality. This is because the mortality rate of children has not the same social significance as the mortality of infants; and the childhood rates of mortality are not widely quoted as a measurement of the community's health and welfare.

The measurement of childhood mortality was as inaccurate as the measurement of all vital events. From 1876, deaths were recorded by six-year age groups in the annual health reports, but by 1885, the more commonly used five-year age groups were shown. Unfortunately this data provides little valuable information. The number of child deaths as a percentage of the total mortality in colonial Burma was plotted for every year from 1885 to 1939, but with sparse results. Too many uncertainties surround the data; for example, it would appear that, between 1903 and 1913, the average female mortality in Upper Burma in the age group one to ten years was lower than that in Lower Burma. The difference is more marked in the five-year age groups; that is, in Upper Burma the one- to four-year age group in those years formed 13.03 per cent of the total female mortality and the five- to ten-year age group formed 5.4 per cent of the total female mortality. In Lower Burma, the figures were 13.44 per cent for the one to four years and 6.81 per cent for the five to ten years. But are these figures an accurate reflection of differential mortality in colonial Burma or are they an example of the variation in the registration of children's deaths? As the figures do not correspond with any known pattern of mortality, it may be that the difference is purely in the degree of registration.

The authors of the annual health reports estimated the crude birth and death rates on several occasions, but only one example of an estimated rate for young children has been found. This was made in 1914 by the sanitary commissioner, C. E. Williams, who estimated that the mortality of one- to two-year olds in Burma was 98 per 1,000.[45] The opinion of an experienced officer should not be ignored but, without further data, this single estimate was not felt to be sufficient evidence.

Therefore, in order to obtain the most accurate possible estimate of childhood mortality, the model life tables were used. Indirect estimates

TABLE 4.5
Estimates of Child Mortality in Burma (from West Model Life Tables)

| Inter-censal Period | Age | Life Table Level | Numbers Dying in Age Interval (per 1,000) | |
			Male	Female
1891–1901	1–5		124.9	132.3
and	5–10	5	27.2	30.7
1901–11	10–15		18.6	22.8
	1–5	3	139.2	149.8
		4	132.2	141.2
1911–21	5–10	3	28.6	33.0
and		4	28.0	31.9
1921–31	10–15	3	19.4	24.2
		4	19.1	23.6

Sources: *Census of Burma*; Coale and Demeny, *Regional Model Life Tables and Stable Populations*, West Model Life Tables, *dx* column.

were made of the mortality in the childhood age groups by taking the figures from the *dx* column of the tables, which shows the numbers of deaths occurring per 1,000 of population in the specified age interval. It must be appreciated that, as with the IMR, these indirect estimations from the life tables are only accurate if Burma's childhood mortality pattern is the same as that shown in the West Model Life Tables. But even with that proviso, the tables offer the best opportunity of estimating the levels of childhood mortality in colonial Burma.

The inter-censal levels of mortality in the study area of Burma were calculated in Chapter Two, which meant that it was only necessary to read the estimates of child mortality from the appropriate life table. The numbers of male and female children estimated to have died in each age interval are shown in Table 4.5. A life table level of 5.0 has been assumed as the best estimate for the inter-censal interval 1891 to 1901, and for the two inter-censal intervals of 1911–21 and 1921–31, two life table mortality levels are shown. This is because the median levels calculated for these two inter-censal intervals were 3.54 and 3.46 respectively, and therefore the estimate of Burmese childhood mortality obviously lies between these two levels of 3 and 4. For example, the

TABLE 4.6

Female Age-specific Mortality per 1,000 (from West Model Life Tables)

Life Table Level	Age	Female
3	1–2	76
	2–3	35
4	1–2	
	2–3	
5	1–2	68
	2–3	30

Sources: Coale and Demeny, *Regional Model Life Tables and Stable Populations,* West Model Life Tables, *lx* column.

mortality level of one- to five-year-old females between 1911 and 1931 was in the range 141 to 150 per 1,000.

As already stated, these estimates are accurate only if the Burmese mortality pattern corresponds to the West Model Life Tables, but if a "broad brush" approach is accepted, then these estimates probably provide a better guide to the mortality than the registration figures. These latter figures have an additional limitation, as they do not give the detailed number of deaths in the important weaning period. The female age-specific data is available in the life tables and is shown in Table 4.6 for the one- to three-year-old period, when a toddler may be supplanted by a new baby, in addition to facing the hazards of weaning.

The data in Table 4.6 suggest that the mortality in the one- to two-year-old age group in colonial Burma was between 68 and 76 per 1,000 for females. This is somewhat below the 98 per 1,000 described above, which was the only estimate found in the health records, but the latter was related to the very high mortality occurring in infants and young children in Mandalay town.[46]

Very few other general comments on childhood mortality appear in the health records. A comment was made in 1918 that the deaths of zero to five year olds was always under suspicion of being incomplete, especially when violent epidemics such as the flu pandemic were present.[47] In 1868, the civil surgeon of Moulmein was quoted as saying that "Burmese children are terribly mismanaged by their mothers",[48] but the detailed comment that appeared about the infant group was lacking for the one- to four-year-old children. Much more information is available about school-age children from a nutrition survey carried out between 1939 and 1941, and from the records of the medical inspection of schoolchildren.

Nutrition of children

Some aspects of nutrition in young children have been touched on in Chapter Two: these were the universal practice of breast-feeding and its duration of approximately two years, and the traditional methods of supplementary feeding up to one year of age. What is needed now is information about the diet of the one- to five-year-old child. Was the diet adequate or was there a weaning crisis? The indications are that there was a protein energy malnutrition (PEM), or protein calorie malnutrition (PCM), crisis but there is very little concrete historical evidence. In 1955, B. P. Sarin, who wrote about child health in Rangoon, said that the condition *Noe Myet* was known to have existed in Burma for a long time.[49] Sarin described it as the condition a weanling gets when the mother becomes pregnant, a classical description of PEM. A severe form of PCM, known as Kwashiorkor, is described as "principally a disease of the second year of life", when breast-feeding is decreasing, the traditional supplementary diet is not adequate, and the non-immune child is exposed to a wide range of bacterial, viral and parasitic infections.[50]

In 1873, a letter to the secretary of the chief commissioner of British Burma about the insanitary state of Prome town was quoted in the annual health report. It stated that "The children of people living in the quarter (Kahthay) are all unhealthy looking, with big abdomens and attenuated limbs."[51] This description of the children and the presence of the local name for a weanling disease suggest that a nutritional crisis occurred in early childhood, but this is still insubstantial evidence on which to base an argument. However, a number of reports have been published since 1956 that describe the incidence of PEM in post-war Burma, and, as many of these studies reveal traditional feeding patterns, they may also be taken as a guide to the pre-war picture.

The papers in the collection (discussed in Chapter Three which were probably from the 1970s) on *Beliefs and Practices about Foods and Feeding* reveal that adult Burmese food with its spice and chilli content is considered unsuitable for small children. Amongst these papers is a report from the Mon state by Dr Daw Ohn Kyi, who stated that only rice, salt and oil is given to young children.[52] A paper from Mandalay district by Dr Ma Ma Tin contains more detail about diets. Dr Tin said that by two to three years of age, the child is given adult food with the exception of spices and chillies, but eggs, meat, milk and fish are withheld until the third birthday.[53] The beliefs that determine this withholding of protein are complex, and are partly due to the faith of the Burmese in the ability of rice to give strength to the child. In addition there is the belief that pulses, beans and milk cause diarrhoea, and that meat and fish are associated with worm infestation.[54] Dr Po Po, who wrote in 1965 on childhood nutrition in Burma, said that children were wholly on the breast until two to three years old, and that if any supplementary feeding occurred, then the majority of children received only rice, salt and oil.[55]

These comments are really a continuation of the argument in Chapter Three, that the diet of the infant was inadequate. It would appear probable, not surprisingly, that this inadequacy continued into young childhood, causing widespread PEM. Two modern reports, written in the 1970s, pinpoint the crisis period for Burmese children as between 24 and 36 months. This is the time when breast-feeding would be declining in quantity or ceasing altogether and before the switch to an adult diet. Dr Kywe Thein and associates, in their study of Rangoon children in 1971, found that the highest incidence of PEM was at 36 months, and that it was associated with low socio-economic status in the parents and medium to large family size.[56] The weaning food was reported to be usually rice and clear soup only. In 1974, Dr Cho Nwe Oo reported on a study of children who lived in the islands of the Mergui archipelago and in Hlegu township. Her findings showed that the severest degree of malnutrition occurred in children aged 24 to 35 months.[57] Another modern paper (probably from the 1970s) showed that the incidence of PCM in Burma was seasonal, and that it occurred chiefly during the cold and rainy season, when the viral diseases of childhood such as measles and whooping cough were also prevalent.[58]

Another post-war finding is that Burmese children grow very slowly between the ages of six months and three years, which emphasises the importance and effect of the low nutritional intake in that period. Dr Postmus, who conducted the WHO Nutrition Survey of Burma, reported in 1957 that the height and weight of Burmese children increased very slowly until the age of three years. "After three years they grow much better than children in other Oriental countries, but not sufficiently to make up arrears, so they are at the age of five years shorter and have less body weight than other Oriental children."[59]

The evidence from modern Burma suggests that many children between the ages of one year and three years are malnourished and that this malnourishment is due to inadequate supplementary feeding. The WHO survey found that very young Burmese children grew more slowly than their counterparts in other countries. In addition, in 1977,

Dr Cho Nwe Oo described finding PCM in 50 per cent of Burmese children under the age of four years.[60] It seems clear that in modern Burma, the inadequate diet of young children was causing up to half of them to exhibit clinical signs of PCM. But does this information help to clarify the inadequate knowledge of the nutritional status of young children in colonial Burma?

I would suggest that there is enough evidence to support the view that PCM was a major problem in one to three year olds in nineteenth- and early twentieth-century Burma. The existence of a traditional name for the weaning crisis, and the considerable body of evidence discussed here and in Chapter Three about the widespread cultural and traditional restrictions on the diet of children all point to a problem that long predates the Second World War. But the concrete evidence for the young child's diet is still lacking, and so the view must remain strong probability and not fact.

In the immediate post Second World War period, B. O. Binns, the author of several papers on food and agriculture in Burma, supplied the government of Burma with food statistics. Amongst these were revised figures relating to an analysis of pre-war diet in Burma, which included an estimation of the calories available by age group for the pre-war population.[61] In this table, Binns suggested that the diet of one to three year olds living in the plains area (that is, not the hill areas) of Burma amounted to 1,130 calories per day, and that four to six year olds received 1,506 calories per day. Dr Cho Nwe Oo, reporting on a survey in Hlegu town in 1974, found that the nutrient intake in weighed food of children aged one to three years was 763 calories, and that of four to five year olds was 1,139 calories.[62] If Binns' estimate is accurate, it suggests that one to three year olds in pre-war Burma enjoyed a diet containing approximately one-third more calories than the diets of Burmese children in the 1970s. But closer examination of Binns' data shows statistical weaknesses. The figures for consumption and the estimates of "Probable Calorie Availability" are based on the "edible portion" of the food. Binns' figures appear to be "based on reliable official statistics of production recorded by experts and checked by close personal experience."[63] This means that the figures are a calculation of the food available per head of population based on the assumption of equal opportunity to acquire the theoretical share. The Hlegu figures, by comparison, are based on the cooked weight of the food actually offered to the child and were found to form only 65 per cent of the required intake of one to three year olds and 70 per cent of the required intake of four to five year olds.[64]

Even if the socio-economic factors are ignored, the distribution of food in the Burmese family was probably unequal. In Burma, as in many other cultures, "the major share of the best food would be set aside for the father who is the bread winner", and he would probably be fed first.[65] This may not have been important in a family where food was plentiful and of high quality, but it would certainly tend to disadvantage children in a poor family where food was scarce. The consumption of food and the entitlement to a fair share of food can only be ascertained with any accuracy by a study within the family, and not by crudely dividing the sum of food production by the size of the population, as calculated by Binns. Therefore even if the quantity of food in colonial Burma was theoretically sufficient for the requirements of all the population, cultural and socio-economic factors probably combined to ensure that the diet of pre-school children was inadequate.[66]

It is not possible to go further and suggest that a specific number of one to four year olds died of malnutrition in colonial Burma. There is a possibility that the West Model Life Tables might understate the mortality in the two- to three-year-old age group, as the modern data for Burma suggests that the weaning crisis occurred between 24 and 36 months.

Much more detailed information is available on the nutrition of Burmese schoolchildren. There are two main sources in the colonial records that discuss the dietary deficiencies of these children, and by far the most informative and authoritative of these is the report by Dr U Maung Gale. Between 1939 and 1941, Dr U Maung Gale conducted the first nutrition survey in Burma, during which he examined the diets of 844 families and clinically examined 3,070 schoolgirls and 3,728 schoolboys between the ages of four and 12 years for signs of malnutrition. He divided the children that were examined into four categories — category 1 for those in a good nutritional state, category 2 for those in a normal state, and categories 3 and 4 for those who were subnormal and bad respectively. Children in the third category were defined as those "Children who are capable of appreciable improvement and children who show clinical signs of deficiency, namely — anaemia, phrynoderma, Bitot's Spots, angular stomatitis and sore tongue, but who would otherwise be classed as 'normal'." In the fourth category were those "Children who are obviously malnourished, and children with severe degrees of clinical signs of deficiency".[67]

Dr U Maung Gale's survey included children from Insein, Bassein, Yamethin, Minbu and Thaton districts, all of which lie within the study area, and his results are shown in Table 4.7. (He also surveyed children in the Mergui district and these results have not been included in the table as the district lies outside the study area. Furthermore, that survey examined the children on the rubber estates and the mining areas of Mergui, and children from two towns, making it atypical.)

TABLE 4.7

Results of the Clinical Examination of Schoolchildren for
Signs of Malnutrition, 1939–41

	Percentage of children in each category				
District	Cat. 1	Cat. 2	Cat. 3	Cat. 4	Total cats. 3 & 4
Insein	4.3	46.6	39.0	10.1	49.1
Bassein	3.0	46.2	41.3	9.5	50.8
Yamethin	3.1	42.6	43.4	10.9	54.3
Minbu	2.0	42.0	44.0	12.0	56.0
Thaton	1.5	48.2	43.8	6.5	50.3

Sources: U Maung Gale, *Reports on the Dietary and Nutritional Surveys.*

This table reveals a surprisingly even level of malnutrition, except
that Upper Burma would appear to be particularly disadvantaged, as
Minbu and Yamethin districts have the highest percentage of children
in category 4 and in the totals of categories 3 and 4. It is also notable that
Minbu district had nearly twice the number of badly malnourished
children as did Thaton district.

All the major areas of Burma are represented in the districts surveyed
— the delta, mid-delta, the dry zone and the rice-growing area of
Thaton. Different socio-economic classes were surveyed in each of the
districts so that a mixture of petty traders, agriculturalists, school-
teachers and labourers were examined in each location. Despite this
mix of socio-economic classes, U Maung Gale found that more than
50 per cent of the children examined showed clinical signs of
malnourishment or were capable of appreciable improvement.

Another very significant finding of the survey was that, of the 811
families examined who ate a rice-based diet, 605, or nearly 75 per cent,
ate machine-milled rice instead of home-pounded rice, with a consequent
loss of proteins and vitamins. (A further 33 families who were examined
ate a more mixed diet, including maize, millet, home-pounded and
machine-milled rice.) It is also notable that in Kyungone village in
Bassein district, where 27 out of 30 families surveyed ate home-pounded
rice, there were no signs of stomatitis or sore tongue amongst the
children.[68]

Many of the children whom Dr U Maung Gale examined and then
listed in category 3 were possibly suffering from only a mild degree of

vitamin deficiency, which could have been remedied by a more balanced diet. But it must also be considered that nearly ten per cent of children showed severe clinical signs of deficiency or malnourishment.

Dr U Maung Gale also examined the diets of the children in several boarding schools in Burma and made various recommendations for improvement. He reported on the diets at the Rangoon Boys Home, St Mary's Anglo-Vernacular High School for Girls (in Rangoon) and the Borstal Training School at Thayetmyo. Criticism was levelled at all three institutions: the diet of the boys' home was reported to be deficient in calcium and Vitamin A,[69] and the diet at the Borstal school was deficient in animal proteins and calcium.[70] Both institutions were advised by U Maung Gale to use more proteins, fruits and vegetables. The findings at the girls' high school were perhaps more surprising, as the calorific content of the diet was only 1,676 per head per day.[71] The recipients of this meagre fare were described as students and teachers, of whom 60 per cent were adult. They usually bought themselves an additional meal each day from street vendors, as the diet provided was deficient both in quantity and in proteins, minerals and vitamins.

The problem of under-nutrition in Burmese schoolchildren was not confined to the poor, and it was perhaps fortunate that the girls at St Mary's high school in Rangoon had enough money to buy themselves another meal. Some degree of malnutrition would appear to have been endemic amongst the children of colonial Burma irrespective of socio-economic status, although the proportion of children with severe malnutrition was highest amongst the very poor. But the existence of deficiency diseases amongst the children of the "better-off" was revealed by the school medical inspections, which were started in 1913.[72] The reports of these school inspections provide the second source of nutritional information that was referred to earlier. These inspections were confined to the Anglo-vernacular and European schools initially, and the examinations were carried out by the local civil surgeon or doctor and paid for by the government. The number of schools examined rose rapidly as the scheme expanded, and by 1931, a total of 301 schools had joined, due to the government recognition of the normal schools, in addition to the European and Anglo-vernacular schools.[73] A report was supposed to be submitted to the sanitary commissioner by the medical inspector of each school examined, but only a proportion reported each year. For example, in 1931 there were 301 schools recognised under the scheme, of which only 229 had actually appointed medical officers; of these 229, only 176 submitted a report.[74] The year 1930 represented the peak of the scheme, as in 1931 the government withdrew all grants as part of the general financial retrenchment, and the number of schools inspected declined rapidly.

Despite the lack of funds, the scheme managed to stagger on to some degree, but the number of children examined dropped each year from the peak of 55,968 in 1930 to 4,307 in 1936.[75] During this period, some medical officers gave their services free of charge to the schools, and other schools raised their own funds for the inspection. In 1936, the sanitary commissioner reported that a scheme had been proposed to the government whereby a full-time medical officer and one or more nurses would be appointed to inspect the schools in the larger towns, but the war intervened before any new posts were funded.[76]

The medical inspectors of schools sometimes reported on the nutritional state of the pupils examined. For example, in 1925, there were 19,574 pupils assessed for their nutritional state, of which 25.38 per cent were said to be in a fair nutritional state and 4.88 per cent in a poor nutritional state.[77] The problem with these figures, as with all the data produced by the school inspections, is that the individual reports were arbitrary in their nature. The sanitary commissioners did not lay down standards of reference for the inspectors to follow, and the nature of the examinations and the clinical standards applied varied wildly. In 1939, this variation was illustrated by the results from two schools in Rangoon. The inspector of the Baptist English High School reported that 46.8 per cent of the children had defective teeth, whereas at the Methodist Burmese Girls High School, a different medical officer found that only 1.2 per cent of the pupils had defective teeth.[78] (Perhaps Baptism leads to an outer cleansing only.) But even if allowance is made for these variations, the average of the school figures provides some guide to the incidence of deficiency-related diseases. Between 1924 and 1939, an average of 4.5 per cent of children examined were reported to have skin disease, and 7.4 per cent were said to have defective eyes. In the same period, an average of 19.9 per cent were said to have bad teeth.

The sanitary commissioners found little comfort in these figures, as the children inspected were those whose families were wealthy enough to pay school fees, and therefore represented an elite. Bisset, the director of public health, remarked in 1927 that there were 350,000 children who attended 5,600 vernacular schools, none of which were examined. He added that the ones who were cared for systematically (28,981 or eight per cent in 1927) were those "who probably require it less than the children of the poorer classes".[79] No treatment was offered to the examined children, but a medical report of the findings was sent to their homes. Some medical officers complained of a lack of co-operation and interest from the parents, but the medical officer of the Cushing High School in Rangoon said that all the parents had acknowledged receipt of their child's report and most had had their children treated.[80]

This discussion of the medical inspection of schoolchildren has digressed a little from the original objective, which was the nutritional standards of the children concerned. However, it is important to describe the background against which the inspections were made and the data collected, especially as references to the inspections will also be made under the section concerning diseases.

The nutritional data collected from the school inspections is of interest despite its bias, as it shows that some malnutrition existed even among the wealthier seven per cent of children in Burma. But under-nutrition or dietary deficiencies were not confined to the European or Anglo-vernacular schools in Burma; cases of beri beri in the mission schools were common. In 1909 and 1910, there were 176 cases of beri beri reported at five American Baptist and Roman Catholic mission schools in Bassein, Insein and Shwegyin districts.[81] More cases of beri beri were reported in 1912 from the American Baptist Mission School at Maubin.[82] At Mawlaik School in the Upper Chindwin district, there were outbreaks of beri beri amongst the pupils in 1923, 1924 and 1925.[83] The quantity of the diet was found to be insufficient and in addition, although hand-pounded rice was used, the rice was often old, damp and subjected to prolonged storage, as Mawlaik town imported its rice from areas which were one to five days' boat journey away.

It is U Maung Gale's systematic report across socio-economic groups that offers the best guide to the nutritional standards of schoolchildren in colonial Burma. He found that approximately 50 per cent of schoolchildren were suffering some degree of malnutrition, and the significance of this lies in the interaction between malnutrition and infection. "The two conditions are synergistic; the presence of one pre-disposes and aggravates the other in a vicious cycle. This predisposition to infection in malnourished subjects is attributable to a defective immune response associated with malnutrition."[84] It is this synergistic effect that makes the findings of malnutrition in children so important; "In malnourished children, therefore, ordinary childhood diseases lead to severe complications and poor outcome. This adverse effect of malnutrition is best exemplified in measles where case fatality rates in the malnourished exceed that in normal children by as much as 189 times."[85] These comments made in 1985 by T. E. Tupasi in a paper on "Nutrition and Acute Respiratory Infection" spell out the significance of malnutrition, especially the significance of the vulnerability of the toddler and the schoolchild to the combination of malnourishment and infection that is present in a tropical country.

In colonial Burma, there was an additional factor at work, and that was the change in the Burmese diet after around 1900, when most of the population switched from the consumption of hand-pounded rice to the eating of machine-milled or white rice. (Dr U Maung Gale found that 75 per cent of the population who ate a rice-based diet were eating machine-milled rice.) During milling, 76 per cent of the thiamine, 56 per cent of the riboflavine and 63 per cent of the niacin content of the husked rice is removed, and the difference between home-pounded rice and machine-milled rice is the reduction of thiamine from levels of between 3.0 to 5.0 micrograms per gram to 1.0 microgram per gram.[86] Deficiencies of the Group B vitamins are some of the inter-related factors predisposing the malnourished individual to infection.[87]

The under- or malnutrition of the child in colonial Burma should therefore not be viewed as a simple and isolated factor, but as part of a pattern of events leading to high mortality at vulnerable periods in the child's life. The other factor in this pattern was disease.

Childhood diseases

Debility and morbidity in the Burmese child was almost certainly polycausal, but it is simpler to discuss the various factors one at a time, while remembering that nutritional deficiencies, parasites and infection form a circle of interaction. This section will look first at the parasites commonly found in Burmese children and then the infectious diseases.

The registration of deaths is of little assistance in any assessment of disease-specific child mortality in colonial Burma. The deaths were registered by age, but these figures were not cross-referenced with disease-specific mortality. The result is that there is no way of estimating the number of child deaths from plague, for example. In that sense, children's deaths are "hidden" in the records and very few specific comments were made about them in the annual health reports. A good example of this is the investigation that was conducted into the problem of intestinal parasites or worms in colonial Burma.

Worms/internal parasites
Between 1911 and 1927, the annual health reports carried comments about the experiments that were taking place among the prison population to assess their parasite burden. *Ankylostoma*, or hookworm, were found in gaol inmates in Burma from Akyab to Mandalay. In 1919, it was reported that 88 per cent of prisoners examined were infected with hookworm,[88] and in 1921, it was reported that of 8,896 prisoners examined in 22 gaols, 5,999 (or 67 per cent) were found to be infected, with many of the gaols declaring a 100 per cent infection rate (although doubts were expressed about the accuracy of these tests since they were conducted, in the main, by the prisoners themselves).[89] In 1926, Dr Asa Crawford Chandler from the Calcutta School of Tropical Medicine

and Hygiene visited Burma in connection with a field enquiry into hookworm. The main conclusions from this field survey were that heavy infections of hookworm existed in some areas of Burma, especially the intermediate zones between the flooded areas of the delta and the dry zone, and that the rate of infection was modified by social behaviour.[90] Some additional detail about Dr Chandler's findings appears in the *Indian Journal of Medical Research* 1926–27.[91] The existence of a high rate of incidence in the intermediate zone was confirmed by Dr Chandler's findings in a village near Prome, that 100 per cent of the population were infected with hookworm.[92] Dr Chandler also reported on the incidence of *Ascaris* (roundworm) and *Trichuris* (whipworm) in Burma, both of which were very common in the delta and coastal regions, where 60 to 85 per cent incidence was reported.[93] In the dry zone of Upper Burma, the incidence was much lower — six to 25 per cent of the population were infected with roundworm and zero to 16 per cent with whipworm.[94] The *Annual Report on Hospitals and Dispensaries* for 1934 also mentions roundworms and hookworms under a list of specific diseases treated, but without further comment.[95]

These reports are interesting and informative, but they reveal nothing about the incidence of parasite infection in children, surely the population that was most at risk. Ascariasis is more common in pre-school and young schoolchildren than other sections of the population, and although hookworm infection may be less prevalent in very young children than in adults, the incidence of infection is important from five years of age due to the possibility of anaemia.

Post-war investigations have paid more attention to the rate of parasite infection in children. Dr Kyaw Win reported in 1976 on an investigation that he had made into helminthic infections in the Mon state. The prevalence rate of hookworm infection in the general community in this study was found to be: in the zero to four-year-old group, 14.4 per cent; among the five to nine years, 32.5 per cent; among the ten to 14 years, 41.4 per cent; and in adults, 40 per cent.[96] Between 1955 and 1960, another field study conducted in Insein district reported on an examination of 3,882 people living in 12 villages and attending three local schools. The study (which examined, among other things, the stools from the schoolchildren) found a 39 per cent incidence of hookworm, a 35 per cent incidence of roundworm, and a 42 per cent incidence of *Ascaris* among the schoolchildren.[97] Foll, the chief medical officer with the Burmah Oil Company, reported in 1954 that roundworm, threadworm and *Giardia* (a flagellate) were commonly found in Upper Burma, but that hookworm, although not infrequently found in adults in Upper Burma, was more prevalent in the delta.[98]

This evidence suggests that hookworm, roundworm and whipworm were endemic in colonial Burma, but that the rate of infection varied regionally, with the dry zone of Upper Burma probably having the lowest incidence. The infection rate in children between the ages of one year and fifteen years was probably at least 30 per cent, and many children would have been hosts to more than one parasite. This conclusion involves making assumptions about the probable rate of incidence in the children of colonial Burma based on the rates of infection found in this age group in modern Burma. But the conclusion does not necessitate making assumptions about the widespread and heavy incidence of the parasites in the general population of colonial Burma, as this was confirmed by the discussion above.

The importance of this finding is not only the simple conclusion that the host species suffers mildly from the invasion of any parasite species, but the proven connections between malnutrition and worm infestation. A study in Bangladesh in 1980 showed that children fed on a rice-and-vegetable-based diet suffered from poor absorption of fats and nitrogen when infected with roundworm. The improvement in these children's absorption after treatment was more than eight per cent of the intake, "which would certainly be of nutritional importance for individuals consuming a diet marginally adequate for protein."[99] Another study of 1,550 Kenyan children between the ages of six months and 16 years, which was published in 1983, found that 25 to 30 per cent of each sex were affected with *ascaris*. This incidence was associated with PEM in young children, as a heavy infection with roundworm limited the full utilisation of nutrients in the diet.[100] Giardiasis in young children is also associated with weight loss, mal-absorption and debility.[101]

The discussion in this chapter about the health of children in colonial Burma has found that approximately 50 per cent suffered some degree of malnutrition. In addition, there is now the view that approximately 30 per cent of children were infected with worms, which can impair the absorption of nutrients. A third factor that should be considered is diarrhoeal disease. Again this is not an unrelated element, as infection with *Giardia* can cause foul diarrhoea, and hookworm infection often manifests as diarrhoea. Also, and most importantly, malnutrition is both a predisposing factor and a result of diarrhoea.[102]

Diarrhoea and bowel complaints
There is very little information in the Burma colonial records about childhood diarrhoeal mortality or morbidity; only three references have been found. In 1868, the civil surgeon from Moulmein listed bowel complaints amongst the principal diseases of children,[103] and in 1880, there was a comment in the Resolution accompanying the annual health

report: "Several of the medical officers are of the opinion that native children suffer from being insufficiently clad and are thereby predisposed to diarrhoeal and bowel complaints."[104] In 1894, this theme was taken up again in the annual health report with another comment linking bowel complaints to insufficient clothing for children.[105]

More specific information is available about childhood diarrhoea in Burma from post-war reports. In 1979, Dr Soe Soe Aye reported on the morbidity of children seen at the Rangoon Children's Hospital and found that gastro-enteritis admissions were 16.9 per cent of the total, second only to respiratory disease.[106] These children were admitted with acute gastro-enteritis, and the category did not include dysentery. Dr Ma Ma Tin made a similar survey of children treated at the Mandalay Hospital in 1972, and again found that gastro-intestinal disorders were second only to respiratory infections in the number of admissions.[107] The WHO published an interim report in 1987 on diarrhoeal diseases in Southeast Asia, including Burma. This showed that 28.3 per cent of the deaths of children between the ages of zero to four years are diarrhoeal associated.[108] The report also estimated that, in 1985, there were 2.7 diarrhoeal episodes per child per year in Burma up to five years of age.[109]

The references to childhood diarrhoea that date from the colonial period are vague and generalised, but are sufficient to confirm the existence of the condition in British Burma. Post-war research in Burma has been a little more enlightening as it has identified diarrhoeal disease as the second most important cause of morbidity in the children of Rangoon and Mandalay, and as a major cause of mortality in zero to four year olds in modern Burma. It is difficult to draw concrete conclusions about the incidence of diarrhoea in the children of colonial Burma, but it should be noted that the case incidence mortality would have been far higher in the pre-war years because oral rehydration therapy was not available, and the level of medical services in the rural areas was poor to non-existent.

Respiratory tract infections

The post-war reports from the Rangoon and Mandalay hospitals had identified respiratory disease as the most important cause of admissions to the children's sections of the hospitals. Dr Soe Soe Aye, author of the Rangoon report, described respiratory tract infection, malnutrition, and gastro-enteritis as a "well known" triad, as the peak incidences of each disease closely followed each other.[110] The peak of gastro-enteritis cases occurred in June, followed very closely by the peak of malnutrition incidence, and the highest number of admissions for the respiratory diseases was in August and December. Obviously the diseases have seasonal incidence and childhood respiratory diseases in modern Rangoon peak towards the end of the rains and in the cold dry season. But was this pattern followed in colonial Burma?

Once again the information from the colonial records is scanty. From 1902, respiratory diseases formed one of the seven major categories under which deaths were registered, but, as stated previously, there is no way of judging how many of the deaths registered under any of these major categories were child deaths. A few references to childhood respiratory infection do appear in the annual health reports, and the earliest one of these was a comment in 1867 by the civil surgeon of Moulmein that croup was a frequent source of mortality amongst children.[111] In the same year, the civil surgeon of Sandoway district described a severe form of bronchitis amongst children.[112] The following year, 1868, the Moulmein district civil surgeon, who perhaps had a particular interest in children, described croup and inflammation of the lungs as one of the principal diseases amongst children.[113] Little more was said in the annual health reports until 1932, when there was a comment from the district health officer of Lower Chindwin. The mortality rates from respiratory disease had risen in the district, and the DHO attributed this rise to the inclusion under this category of the deaths of infants and children. These deaths, in previous years, had been returned as *Thungena*, the local name for a childhood disease.[114]

These references to respiratory disease amongst children give no guide to the incidence or the extent of the mortality from the disease. Once again the only guide to the possible incidence comes from modern, post-war data. In the children's department of Mandalay Hospital, 5,166 children were admitted suffering from respiratory disease between 1966 and 1970. The majority of these children, 3,189, were admitted with broncho-pneumonia, a further 1,626 were admitted with upper respiratory tract infections and 137 with bronchitis. The other two major respiratory diseases were pulmonary tuberculosis, with 97 admissions, and acute laryngo-tracheo bronchitis, with 59 admissions.[115] The very high incidence of broncho-pneumonia (more than 60 per cent of the admissions) is of particular interest, as there seems no reason why the incidence should be higher in post-war Burma than it was in colonial Burma, leaving therefore a strong suggestion that childhood mortality from pneumonia would have been very important in the pre-war years. The chances of a child recovering from a major chest infection without the aid of modern antibiotics would have been very poor.

Another item of interest in the Mandalay Hospital report is that nearly two per cent of admissions resulted from pulmonary tuberculosis. This disease attracted a lot of comment in the annual health reports in the later years of the British administration, but its true incidence remained unclear. The highest mortality appears to have occurred in the adult age group, particularly the higher ages of 40 to 50 years, whereas under 15 years of age the mortality was said to be insignificant.[116] But the overall lack of comment on childhood mortality, which was presumably due to a dearth of official information, means there is still a doubt as to whether the deaths from tuberculosis were really insignificant or merely unobserved. In 1910, it was suggested that certified sanitary inspectors should be appointed to examine the schoolchildren and that tuberculosis should be made a notifiable disease in Burma. This was proposed in a paper by W. G. King, a former sanitary commissioner of Burma, at a BMA conference in Burma, which discussed the spread of tuberculosis in the province.

In 1939, Professor S. Lyle Cummins spent 12 weeks in Burma assessing the tuberculosis incidence in the country. He reported finding a high tuberculosis index in Rangoon but a very low incidence in Upper Burma. Schoolchildren under 15 years of age were tested in the towns of Mandalay, Shwebo, Maymyo, Akyab, Moulmein, Bassein and Rangoon. The results of these tests showed far more positive reactions in the Lower Burma towns than in Upper Burma, with the highest incidence in Rangoon.[117]

There is no doubt that tuberculosis existed in the towns of colonial Burma, but was there a widespread incidence in the rural population that was causing mortality amongst the children? A cautious assessment would be that there is no evidence to suggest this and in fact Professor Cummins' opinion was that "The conditions found in Burma convinced me that, apart from the larger towns, the disease is a relatively new one to the population."[118]

Two other common and important respiratory diseases are measles and whooping cough. Once again there is no guide to the incidence of these diseases amongst the children of colonial Burma and little information about mortality. Scattered references to measles do appear in the annual health reports, and from 1921, the disease was separately registered as a cause of death in larger towns, but without any age-specific data. This is frustrating because the infection was almost certainly an important contributor to the death rate among young Burmese children, especially in the dry zone. But with only very limited and non-age related data from some towns, it is impossible to estimate childhood mortality.

The earliest reference to childhood measles appeared in the annual health report of 1868, and was once again from the civil surgeon at Moulmein, who described measles as a principal disease of children.[119] In the same year, whooping cough was described as "appearing epidemically amongst children" in Sandoway district during March

and April.[120] Neither of these references mentions mortality from the
diseases and a report in the previous year, 1867, which stated that
measles was epidemic in Rangoon and had caused 158 deaths, omitted
any mention of children.[121] That must have been a bad year for measles,
as MacDonald, the civil surgeon from Prome, also discussed the disease
in his report, but interestingly he attributed the epidemic in Prome
to "natives of Upper Burmah who come down here annually in search
of labour, and must have brought the disease along with them."[122]
This may be a partial attempt to blame the spread of disease on the
independent kingdom of Burma, or it may have reflected the probability
that respiratory disease was more common in the dry zone than in the
more humid delta.

One reference to childhood mortality from measles appeared in the
annual health report of 1868. The health officer of Rangoon reported
that there had been 58 deaths from measles in Rangoon, 43 of which
had been children under five years of age.[123] This illustrates quite
clearly how vulnerable young children are to the virus compared to
adults. The only other reference to childhood deaths from measles
appeared in the annual health report of 1910, when an epidemic of
measles in Kyingyan and Pakokku was said to have "caused the deaths
of many children".[124]

These historical references can provide only a glimpse into the
extent of measles incidence in colonial Burma, and for a more
authoritative guide, the modern data is the only source. A measles
survey, undertaken by P. C. Banerjee in Sagaing town between January
and June 1966, found that 98 per cent of the population had had frank
measles, usually between the ages of one and nine years.[125] The case
incidence mortality rate in this age group was just over two per cent,
but it should be noted that this mortality was very much reduced by
access to medical care. The report stated that the case mortality rate was
high when the children were not attended by trained medical personnel,
when their environmental sanitation was poor, and when their resistance
was low due to malnourishment.[126]

Two aspects of this report are of particular interest in any assessment of measles in colonial Burma. First is the very high case incidence,
which implies that the great majority of children in colonial Burma
would also have faced a measles attack. The other pertinent factor is
the increased case mortality in the malnourished child, which was
probably due to the measles infection precipitating PEM. (The lack of
access to trained medical care and poor environmental sanitation can
be assumed for most of colonial Burma's children.) Among the common
complications of measles are protracted diarrhoea and broncho-
pneumonia; the former frequently leads to severe clinical PEM with a

high case mortality rate, and the importance of the latter was seen in the Mandalay Hospital report, where more than 60 per cent of the child respiratory admissions were for broncho-pneumonia.

Measles must therefore be judged one of the major contributors to child mortality in colonial Burma, but its incidence and case mortality rate are hidden in the deaths from respiratory diseases, diarrhoea and "All Other Causes". The chief importance of measles probably lies in its synergistic relationship with malnourishment. The child who is mildly malnourished, who has in addition a parasite burden, is far more likely to die of secondary infection or acute PEM following a measles attack than a healthy, well nourished child.

Epidemic and other diseases

No doubt there were numerous other infections from which Burmese children could, and did, die: enteric fever, meningitis and dengue all took lives. The major epidemic diseases of plague, smallpox and cholera must have killed children as well as adults, but with the exception of smallpox, very little information about child deaths from these diseases can be traced in the colonial records. This is not to suggest that the authorities ignored plague or cholera, indeed in the 1911 annual health report, 13 pages were devoted to a description of plague measures, but without a mention of children. In the years 1905 to 1911, when plague mortality in Burma was at its highest, the average number of deaths per year was more than 7,000. Children under the age of 15 years formed just under 40 per cent of the total population at that time, but there is little means of judging whether they also provided 40 per cent of the plague mortality. Probably they did not, because the implication is that the plague mortality fell most heavily on workers such as bazaar sellers and coolies. If it is estimated very approximately that child deaths were 25 per cent of the total plague deaths, then it follows that plague was not a major cause of child mortality but formed, for example, only four per cent of the total child mortality in 1905.

The British administration recorded the incidence and mortality from cholera in a very similar way to that of plague. The incidence of cholera was recorded for many years by the number of cases in each administrative circle; and in 1888, the annual health report devoted 15 pages to comment on the disease. But, despite this detail, it is not possible even to estimate the child mortality from cholera. Probably it was not significant, except in one or two epidemic years such as 1888 and 1915. In contrast to this lack of information, smallpox deaths were recorded in the annual health reports with age-specific data for most years. By the late 1930s, the one- to ten-year-old age group was a declining percentage of the total smallpox mortality, from approximately

30 per cent in the 1920s to 15 per cent in 1939. In addition, the total smallpox deaths in Burma had declined from 8,540 in 1906 to an average per year of 1,244 deaths between 1932 and 1939. To put this in some perspective, the total average mortality per year was 263,952 between 1932 and 1939. Smallpox, therefore, became progressively less important as a cause of child mortality in twentieth-century Burma, even when allowance is made for under-registration. The success of the smallpox vaccination programme was confirmed by the number of schoolchildren vaccinated. From 1917, at least 95 per cent of the children examined in the school inspection scheme had received a primary dose of vaccine. For full protection from the disease, a second dose of vaccine was considered necessary, and in 1931, only 30 per cent of the schoolchildren inspected had been revaccinated, but by 1937, the number had grown to more than 50 per cent.

One other disease that should be mentioned in connection with the children of colonial Burma is yaws. This is not a disease that causes a high mortality, but it appears to have had a widespread distribution in Burma. In 1910, an investigation was made into the incidence of yaws in the Lower Chindwin district. The report stated that the disease was common in children, and that in the later stages of the disease, the long bones of the children's legs and arms were affected.[127] The annual health report of 1912 said that yaws had a wide distribution in Burma; it was found in Henzada, the Lower Chindwin, Mergui, Kyaukse and Pakokku districts.[128] The disease is contagious and is "caused by bacteria that are transmitted primarily by direct contact among children living in unhygienic conditions."[129] Yaws undoubtedly existed in Burma prior to 1910 but until that date, the disease attracted no attention or comment in the health records, and then suddenly it became a topic for comment and a recognised health problem.

The discussion of childhood disease in Burma has ranged over a variety of problems, but has attempted to establish and stress the links between nutritional deficiencies, diarrhoeal and respiratory diseases, and intestinal parasites as the main and synergistic causes of childhood deaths in colonial Burma. The major epidemic diseases of cholera, plague and smallpox also played a role in the earlier years of the British administration; but from 1912, the incidence of these diseases declined in Burma and the proportion of total mortality attributed to them also declined. These changes coincided with the decline (in the short term) of the proportion of children in the total population after 1911. This obviously requires explanation, as the decline in smallpox, in particular, should have resulted in an increased survival rate in young children, and not, as implied, an increased mortality rate.

Three factors may have contributed to this decline in the proportion of children in the population. First was the flu pandemic, which caused heavy crisis mortality in 1918 and increased the mortality levels in 1919 and 1920. But this was short term only, and recovery in the proportion of children would have been expected by 1931. Instead, the percentage of children, especially male children, was still low in 1931, and this may have been due to two other factors: the increased incidence of malaria, and a decline in the nutritional value of the Burmese diet. The nutritional changes were the result of the increase in the use of machine-milled rice after 1900 by the general population of Burma, and the dietary change spread with the development of small, upcountry rice mills.[130] This was confirmed by U Maung Gale's findings, between 1939 and 1941, that 77 per cent of the population examined were eating machine-milled rice. The nutritional loss is major, as 70 per cent of the thiamine content is lost with machine milling, and also proteins, niacin and riboflavin. These nutritional changes were discussed in Chapter Three, and will be discussed further in Chapter Six. Therefore the concentration now will be on the importance of the flu pandemic, and then malaria, in the mortality of Burmese children.

Influenza and malaria

The total mortality from the flu pandemic was estimated by the health authorities in Burma to be 200,000 in 1918 alone, with another 100,000 to 150,000 excess deaths in the following two years. Some of this excess mortality would be directly attributable to the flu, and some would be due to secondary respiratory infections caused by the pandemic.[131] How much of this excess mortality was child mortality? The recorded child mortality rates for 1918 show a massive increase when compared to the mean of the previous five years: this was an increase of 50 per cent in the mortality of male and female zero to five year olds, and nearly 100 per cent increase in the mortality of both sexes in the five- to 15-year-old age group.[132] There are variations within these broad figures, for example, proportionately more girls appeared to die in the ten to 15 year age group than in the five to ten year age group. This may be an anomaly in the registration, reflecting an exaggeration in the declared age of girls in Burma, or it may accurately reflect a real mortality differential.

Assuming that a high degree of under-registration existed in the zero to five-year-old age group, it is probably safe to say that two children died in 1918 for every child's death in a "non-crisis" year. In addition to these losses, the health officials considered that mortality was particularly heavy among pregnant and parturient women, and that abortions and miscarriages "were common during the course of the disease".[133] The number of registered births dropped from 33.0 in 1918 to 29.9 in 1919, but although a sharp drop in births during a pandemic is expected, the recorded drop is insignificant compared to the difference between the recorded births and the estimated crude birth rate for 1911 to 1921 of approximately 45 per 1,000.

It is impossible, therefore, to make an accurate estimate of child mortality during the flu pandemic, or to calculate the additional losses that occurred due to a rise in the stillbirth and miscarriage rates. It would have been rewarding to calculate the real infant and child losses caused by the pandemic, but with the inherent faults already in the registration system and the additional strain arising from the pandemic, a closer attempt to quantify the losses from the registration figures must be dangerous.

Malaria poses an equal problem. The health records suggest that malaria was a major killer of children in some districts, but if it is to be argued convincingly that malaria, and deaths due in a secondary way to malaria, were the main cause of the sustained mortality after 1921, then more concrete evidence is needed. One way of obtaining some quantitative evidence is through the child/woman ratio. It was established in the first section of this chapter that the child/woman ratio dropped from just under 2.0 up to and including 1911, to 1.10 in 1921, and 1.11 in 1931. The individual district ratios for 1921 and 1931 were calculated to see if there were regional differences within the study area. The results are shown in Table 4.8 and reveal quite startling differences in the different regions of Burma. Only districts with a ratio of less than 1.0 in 1921 are shown in the table, and this has excluded seven of the ten Lower Burma districts, leaving only Hanthawaddy, Henzada and Bassein. The three mid-Burma districts of Prome, Toungoo and Thayetmyo all fell below a ratio of 1.0 in 1921, as did nine of the 12 Upper Burma districts. Only Pakokku, Sagaing and Katha districts in Upper Burma had a ratio of 1.0 or more in 1921. The fourth column of the table shows the child/woman ratio of these districts in 1931, and this shows a comparative recovery in the Lower Burma districts but only a marginal recovery in mid-Burma, with Prome district still below a ratio of 1.0. In Upper Burma, four of the nine districts were still below a ratio of 1.0 and of these, three were irrigated districts.

The calculations were made from census data, using Buddhist data for the 1921 figures and Burmese data for 1931, due to the change in the arrangement of the census tables. The ratios will be slightly depressed due to the calculations being based on women between the age of 15 and 50 years, instead of the more conventional 15 to 45 years. This was necessary, as only ten-year age groups were available in the 1921 census

TABLE 4.8
Child/Woman Ratios in Selected Districts of Burma

District	District Location	Child/woman Ratio (All Children 0–9/Females 15–50)	
		1921	1931
Hanthawaddy	Lower Burma	0.87	1.13
Henzada	Lower Burma	0.98	1.04
Bassein	Lower Burma	0.99	1.03
Thayetmyo	Mid-Burma	0.97	1.00
Toungoo	Mid-Burma	0.98	1.00
Prome	Mid-Burma	0.89	0.94
Magwe	Upper Burma	0.99	1.04
Yamethin	Upper Burma	0.99	1.07
Meiktila	Upper Burma	0.90	1.01
Myingyan	Upper Burma	0.98	0.98
L. Chindwin	Upper Burma	0.98	1.03
Shwebo	Upper Burma, irrigated	0.96	1.02
Kyaukse	Upper Burma, irrigated	0.83	0.96
Mandalay	Upper Burma, irrigated	0.77	0.86
Minbu	Upper Burma, irrigated	0.92	0.93

Sources: *Census of Burma*, 1921 and 1931.

data; but as the figures are for comparisons of the districts within that census and with the 1931 census, the extra five years makes little difference, probably less than five per cent.

It must be concluded from this table that the Upper Burma districts suffered disproportionately from the flu pandemic, and also that their child mortality remained much higher than the average mortality experienced in the rest of the study area. The figures in the table are not highly accurate, but they are comparatively accurate; since each census year is based on the same system of recording, the figures can be used to show differences between the districts with some degree of confidence.

It can be seen from the table that four of the Upper Burma districts with a ratio below 1.0 in 1921 were irrigated districts, and that three out of the four had a ratio of less than 1.0 in 1931. It was suggested in Chapter Three that the incidence of malaria was higher in the irrigated districts of the dry zone, and this view is supported by the child/woman ratios. The health authorities accepted that there was a connection in Burma between the extension of irrigation channels and epidemic malaria, but no age- and disease-specific mortality figures were collected.

The clearest example of the connection between irrigation and epidemic malaria and its effect on the local children was shown in one of the first outbreaks to be investigated in Burma. In July 1911, the new Mon Canal was opened in Minbu district. By December 1911, the death rates in some of the administration circles near the canal had soared to over 200 per 1,000. In Legaing circle, which had a population of 10,000, the mortality "ratio in December was 306 per mille."[134] Investigations that were carried out in December 1911 and January 1912 "disclosed the fact that the vast majority of the children in the infected villages had enlarged spleens, and a spleen rate little short of 100 per cent was frequently met with even as late as the end of January."[135] The appearance of the children was described as extremely dirty in their persons and clothing, most of them were anaemic, "in a low state of health generally, and an advanced condition of itch was universal."[136]

This is an unusual report, as it is one of only two reports in the Burma health records that describe the secondary effects of malaria in children. The second comment occurred in the annual health report of 1915, in a discussion of the prevalence of malaria on the borders of the Shan states and Mandalay and Kyaukse districts. The sanitary commissioner said that the effects of malaria were very apparent, "The children are few and stunted, and the spleen index is very high."[137]

Despite the increasing recognition in the annual health reports of the importance of malaria, little attention was given to the malaria mortality of children, especially in the rural areas. Two annual health reports, those of 1916 and 1917, discussed the effect of malaria on the age distribution of the population in the irrigated districts, but these were abstract debates that paid little attention to the health of the surviving children. However, the discussions were of interest because the health authorities found that the irrigated districts of Mandalay and Kyaukse had a lower child/woman ratio than comparable, but non-irrigated, districts. A survey of Madaya township in Mandalay district had revealed a considerable amount of detail about the demographic structure of the population in the affected area. A total of 337 villages in Madaya township and parts of the adjacent townships were visited, and enquiries were made into the number of children in the households. The health authorities estimated that the zero to 15-year-old child population should have formed 39.84 per cent of the total population (which is very close to my calculation of 39.9 per cent for Buddhists in the study area in 1911). The health authorities estimated that in the 337 villages surveyed, "there was a deficit of child population" of between 25 and 33 per cent.[138] A survey of the spleen indexes — that is, the percentage of children with enlarged spleens — in these villages showed that in 161 villages examined, the index was between 50 and 100 per cent; in 33 villages, it was between 25 and 50 per cent, and in 26 villages, it was between ten and 25 per cent.[139]

The authorities were in no doubt that these dismaying statistics were due to malaria in the irrigated districts, but despite this, the only response of the administration was to provide a travelling dispensary equipped with quinine tablets, when the situation really required a major programme of research and preventative measures. This was admitted in 1917 by C. E. Williams, the sanitary commissioner, who wrote that "a much greater saving of life and suffering would result from expenditure" on rural sanitation to prevent malaria than "by many times the equivalent sum spent on the construction and equipment of stationary hospitals at the larger centres of the population, which are rarely visited by the outlying populations, and almost never by their children."[140] Williams was an enlightened sanitary commissioner, but despite his recognition of priorities, the political and economic pressures continued to ensure that the major schemes for the prevention of malaria were confined to the towns, the military police and the industrial centres.

The emphasis here on the irrigated areas should not disguise the fact that other districts had major malarial problems. It was reported that "malaria is an outstanding public health problem in the centre area" of Yamethin district in 1939.[141] The districts that formed the axis of mid-Burma — Prome, Toungoo and Thayetmyo — also had malarial areas, and it should be remembered that they were also noted as having a very high hookworm incidence.

It was often a combination of diseases that killed children. When malaria was epidemic, the children would die, but they would also die when endemic malaria complicated other diseases. It was noted in Myitkyina district in 1936 "that malaria complicates many other diseases such as pneumonia, typhoid, ankylostomiasis, dysentery, etc."[142] Sinton's research in India into the connection between malaria and other diseases had noted a rise in the death rate from respiratory diseases, including pneumonia, in malarious areas.[143] A modern study in East Malaysia noted that the children in malaria endemic villages who had a positive infection tended to be more retarded in growth and more anaemic than those children who showed no evidence of parasitaemia or measurable spleen enlargement.[144] This study reported that 37 per cent of the children in these villages had conditions between chronic PEM and severe to chronic PEM with stunting and wasting.[145]

Conclusions

What conclusions can be drawn from this discussion about the family and childhood in Burma? The data has revealed factual evidence, such as the age of marriage and the number of children born, but equally significant, perhaps, are the deductions that can be drawn on the cultural influences on family life. Many of these, such as prolonged breast-feeding and the non-universality of marriage, will have had a marked downward pressure on demographic growth. There is also the possibility that the cultural food preferences displayed by pregnant and lactating women and the restricted diet offered to young children may have contributed to population control.

It has been established that measles was one of the major contributors to child mortality. Young and malnourished children were particularly vulnerable to the disease, especially when it was in combination with malnourishment and the parasite burden, but quantification of the mortality rate has not been possible because such deaths were often registered under different categories. Some evidence has been provided from analysis of the child/woman ratio to confirm the suggestion, made in Chapter Three, that the incidence of malaria was higher in the irrigated districts of the dry zone.

The child in colonial Burma therefore faced an uncertain future. Having survived the rigours of birth and weaning, the young were then faced with the triad of a parasite burden, malnutrition and infectious disease. These, of course, were not new problems, but they were given greater impact in the colonial period by the damaging dietary shift to polished white rice and the high rates of malarial disease.

5 Adult morbidity and mortality and the development of public health in Burma

Norman Owen introduced his essay "Measuring Mortality in the Nineteenth Century Philippines" by saying that "Death is ubiquitous in the Southeast Asian past."[1] This ubiquity is one of the great gulfs that separates the modern western historian from even the recent past in Southeast Asia, as it is difficult to make the imaginative leap into a society where death is "everywhere pervasively present",[2] and not comfortably removed to an extreme old age. The point to be made here is that surviving childhood in colonial Burma was not a guarantee of a long life; mortality in all the adult age periods was high, and death by disease or accident was never far away.

What diseases killed adults in colonial Burma? Undoubtedly the major epidemic diseases — cholera, plague and smallpox — took a heavy toll in some years, but the respiratory and diarrhoeal diseases, including enteric fever and tuberculosis in the urban areas, were also major killers, as was malaria. The number of accidental deaths was high, and snake bite, rabies and venereal diseases exacted a steady loss of life. The object of this chapter is to examine the adult mortality, to measure it as far as possible, and to discuss the impact of the British administration's sanitary policies on the health of the adult population. It will not be possible to write a full history of the development of the public health services in Burma, but aspects of the administration's attempts to control the spread of disease and to improve rural and urban hygiene will be touched on as part of the epidemiological discussion.

One other question that this chapter will attempt to address is the role of the Indian migrant in the history of disease in colonial Burma. Were the casual labourers in the migrant community the focus and agents of infectious disease, or were they vulnerable to contagion through poverty and poor living conditions?

TABLE 5.1

Adult Mortality as Percentage of the Total Mortality and the
Number of Adults as Percentage of the Total Population of Burma

Census Year	Proportion of Adults in Total Population (%)		Proportion of Adults in Total Mortality* (%)	
	Male	Female	Male	Female
1891	60.4	62.5	53.3	55.8
1901	60.6	61.3	53.3	55.8
1911	60.1	61.1	53.3	55.8
1921	62.2	62.7	46.1	48.7
1931	62.1	62.0	46.1	48.7

Notes: *The figures shown in these columns of mortality are taken from the West Model Life Tables Level 5 for 1891, 1901 and 1911, and Level 3 for 1921 and 1931.

Sources: *Census of Burma;* Coale and Demeny, *Regional Model Life Tables and Stable Populations*, West Model Life Tables.

Before any of these questions can be discussed, the adult mortality in the colonial period must be defined in terms of numbers. Approximately 60 per cent of the population in the colonial period were over 15 years of age but deaths among this adult population formed less than 60 per cent of the total mortality. This calculation is based on information from the West Model Life Table levels, which were calculated in Chapter Two. Table 5.1 illustrates this point by comparing the percentage of adult mortality to the percentage of adults in the population of Burma.

The figures showing the percentage of total mortality by age in Table 5.1 have not been adjusted to the precise life table levels that were calculated in Chapter Two, e.g. 5.15 for the inter-censal period of 1901 to 1911 and 3.54 for 1911 to 1921. Instead the "flat rate" levels of 3 and 5 have been used, as the comparison needs a "broad brush" approach. However, the table suggests that the adult population, although making up 60 to 62 per cent of the population of colonial Burma, accounted for only an estimated 46 to 55 per cent of the total mortality. It is also apparent that after 1911 the imbalance was greatest, as over 62 per cent of the population accounted for only 46 to 48 per cent of the mortality.

This imbalance reveals the increased child mortality that occurred after 1911 and was discussed in Chapter Four.

Another useful way of examining mortality is to look at the seasonality of the deaths; that is, the months in which the highest number of deaths occurred year by year. Obviously there is a potential problem with the Burma data as only the deaths that were registered can be used in a seasonality study, and 25 to 33 per cent of the mortality was apparently not registered. But there is no reason to suppose that the inaccuracy of the registration was itself affected by seasonality. Therefore any change in the long-term pattern of mortality would be real.

The Burma data was examined by plotting for each year, from 1885 to 1939, the three months in which the highest numbers of deaths were registered. The results of this are shown in Figure 5.1 in a series of histograms labelled a to f, each of which is based on the mortality from a ten-year period, except for f, which is based on five years only. From 1885 to 1904, the data is for Lower Burma only, and from 1933 onwards, the data is rural only, as the figures were no longer available for the whole of Burma. But these two changes in the statistical base do not appear to have had any effect on the general trend of the seasonality, which shows a marked and continuous shift from a summer peak (on a July/August/September axis) to an autumn/winter peak. The second histogram, b, illustrates the fact that this process was already underway by the decade from 1895 to 1904, although the data came from Lower Burma only. The shift continued until the mortality peak had changed to October/November/December, seen in the 1925 to 1934 histogram.

Such a change in the seasonality of mortality would not be of great significance if it were an isolated piece of evidence, as it could be argued that the data was too unreliable or the method not precise enough to bear interpretation. But when this is viewed with the other accumulated data, such as the decline in the child/woman ratio after 1911, the decline in the proportion of children in the population after 1911, and the suggestion, already made, that as the epidemic diseases declined, malaria increased, then it becomes very significant.

The summer peaks of mortality were associated with a rise in the incidence of diarrhoeal diseases, commonly linked with flies, rain and inundation. It could be argued that the British attempts to improve sanitation and water supplies in the major towns had so effectively reduced diarrhoea incidence that a change occurred in the seasonality of mortality. However, that should have produced a lowering of overall mortality, which did not occur. Another factor to be considered is whether there was a change in the proportion of the population which was urban, as a rising urban population would have meant that

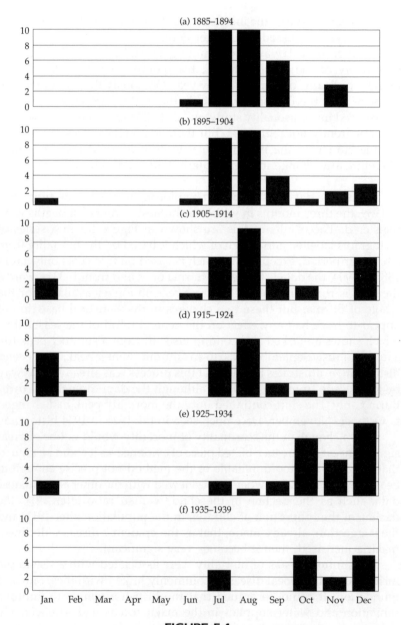

FIGURE 5.1

Seasonality of Mortality in Burma 1885–1939

For each year of the specified period, each of the three months in which the total registered mortality was highest have been counted as one occurrence for that period and plotted on the histogram. Upper Burma is excluded before 1909.

TABLE 5.2

Urban Population as a Percentage of the Total Population

Census Year	Urban Population in Total Population (%)
1891*	12.44
1901	9.44
1911	9.31
1921	9.77
1931	10.36

Notes: * The high figure for 1891 probably indicates under-enumeration in the rural areas.

Sources: *Census of Burma.*

proportionately more people were being affected by changes in the sanitation of towns. The percentage of the total population that was described as urban in the census records is shown in the Table 5.2.

The table shows that the increase in the proportion which was urban in Burma prior to the Second World War was marginal, perhaps one per cent, and that approximately nine-tenths of the population remained in the rural areas. If urbanisation was not a factor, then what did cause the change in the seasonality of mortality in colonial Burma?

Epidemic diseases and their effects on the public health service

In the nineteenth century, the major epidemic diseases of cholera, smallpox and plague haunted the Burmese and were regarded with terror. Yet, if we were to study the actual mortality rate of these diseases, we will see that, at the beginning of the twentieth century in Burma, they contributed to less than ten per cent of the total registered mortality, and the figure declined as a percentage of the total mortality so that by 1940, it was about two per cent. Consequently, these diseases could not be solely responsible for the changing disease patterns. The incidence of these diseases is illustrated in Table 5.3. These three epidemic diseases will be discussed in an attempt to assess their overall significance in the history of health in Burma, and the effectiveness of the colonial government's response to the diseases.

The history of cholera and plague epidemics, despite a high level of research and interest, still holds unanswered questions. Why, for

TABLE 5.3
Epidemic Disease as a Percentage of the Total Registered Mortality

Period	Cholera	Plague	Smallpox
1902–11	2.9	3.2	1.5
1912–21	2.1	2.1	0.8
1922–31	1.8	1.7	0.9
1932–39	0.7	0.8	0.5

Sources: Annual health reports.

example, did cholera and plague explode into pandemics in 1818 and 1894, and why did they subsequently decline? Who died of the diseases and why?

The history of cholera in Burma is of particular interest, as it seems probable that the disease was endemic in the delta before 1818. It was also "mishandled" in the early years between 1855 and 1892[3] by the health authorities, as it happened to fall into the limbo period between the first identification of bacillus by Louis Pasteur and Robert Koch and acceptance of the fact that these germs were the cause of illnesses. Scientists and doctors of that time clung to their "miasmic" theory, which ascribed disease to transmission through the air and the earth; which is why many of the health reports were scathing about filthy practices and insanitary conditions.

Cholera

The number of cholera deaths registered in Burma between 1868 and 1939 was 324,000. When these deaths are calculated as an average of 4,500 per year, they appear almost insignificant compared to the probable number of deaths from malaria, but an averaged figure cannot convey the terror that was inspired by the sporadic ferocity of the cholera epidemics. These outbreaks could kill high numbers of people very rapidly, leading in 1888 to death rates of over 500 per 1,000 in eight circles of registration in Lower Burma.[4]

The bacillus responsible for the disease, *Vibrio cholerae*, acts on the small intestine, and causes withdrawals of fluids and salts from the body cells into the gut lumen. In its most extreme manifestation, cholera is one of the most rapidly fatal illnesses known,[5] and can kill an apparently healthy person within three to four hours of the onset of symptoms.[6] A more common pattern for the disease is death following 18 hours to several days after the onset of untreated symptoms. It was the rapidity of the decline and the very high fatality rate that caused the disease to be regarded with such fear by both the British and the Burmese.

When did cholera first enter Burma? The date is not known but it is probable that cholera was well known in Burma before the pandemic of 1817–20. As William McNeill wrote, the "disease had long been endemic in Bengal, and spread thence in epidemic fashion to other parts of India and adjacent regions from time to time."[7] The existing overland route from Bengal to Burma by way of Chittagong and Arakan makes previous outbreaks in Burma likely. Father Sangermano, who lived in Burma between 1783 and 1808, described a disease "called by the Portuguese, mordazzino", which caused "what the physicians call cholera." This disease was not confined to Burma, but was "spread all over India". This is not sufficient to identify the disease as cholera, but Sangermano's description of the course of the disease is diagnostic: "The continual evacuation both by vomit and stool will reduce a man in a few hours to such a state of exhaustion that he is scarcely to be recognised for the same person."[8]

This all too vivid description of the disease would appear to confirm the presence of cholera in Burma prior to 1817. It also raises the interesting possibility that the Irrawaddy delta may have been a reservoir of infection. The epidemiology of cholera is still a subject of research, and papers in *The Lancet* in 1985 and in *The American Journal of Epidemiology* in 1982 argue that the identification of the principal reservoir of infection is not yet clear.[9] The previous assumption was that there were human carriers whose asymptomatic infection provided a low-level continuous transmission. More recently, epidemiological research has turned to the possibility of aquatic reservoirs of infection in the saline waters of estuaries and deltas.[10] More research would be needed before this possibility of a reservoir of infection in the Irrawaddy delta could be established, but confirmation of the existence of Asian cholera in Burma prior to 1800 might well be significant in disease incidence during wars and population decline in the delta.[11]

The first British report of cholera in Burma was when their troops died of the disease during the first Britain–Burma War of 1824–26. The Eighty-ninth Regiment, who were camped near Prome, were said to have lost 30 men in one week, and Prome was crowded with dead and dying Burmese, both soldiers and civilians.[12] It is not clear whether the cholera was imported from Bengal with the British troops or whether it was contracted in Burma. After the second Britain–Burma War in the 1850s,[13] the disease was recorded in the annual health reports in some detail, and therefore it is possible to examine the seasonality of cholera, its racial and sexual proclivity and the location of the heaviest mortality.

The incidence of cholera had a marked seasonal pattern, although isolated and sporadic outbreaks occurred throughout the year. The peak of the cholera mortality came between March and August, the hottest months of the year. This period marked the end of the dry season and the beginning of the rains, which came between May and August. The histograms in Figure 5 show that, until 1914, July and August were the months when the heaviest mortality from all causes occurred. It should be noted that the cholera mortality discussed here, like the mortality shown in the histograms, is the total registered mortality and not the registered adult mortality only.

The cholera mortality reveals a racial and sexual bias, as a disproportionate number of the victims were male, immigrant Indians. The exact extent of the racial bias is not recorded, but the migrant labourers were consistently identified in the health records as victims of cholera. The sexual bias in the recorded deaths is simpler to determine; for example, between 1914 and 1939, there were 100 male cholera deaths registered for every 69 female cholera deaths.

The geographical location of the disease is harder to define. The heaviest mortality was often registered in the rural districts, but the sources of the outbreaks were usually traced to civil engineering or industrial projects such as sawmills, rice mills, brickfields, forest camps, railway repairs, railway building, or the petroleum industry.[14] The common factor linking these sources was the employment of cheap labour.

The discussion so far has referred to registered cholera deaths, but the registration of total deaths has been estimated to omit 25 to 33 per cent of the mortality. However, the registration of cholera, plague and smallpox was probably sufficiently accurate to enable the figures to be used as a guide to the mortality. Such a large proportion of the health officials' time was devoted to the reporting of cholera and plague that the mortality rates recorded for these diseases must have been more accurate than the general registration. It is easy to be too critical of the amount of time that the health officials devoted to cholera and plague, to the neglect of other diseases, as obviously one of the most vital jobs of a public health official is to contain epidemic disease. But the disproportionate amount of attention that cholera received must be seen as an indication of the fear that the disease inspired. For example, from 1893 to 1899, between six and nine pages of an annual health report averaging 38 pages was devoted to an analysis of cholera deaths. The report included the number of cholera deaths by administrative circle, the dates of the first notified deaths, the meteorological conditions accompanying the outbreaks, cholera maps and case descriptions. During this seven-year period, the average number of cholera deaths was 4,500 per annum, while in the same period, approximately half a page of text was used to discuss the 50,000 deaths per annum attributed to "Fevers".

Ironically, the efforts of the health administration to contain cholera sometimes led to the under-registration of the deaths. Headmen occasionally suppressed the evidence of cholera deaths to evade the disinfection and enquiries that followed a death from a notifiable disease.[15] In 1918, a woman fled from a cholera-infected village in the Lower Chindwin district to Toungoo district, where she died of the disease. The death was registered as *Mi-Yat*, or "woman's disease", and it was reported that the subsequent funeral feast disseminated the infection through the district.[16] Under-registration could also occur when panic caused the evacuation of villages. In 1883, the sanitary commissioner complained that the friends and relatives of cholera victims frequently ran away, leaving the corpses unburied and decomposing.[17] There was some crude counter-balancing of the under-registration, as British officials believed that some deaths were wrongly attributed to cholera. In 1875, the civil surgeon of Rangoon said: "the majority of the deaths attributed to cholera were cases of chronic diarrhoea in ill-fed, filthy coolies."[18] Despite these vagaries, the registration of cholera deaths was probably accurate enough to indicate the actual trend of the mortality, and this, as a percentage of the total registered mortality, was clearly downward after 1900.

TABLE 5.4

Average Number of Cholera Deaths per Annum, and Expressed as a Percentage of the Average Total Mortality

Period	Average Cholera Deaths per Annum	Cholera Deaths as a Percentage of Total Mortality
1876–81	4,570	9.0
1882–91	5,200	7.5
1892–1901	4,758	4.9
1902–11	6,400	2.9
1912–21	6,000	2.1
1922–31	4,300	1.8
1932–39	2,000	0.7

Sources: Annual health reports.

Table 5.4 shows a very high percentage of cholera deaths in the total registered mortality between 1876 and 1891. This may indicate that the registration of cholera deaths was more efficient than that of deaths from other diseases. But the steady decline in the cholera deaths, as a percentage of the mortality, was real, and was accompanied by a similar decline in the deaths from plague and smallpox after 1911.

The question posed just before the beginning of this section on cholera was who died and why. It was then suggested that the mortality had a racial bias; that migrant Indian labourers died disproportionately from the disease. Most of these labourers were Hindu, single, male and between 15 and 40 years of age. Theoretically the death rate of such a group should have been lower than the Burmese death rate, as it would exclude the infant, child and aged mortality. But until 1910, the registered Hindu mortality was higher than the provincial rate. This is illustrated in Table 5.5, which shows ten-year averages of the death rates from 1885.

The mortality of Indian migrants in Burma needs to be examined, despite the overall emphasis in this book on the indigenous community, as these migrants played an important role in the disease pattern of colonial Burma. The emphasis in this section on cholera, is not meant to suggest that the disease was solely responsible for the high Hindu death rate; other factors such as poor nutrition, plague, and other bacterial and viral diseases also contributed. The migrants also played a role in the Burma health records as a "whipping boy", a group on whom the spread of epidemic diseases could be blamed.

Prior to 1885, cholera epidemics were often attributed to migrant labour from Upper Burma,[19] but once this area formed part of British Burma, then the blame was persistently laid on coolies coming overland from Chittagong or arriving by sea from Orissa. The Chittagong coolies came to Burma in February to work in the rice mills or help with the

TABLE 5.5
Comparison of the Registered Hindu and Provincial Death Rates (per 1,000)

Period	Average Hindu Death Rate	Average Provincial Death Rate
1885–94	27.14	19.07
1895–1904	28.77	24.26
1905–14	27.74	26.61
1915–24	22.42	26.05

Sources: Annual health reports.

harvest, and they were linked in the health reports with cholera outbreaks in Akyab in 1876, 1877, 1878, 1892, 1894, 1898, 1923, 1931, and 1932.

In the 1878 outbreak at Akyab, 90 per cent of the 853 cholera victims in the town and surrounding districts were Indian migrants, "who are very filthy in their personal habits."[20] That same annual report documented 1,183 cholera deaths in Rangoon town and district, and natives of India were said to be principally affected due to "overcrowding, dirt and impure water". Likewise, an outbreak in Tharrawaddy district was attributed to a gang of Bengal coolies who were employed by the Irrawaddy Valley (State) Railway. The sanitary commissioner, W. P. Kelly, complained in that health report that the rail coolies were spreading disease amongst the inhabitants of the country.[21] In 1908, there were more than 11,000 cholera deaths and Indian coolies "fell victim to the disease in large numbers", when the railway borrow pits that they used for bathing and domestic water became contaminated.[22]

These descriptions of the way in which the migrants succumbed to cholera are representative of the comments that appeared almost every year in the health reports. The way in which the deaths were reported is also significant — the blame for the deaths was laid on the victims, attributed to their "filthy habits". The links between cholera and Indian migrants were reported until the 1930s, and so was the health authorities' insistence that cholera infection was introduced from endemic centres in India.[23] This was despite the blame put on the workers from Upper Burma prior to annexation. Even if the prejudice displayed in the reports is ignored, the consistency of the links between Indian migrants and cholera cannot be.[24]

It is perhaps salutary to remember that, amidst British criticism of the "filthy habits" of coolies, these migrants were encouraged to come to Burma by the British authorities to provide a cheap labour force. Once the migrants had passed through the ports, the authorities took no further responsibility for them, and their needs for housing, sanitation and supplies of drinking water were the responsibility of neither the government nor their employers. The resulting situation was described by C E. Williams, the sanitary commissioner, in his report of 1907. He stated that the outbreaks of cholera in Rangoon were practically confined to boat people or those who lived on the banks of rivers or creeks. This mortality was heaviest in the Muslim population of launches and riverboats, and amongst the Hindu coolies that worked at the rice mills. Both of these groups drew their drinking water from the river, which, Williams suggested, at a "modest estimate" took the excreta from the 50,000 labourers employed on the boats or in the mills, via latrines that overhung the river.[25]

An objective view of the position of the Indian migrant in colonial Burma was provided by the 1931 report of the Royal Commission on Labour in India. The report was very critical of the "maistrie" system, whereby an intermediary was contracted to supply labour from India for a project in Burma, which meant that the employer in Burma had no direct contractual relationship with their employees.[26] The commission found that "no one is responsible for the welfare or protection of immigrants after they have actually landed".[27] The result was that a pool of under-employed labour was formed, often living in overcrowded lodging houses or barracks, with no sanitation or clean water supplies.[28] The report stated quite clearly that the system was creating a health problem: "the poor physique and low standard of health of the average immigrant are such as readily to lay him open to attack from disease, especially under the conditions facing him on arrival",[29] and that "the maintenance of a large mass of labour which is inadequately protected, is bound to lower the general standard of life and health; and the interests of Burma, no less than that of the immigrants, demands that their welfare should be a constant care."[30]

The commission estimated that two-thirds of the labour employed in factories, mines, oilfields, railways and plantations was Indian, and it is notable that all of these places of employment (with the exception of plantations) were identified in the health reports as foci of cholera epidemics. There were two reasons for this: firstly, the appalling sanitary conditions under which these men were expected to live while they were working, and secondly, when the contract was finished, there was no provision in the maistrie system for returning the men to India. This meant that groups of unemployed workers had to make their way back to the docks from as far away as northern Burma or the Shan states. The commission suggested that industrialists must accept responsibility for their own workers' repatriation, instead of leaving them "in a foreign country without the means of subsistence after a short period."[31]

The evidence from the Royal Commission and from the health reports implies that the migrants were the victims of cholera and other diseases, largely due to their terms of employment. The annual health report of 1878 describes the conditions under which these men lived and died. At Konityua in Tharrawaddy district, 54 migrants were found living in a hut that had room for only 30. The men, who were employed by the railway company, had contracted cholera and six of them had died. Another man was dying under the raised floor of the hut, and the bowel evacuations of the cholera victims were in the grass next to the hut.[32] This incident also highlights the links between the development of transport and the spread of disease through the use of cheap labour, which is not only vulnerable to infection but becomes the focus of transmission to the indigenous population. In the previous year, 1877, merchants and mill owners at Akyab became "convinced of the absolute necessity for improving the barracks" in which their mill employees lived, following an outbreak of cholera. Several of the mills had had to stop working due to the loss of life and there was "considerable pecuniary loss" to the employers.[33]

The discussion so far has attempted to address the question of who died and why. Emphasis has been placed on the role of the migrant Indians as victims and effective agents of the disease, but this should not be allowed to obscure the losses amongst the rural population. In 1919, there were 360 cholera deaths in the Upper Chindwin district and 412 in the Chin Hills, where "The ignorance and savage habits of the natives served to cause a rapid spread of the disease".[34]

Role of the authorities: improved sanitation and water supply
The second question that was posed was, what caused the disease to decline? An attempt to answer this must involve a review of the measures used by the health officials to contain cholera. Before these measures can be judged, however, more detail is needed about the transmission of the disease. It has already been stated that cholera existed in Burma prior to the colonial period, and it has also been suggested that the delta may possibly have been a reservoir of infection. The other accepted form of transmission is through active infection or by asymptomatic carriers, and this was the link that the British would seem to have unwittingly forged through the migrant route from Bengal to Burma. One way of testing endemicity is by looking at the number of cholera cases that were detected at the ports of entry, although this of course excludes the asymptomatic carriers and also the migrants who entered Burma by the overland route.

The majority of Indian migrants who arrived by sea entered Burma through the port of Rangoon, where the health authorities inspected all the vessels that had declared cases of infectious disease. Spot checks were also made on other vessels. (The figures given for the migrants in the following discussion are rounded, due to the occasional confusion in the records. In some years the numbers of migrants recorded included those entering at the Akyab and Bassein ports, but not always.)

Between 1913 and 1922, more than two and a half million migrants entered Burma through the ports. From this huge number, only 331 cases of cholera were reported or detected throughout that period, 87 of whom had died at sea. The highest number of cases (242) was in the years 1918 to 1921, which coincided significantly with the flu pandemic. There was epidemic cholera in Burma in 1919, and the mortality in that year reached four per cent of the total mortality, but in 1915, when the cholera epidemic was responsible for 6.4 per cent of the total mortality, only 20 cases of cholera were notified at the ports.

In the ten-year period 1923 to 1932, an average of 300,000 migrants a year were entering through the ports, but a total of only 81 cases of cholera were identified or notified on incoming vessels throughout that period.[35] In the same period, 106 cases of smallpox, 101 cases of measles, 388 cases of chickenpox and 167 cases of leprosy were notified or found. There can be no doubt that disease, including cholera, was entering Burma with the Indian migrants, but there must be strong doubts about whether sufficient cases of cholera were entering through the ports to account for the constant incidence of the disease. There remains, however, the asymptomatic carrier as the possible agent of transmission; this will be considered in conjunction with the health authorities' response to outbreaks.

The health authorities' measures were essentially reactions to outbreaks rather than preventative actions, which would of course have been expensive. No attempt was made to examine all the migrants entering by the ports until plague threatened Burma, and even then, no checks were put on the overland route from Chittagong. Water supplies were checked when outbreaks of cholera occurred; then the wells were treated with potassium permanganate, suspect wells and tanks were closed, and advice was given to villagers via the headmen.[36] The evidence of a lack of a clear policy to control outbreaks was well illustrated in the health report of 1908, when C. E. Williams, the sanitary commissioner, wrote that probably the "best results were those following the voluntary and spontaneous evacuation by the inhabitants of an infected village, of their habitations until the epidemic had ceased."[37] But earlier in the same report, Williams wrote that infections were carried from one point in a district to another "by the movement of population, and by refugees from the first infected places."[38]

More positive action was displayed in 1918 when an outbreak occurred amongst labourers working on a Public Works Department road from Hsipaw to Nawngtehio in the northern Shan states. The spread of infection was controlled by the "picketing of roads, railway, sources of water-supply, etc., and the formation of segregation camps."[39] Despite these measures, 418 deaths were reported and more suspected.

By the 1920s, the health authorities were practising mass cholera inoculations where outbreaks had occurred in attempts to limit the infection. The authorities believed that inoculation was a very effective form of prevention and protection, but it was not until 1930 that the Irrawaddy Flotilla Company arranged to inoculate their crews annually.[40] As transmission by boatmen had been recognised since 1894, this reluctance on the part of the employers to act responsibly to check cholera illustrates perfectly the characteristic lack of foresight and meanness of those who employed cheap labour.

Periodically, cholera sheds were erected in which patients could be isolated from the rest of the community. In 1876, the victims of the outbreak in Akyab were housed in temporary shedding. Three hundred and sixty-six people died during the epidemic and the annual health report noted, somewhat pessimistically, that the sheds were erected "not very far from the burial ground".[41] The housing of the coolies at Akyab was appalling; in 1872, they were reported to be living packed in sheds, and defaecating behind these living quarters.[42] A modern medical textbook notes that "the communities attacked [with cholera] are poor, crowded, and characteristically without adequate disposal of human wastes."[43]

A shortage of resources was the reason generally advanced in the annual health reports to explain sanitary deficiencies. The problem was that, as the towns and population grew in Burma, the towns rapidly outran the provisions for the disposal of night-soil or the provisions for drinking water, and money was seldom available to remedy the situation. In the 1920s, an interesting dispute affecting the cleanliness of towns caused a lot of comment in the annual health reports. Several of the municipalities in Burma had decided that it would be more efficient and cost effective to privatise the disposal of night-soil and rubbish from their towns. This was opposed by the health authorities, who believed that cost cutting in such a field would tend to increase the insanitary state of the towns. In 1924, the sanitary commissioner firmly stated: "The contract system of removal of rubbish has proved a failure wherever adopted as was only to be expected since such contractors naturally do the minimum amount of work that will be tolerated. The contract system as worked at Prome was little short of a scandal, and in this respect the late committee left an undesirable legacy to its successors."[44]

Prome was also the subject of comment in the earlier health reports, as the town was inadequately drained and some areas became heavily water-logged during the rains. In 1899, an extensive programme of drainage was started, and 57,000 feet of masonry drains had been built by 1902.[45] By 1903, half the town was served by these drains and new pumping machinery and filter plants had improved the water supply.[46]

The water supply in Prome provides a good example of some of the difficulties experienced. The town took its drinking water from the Irrawaddy, and the intake pipe for the supply was situated in a shallow backwater not far from the steamer anchorage.[47] Theoretically the river water was then filtered, but a note in the 1895 annual health report said that the filter gallery and pumping station, abandoned for nine years, was now working.[48] But by 1896 the filters had again given trouble, and the river water was being strained only. The provision of clean drinking water in the towns usually depended on government funds rather than municipal money, and the former was chronically in short supply. In 1938, it was admitted that of the 14 major towns in Burma with populations of 20,000 or over, only seven had a piped-water supply.[49] The situation in the rural areas was, of course, much worse.

The League of Nations Health Organisation arranged an Inter-governmental Conference of Far-Eastern Countries on Rural Hygiene in 1937, and some of the recommendations from the conference were that village committees should be formed with specific responsibilities for hygiene and sanitation. Partly in response to this, a grant of 1,70,000 rupees was made in 1938 to attempt some alleviation of the chronic water shortages in the dry districts of Upper Burma. This grant was a contribution of two-thirds of the cost of a number of small projects, such as the digging of new tanks and wells and the repairing of old ones.[50] Conservancy in the villages was generally non-existent, but bored hole latrines, first used experimentally in the Rural Health Unit at Hlegu, were being installed in other parts of the country by 1938. The 5,000 latrines installed were a beginning, but rural sanitary provision was still negligible when the Second World War temporarily ended any hope of development.[51]

The decline of cholera mortality in Burma coincided with the decline of the disease in India. David Arnold, in his essay "Cholera Mortality in British India, 1817–1947", attributes the decline in India to a number of factors. These include the possibility of bacteriological change and, more importantly, the decline in the severity of famine. But he also saw the intervention by the sanitary and medical staff as an important factor, not in isolation, but as part of a number of changes that broke "the links in the epidemiological chain".[52] This would also seem the most rational explanation for the decline of the disease in Burma. No single factor was probably enough to limit the disease, but the improvements in piped water and drainage in some major cities, the sanitary arrangements at festivals, the inoculation programme and some slight improvements in the social conditions of labourers probably eventually had a cumulative effect. The more interventionist policy of the health officials, which developed during the plague epidemic, and the training of sanitary inspectors and health officers for work in the towns also contributed to the drop in the incidence of cholera. The decline in India may have had some effect on the incidence in Burma also, if it meant a decline in the number of asymptomatic carriers entering the country as migrants.

Plague

In 1899, a ship arrived at Rangoon carrying two men who were dying of plague. The arrival of this ship set in motion a series of regulations, some of them draconian, which were eventually to establish the beginnings of a proper public health inspectorate in Burma. Between 1905 (the first year of epidemic mortality) and 1939, the number of registered plague deaths in Burma was 161,951 or just over 4,600 per year. During this period, the average number of registered deaths per annum in Burma was 244,000, of which only 1.9 per cent approximately was due to plague. So why did plague have such a disproportionate effect on the history of medicine and sanitary developments in Burma?

The plague bacillus, or *Pasteurella pestis*, reached Canton (Guangzhou) and Hong Kong in 1894, having left Yunnan in 1855 and travelled across the Chinese interior.[53] By 1894, even the most conservative members of the medical profession had to abandon the miasmatic theory of the transmission of disease and accept the germ theory. When the outbreaks of plague were reported that year, international teams of bacteriologists arrived in Hong Kong and, within weeks, the discovery of *Pasteurella pestis* was reported.[54] It was many years before the epidemiology of plague was fully understood, but the basis of comprehension was reached internationally before the disease arrived in Bombay in 1898 and Rangoon in 1899.

Undoubtedly the response of western medicine to plague in Asia was governed by the folk memories of earlier plagues in Europe. This explains the dramatic mobilisation of resources that took place in Burma, India and other Asian countries. Terence Hull (1987) wrote that "the outbreak of plague in East Java called forth the mobilisation of financial and organisational resources unprecedented in the public health services of the colony."[55] The outbreak in Java was traced to rat fleas from vessels trading with Burma; the Burmese source was Calcutta.

The questions that need to be asked about plague in Burma are similar to those posed about cholera — how many died and who was chiefly affected, how did the colonial authorities respond to the plague epidemic and what caused the disease to decline in Burma? The total number of registered plague deaths in Burma has already been mentioned, but Table 5.6 shows the average number of deaths from the disease in each ten-year period from 1905, and expresses those figures as percentages of the total mortality. Prior to 1905, the number of deaths was minimal, two in 1900, three in 1901, one in 1902, nine in 1903, and three in 1904.

The registered plague deaths were not, of course, solely adult deaths, but included children. It was estimated in Chapter Four that child

TABLE 5.6

Average Number of Plague Deaths per Annum, and Expressed as a
Percentage of the Average Total Mortality

Period	Average Plague Deaths per Annum	Plague Deaths as a Percentage of Total Mortality
1905–11	7,012	3.2
1912–21	5,680	2.1
1922–31	3,829	1.7
1932–39	2,222	0.8

Sources: Annual health reports.

mortality probably formed, very approximately, 25 per cent of the total plague mortality and that the over 15-year-old age group formed the remaining 75 per cent. The mortality was concentrated in the urban areas of Burma, and with the exception of 1909, the mortality was always higher in Lower Burma than in Upper Burma. For some reason that is not as yet quite clear, proportionately more rural deaths seemed to occur in Upper Burma than in Lower Burma. It is possible that townspeople in Upper Burma were more likely to flee to relatives in the villages when an outbreak occurred, thus spreading the infection to the rural areas. It was estimated that the 1911 census enumeration was affected by plague in Mandalay town, as 10,000 of the townspeople were thought to be temporarily absent due to the plague outbreak.[56] The years when epidemic plague was at its height in Burma were 1906 (8,637 deaths) and 1907 (9,249 deaths). In 1918, another peak occurred and 8,840 deaths were registered, presumably due partly to the overwhelming of the sanitary services by the flu pandemic and, more importantly, by the movements of people trying to escape the pandemic.

The accuracy of the registration of plague deaths was in doubt in the early years. In 1907, the annual health report notes rises in the non-epidemic death rate (which may have concealed plague deaths) of Prome, Minhla, Henzada, Lemyethna and Bassein towns.[57] In the 1908 annual health report, it was suggested that plague mortality was concealed in the fever death rate of seven Lower Burma towns.[58] By 1910, the mobilisation of the health staff ensured that large-scale concealment of plague deaths in the towns no longer occurred. Some minor infringements still took place, usually in an attempt to avoid the attention of the public health staff, but the overall registration of plague deaths was probably accurate enough to reflect the trend of the disease.

Plague in Burma was reported to have a definite seasonal incidence. The health authorities said that the highest number of deaths occurred between December and April each year; from April the number of deaths declined until the following November or December, when the cycle started again.[59] This made the reporting of "the epidemic season" difficult for the authorities, as the annual health report covered a calendar year from January to December. In the first few years, the health officials divided the registered plague mortality into indigenous and imported incidence: the latter was the death of migrants who had been incubating the disease when they entered Burma. There is no doubt that Indian migrants or their ships brought plague to Burma, but equally there can be no doubt that once Burma had become part of the world trading pattern, there was little chance of escaping the infection even without the incoming migrants.

The question of who died of plague in colonial Burma is not easy to answer with any precision, due to lack of detail in the registration records. In contrast to cholera deaths, which were consistently linked to Indian coolies in the health records, little information was given about the identity of plague victims. Some fairly accurate speculation about the identity of these victims can be made from the areas of the towns most commonly affected by plague. These areas were connected with food storage or processing, and were therefore irresistibly attractive to rats. The 1923 health report stated that "Plague in Rangoon is closely connected with the rice industry and the numerous rice mills are very heavily infested with rats."[60] Because of their heavy involvement with the rice industry, Indian migrants would therefore have provided many of the plague victims. In many towns, it was the bazaars that were identified as the plague foci.[61] In 1930, there were 1,962 registered plague deaths in Burma, of which 958 occurred in Mandalay, mostly in the Thirimala Quarter in the neighbourhood of bazaars, rice mills and paddy godowns.[62] In 1933, travelling bazaar sellers were said to have introduced plague to Magwe town.[63] Occasionally the introduction of infection was linked to the clothing industry. An example of this was the introduction of plague to Sague town in Minbu district, which was attributed to the dead rats found in clothing boxes sent from Rangoon.[64] Even the meritorious deed of dying a *pongyi*'s robe could transmit the infection: plague was introduced to Sagaing twice through the medium of robes sent to Rangoon to be dyed.[65]

The implication from this evidence is that people who were involved in any way with food storage or processing were likely to be the initial victims of plague in an outbreak. The other most vulnerable group were those industrial workers who handled storage or packaging that could provide shelter for rats.

The discussion so far has considered the plague mortality in Burma and has attempted to identify the likely victims. The other two questions posed are why did the incidence of the disease decline, and was this due to the health authorities' efforts to contain it?

Role of the authorities: inspections, inoculations, rat drives and regulations
In 1897, prior to the arrival of plague in Burma, a Plague Council was formed "to advise Local Government concerning the measures to be taken for preventing the appearance of the bubonic plague in Rangoon, to consider and report where cases of plague, in the event of the disease appearing, should be isolated and treated, and to frame and submit a code of regulations which might be promulgated in Rangoon, or in any other Municipality, on the necessity arising in consequence of the appearance of the plague."[66] This committee met seven times in 1897 and 12 times in 1898. By the end of 1898, the committee had produced regulations for Rangoon and recommendations that included the examination of immigrants at the ports, quarantine measures and disinfection of luggage.

It was obvious that the greatest danger of infection lay in the contacts with India. Under the new regulations, as ships arrived from Calcutta, all the passengers were examined by a medical officer, and those that had no "satisfactory destination", namely casual labourers, were put into a quarantine camp for ten days. Others, that is first- and second-class passengers and "those with reliable addresses", were subject to a ten-day period of surveillance with a "passport".[67] All deck passengers had their clothing and property disinfected also. This contrasts with the previous regulations, when only those ships declaring the presence of infectious disease were examined, with the occasional spot check on others. Probably it was a passenger with a surveillance passport who was responsible for infecting the first "indigenous" case in Burma, which appeared in February 1905.

Under these regulations, a person wishing to travel from an infected area in Burma was allowed to move on the condition that he carried a "plague passport". This meant that the traveller had to submit to regular medical supervision in any town or village that he visited during the period of incubation. But this control was abandoned after only a few months, "largely due to representations by the commercial communities that the method would trammel trade in the Province."[68] The sanitary commissioners pointed out that trade would suffer far more from a plague outbreak than from a passporting system, but they were over-ruled.

In 1906, when 8,637 plague deaths were registered in Burma, the foundation of the future public health service in Burma was laid when Captain Williams was seconded from India and made special plague officer for Burma.[69] Under his supervision temporary plague inspectors were trained to supervise the disinfection and rat drives in the towns. These inspectors were the forerunners of the sanitary inspectors, who were eventually appointed in most towns in Burma. The proposal to train sanitary inspectors was first made in 1905,[70] and was approved in principle by the government in 1906.[71] Unfortunately, although the decision to establish the training class had been taken, no money was budgeted for this until 1908/09.[72] The scheme for training these inspectors is in many ways representative of many of the initiatives produced by the sanitary commissioners — a story of delay, financial stringency and in 1909, further delay as no money could be made available for the training class.[73]

It was not until 1913 that the first training class for sanitary inspectors was inaugurated, eight years after the need was described as urgent. The classes were held in Rangoon and were organised as bi-annual six-month courses under the auspices of the Royal Sanitary Institute of London. The sanitary commissioners hoped eventually to stipulate that one sanitary inspector should be appointed for every 15,000 people, and that provision should also be made for the inspection of schools and prisons.[74] The health authorities found it difficult, from the beginning of the scheme, to attract Burmese of a high enough educational standard, and they were aware also that training Indians as inspectors would create additional problems.[75] (The health authorities had already made that mistake in 1870 when Indians were trained as subordinate medical staff and were then found to be unacceptable to the Burmese.[76])

The methods that the health authorities employed to deal with plague changed considerably over time. In 1905, the response to notified cases was to burn all the victim's clothes and dressings, to segregate the family and those nearby, and to chemically disinfect the victim's house. In addition, the family and the neighbours received prophylactic inoculation and the house and surrounding area were "ratted". (In 1918, the inhabitants of Moulmein were given eight annas per head for agreeing to be inoculated.[77]) Plague control by rat destruction was very popular amongst the British doctors in Burma, and an astonishing number of rats were killed (4,366,869 in 1906) even in the early years.[78] There was much controversy over these rat drives, as medical opinion was divided as to whether they should be a response to reported infection or whether ratting was an efficient preventative measure. In 1909, Captain Brayne, whose previous experience was in the Punjab, was seconded for plague duty in Prome town. He organised a major programme of demolition and reconstruction of houses and other buildings in the town, overcoming in this process "the obstacles presented by social and racial prejudices".[79] Brayne was said to have carried out his programme of cleaning, remodelling dwellings and rat destruction "with unfaltering sternness".[80]

Part of the problem was the design and the construction materials of the traditional Burmese house. Both town and village houses had a thatched roof supported on rafters, either with no ceiling or with a mat ceiling. The floors in the town houses were usually raised and boarded, providing access for rats under the floor as well as in the roof. In many Burmese towns, the houses were surrounded by pools of mud as drainage in poorer areas was non-existent, the night-soil disposal was inadequate and refuse heaps were found close to the houses. These conditions had existed for many years without attracting more attention than an occasional admonishment in the annual health reports, but when plague threatened, sufficient energy and money were found to attempt some alleviation of the insanitary conditions of the poorer areas.

In Pegu town in 1910, rat drives were "systemised" by mapping the town and dividing it into trapping squares each of 2,000 inhabitants. During the rat drives, each house was treated as a source of infection; the floors were taken up, the ceilings partially removed and the corners of the roofs opened. All the furniture and the contents of the houses were removed "and the place thoroughly ratted by coolies".[81] The first of many changes in the health official's policies was also coming into effect; disinfection was abandoned and instead evacuation, inoculation and rat trapping were seen as the major weapons in the plague war. But by 1911, evacuation was admitted to be rarely adopted in towns, usually, and not surprisingly, because of the difficulties of convincing the population that they had to move.[82]

The year 1911 also saw the beginning of the Divisional Plague Scheme, whereby in the Pegu, Irrawaddy, Sagaing, and Meiktila divisions, the plague staff were appointed on a division level to respond to outbreaks of plague and to apply preventative measures in the division. Funds from the districts and towns in the division were pooled to employ a special plague officer, assistant plague officers, sanitary inspectors and a staff of trained coolies for sanitary work and rat destruction. This new scheme resulted in some much-needed sanitary improvements, which were reviewed in the 1911 annual health report. In Bassein, the byelaws which controlled the lodging houses, the eating-houses and bakeries were revised; the building byelaws were strengthened and the latrines and drains improved.[83] In Henzada town, 1,200 houses were reconstructed in whole or in part[84] and in Myaungmya town, 650 houses were improved.[85] Many of the 198 lodging houses in

Prome town were also improved — 92 were rebuilt and 70 were converted to other purposes or left empty.[86] The sanitary commissioner summarised his 1911 report by saying that the "stimulus given to general sanitary improvement under this system (rat destruction methods) is enormous and unprecedented in this Province."[87]

By 1913, more emphasis was being put on sanitary improvements and the inoculation of the population, as medical faith in the efficiency and effectiveness of continuous rat drives faltered and the large rat-catching gangs were disbanded.[88] The numbers inoculated each year varied from, for example, over 75,000 in 1917[89] to only 55,000 in 1926.[90]

The overbearing methods that were sometimes used by the health authorities provoked a political response in the 1920s. The *Wunthanu Athins*, or "own race associations", encouraged boycotts of the medical services in some areas, as well as the non-payment of taxes.[91] In 1928, villagers in Meiktila district resisted the efforts of the health staff to inoculate them[92] and six years prior to this, the annual health report noted that a chief officer of the *Athins* had carried a dead plague rat on his head to disprove the connection between plague and rats. The sanitary commissioner wrote: "One may be excused some satisfaction in noting that he is said to have died of plague soon after."[93]

It is not surprising that some resentment was provoked by the health authorities' activities. People's houses were destroyed, their lives were disrupted by the rat drives and sometimes they were forcibly evacuated from their homes.[94] But in return there was at least a temporary improvement in the sanitation of some towns, and a review of the numbers and the quality of the health staff needed in the province. From 1913, assistant surgeons were posted to sanitary and epidemic duty in the districts of the Pegu and Irrawaddy divisions. These men were military assistant surgeons who had previously been employed on plague duties and were now to perform a similar function in the urban areas, but under the district civil surgeons. Twelve men were allotted initially to the Lower Burma districts and three reserve officers were temporarily posted to Upper Burma, from where they could be posted to deal with epidemics in urban or rural areas.[95] These postings took place just before the outbreak of the First World War, and by 1915 the scheme was in abeyance, as most of the military assistant surgeons had been recalled by the army. Once again, the plans of the sanitary commissioners to improve the sparse public health services were frustrated, this time by war, not economics.

Laying the framework for a public health service
Plans for a service were gradually emerging (although never fulfilled in the colonial period) and were to consist of first- and second-class medically qualified officers in each of the larger towns, and a force of

sub-assistant surgeons to be posted at need throughout the country. The health officers (HO) were to be employed by the municipalities, and the qualifications and numbers employed were supposedly related to the size of the town population. For example, the annual health report of 1928 proposed that towns with a population of 100,000 should have two health officers — one first-class and one second-class. (The difference was the quality of post-graduate training: a first-class officer held a Diploma in Public Health and a second-class officer, a Government Licence in Hygiene.) Towns with a population of between 20,000 and 100,000 were to appoint a first-class officer, and smaller towns a second-class officer or a part-time officer. In addition, each district council was to appoint a first-class officer and, under this scheme, the government offered to pay half the salary of the health officers in both towns and districts.[96] But like so many health improvement schemes in Burma, this initiative faltered through insufficient funds, in this case, a lack of municipal and district funds. The proposal for the districts was put into abeyance, and only six councils accepted the municipal scheme.[97]

In 1931, the new Burma Municipal (Public Health) Amendment Act was brought into force; this envisaged the appointment of health officers in the towns, and laid down rules governing their pay, qualifications and appointment.[98] The basic flaws in this scheme were acknowledged in the health report of 1939. The health officer could find that he was jeopardising his appointment by forcing his employers, the municipality, to enforce unpopular byelaws; for this reason the posts were unpopular. The sanitary commissioner stated that the "Government of Burma has been approached to provincialise the Municipal Health Officers" but, due to the Second World War, the scheme was in abeyance![99]

What could truthfully be described as the "backbone" of the sparse basic medical care and epidemic control that existed in the rural areas of colonial Burma was supplied by a cadre of sub-assistant surgeons. These men had taken the shorter medical training course in Burma and were licentiates, not graduates. They were paid 50 per cent more salary in the Public Health Service than they would have received in the medical service, but even so were hard to recruit.[100] They worked for long periods away from home in response to epidemic or crisis, such as the 1936 cyclone that was estimated to have killed 1,000 people in Sandoway and Kyaukpyu districts.[101] By 1938, the Public Health Department had 36 of these sub-assistant surgeons in their employment, but not all of them were available for epidemic duties. For example, the role of hygiene publicity officer was taken over by a sub-assistant surgeon in 1932, when the post was abolished due to financial stringency.[102] They were also frequently seconded to special duties, such as campaigns against yaws and goitre.[103]

The idea of a cadre of sub-assistant surgeons arose from the need for a force that could respond to epidemics, originally perceived when plague broke out. The forerunners of these men were the military assistant surgeons who were first posted to Burma in 1912. Therefore, plague in Burma was responsible for more than the deaths of many of the population. The disease was also largely responsible for the creation of the force of sanitary inspectors (later called public health inspectors), some much-needed attention to the planning and sanitary state of the towns in Burma, and also the enlargement of the public health services in the shape of sub-assistant surgeons and public health officers. Perhaps these developments would have occurred anyway, but there is no doubt that it was the imminence and then the outbreak of plague that stimulated the government and health authorities into action.

Smallpox

Smallpox had an extensive history in Southeast Asia, and in adjacent India, its importance had been recognised long enough for a Hindu deity of the disease to exist.[104] McNeill estimated that smallpox and measles arrived in China between AD 37 and AD 653, and suggested that the impact of the disease contributed to the political fragmentation and heavy loss of population that occurred in that period.[105] Barend Jan Terwiel referred to epidemic outbreaks in fifteenth- and sixteenth-century Siam that were believed to be smallpox,[106] and the disease would appear to have been established in Java by the eighteenth century.[107] Balinese mythology implies that smallpox was brought to the island in the fifteenth century by King Majapahit, who came to Bali seeking subjects.[108] Ann Jannetta suggested that the epidemic of smallpox in Japan between AD 735 and AD 737 was the first authenticated Japanese outbreak of the disease, although it probably had a much earlier history there.[109]

When did smallpox arrive in Burma? It was reported to be epidemic during the Toungoo Empire (c. 1580–1635), but the close proximity of China and India with their long history of the disease, suggests a much earlier arrival.[110] The practice of inoculation was well established in Lower Burma before the arrival of the British, which would also imply a familiarity with the disease. (The inoculation process uses live smallpox virus whereas vaccine is made from the lymph of healthy calves previously infected with smallpox.)[111] Further research will probably reveal earlier references to smallpox, but at the present time, it can only be said that in Burma, as in Thailand, the disease is recorded from the sixteenth century and that its history may well be much older.

190

Disease and Demography in Colonial Burma

TABLE 5.7
Registered Deaths from Cholera, Plague and Smallpox

Period	Cholera		Plague		Smallpox	
	No.	Av. D.R. (1,000s)	No.	Av. D.R. (1,000s)	No.	Av. D.R. (1,000s)
1902–11	64,222	6.4	49,081*	7.0*	33,407	3.3
1912–21	59,498	6.0	56,801	5.7	21,023	2.1
1922–31	43,634	4.3	38,291	3.8	20,758	2.1
1932–39	15,465	1.9	17,778	2.2	9,956	1.2

Notes: * 1905–11.

Sources: Annual health reports.

How important was smallpox as a cause of mortality in Burma? The usual problems of assessing the accuracy of the registration data complicate definite conclusions, but, as with cholera and plague, the majority of smallpox deaths were probably registered. The total smallpox mortality as a percentage of the total mortality in Burma was shown earlier in Table 5.3. Table 5.7 shows clearly that between 1902 and 1939, the number of deaths from smallpox were only half those from either plague or cholera, and it also illustrates the declining importance of all three epidemic diseases by the 1930s.

How accurate was the diagnosis and recording of smallpox in colonial Burma? The long history of the disease in the country ensured that the headmen were familiar with the commonest symptoms, but the course of smallpox could vary, which hinders diagnosis. The first few days following the onset of symptoms, the prodromal stage, could produce convulsions, delirium, haemorrhage and death before any skin eruptions occurred. Jannetta suggested that smallpox was likely to be understated in historical records because the victim could die before the familiar and diagnostic eruptions occurred.[112]

In addition to this possibility of under-registration through misdiagnosis, there was also some evasion of the registration of smallpox deaths in the early days of the British administration. This was due to a policy of segregation, which operated for a time in Lower Burma. Doctor Johnstone, the civil surgeon of Rangoon, stated in 1879 that people kept smallpox outbreaks secret from the authorities for fear of being sent to the smallpox hospital.[113] The civil surgeon of Prome commented in the same year that people resented segregation in smallpox huts and said that "where force could not be justified by law, persuasion was adopted" to segregate the infected from the non-infected.[114] The attempts to enforce the policy were presumably unsatisfactory, as the references in the annual health reports to the isolation units ceased. It is probable that the majority of victims were young children for whom the use of isolation units was impractical.

The high incidence of the disease amongst young children is confirmed by the cyclical patterns of the smallpox epidemics, which peaked at three- to five-year intervals. Between these peaks of mortality, the number of deaths declined, in some years to almost insignificant levels. The low proportion of adult deaths to child deaths suggests that most of the adult population had a degree of immunity to the disease derived from an earlier contact, and that smallpox was therefore endemic to Burma. The population most at risk were the children and those adults who, due to a remote habitat, were lacking in immunity. If contact with major population centres is avoided, then it is possible for a generation to reach maturity without immunity to smallpox and they would thus be very vulnerable if an outbreak of the disease should occur. Of course, as with all the Burma data, there are problems of under-registration and probable mis-registration (such as infant deaths possibly being registered as "Fever" deaths), but even when allowance is made for this, it is still quite clear that smallpox was a predominantly childhood disease in Burma.

The British authorities attributed many outbreaks of the disease to infection brought in by Indian migrants. In 1897, an epidemic in Moulmein and Rangoon was blamed on unvaccinated Corringee coolies,[115] and again in 1915 and 1916, the initial outbreaks of the disease were attributed to poor, migrant Indians, many of whom were not vaccinated.[116] There is no doubt that some Indians were infected with smallpox; it was mentioned during the earlier discussion on cholera that 106 cases of smallpox in migrants were identified at the ports between 1923 and 1932. But to blame such migrants for causing epidemics in a country where the disease was already endemic was far too simplistic; but as with plague and cholera, the Indians served as "whipping boys".

The British authorities also suggested that smallpox was spread through the communication lines of the railways and rivers on a south-to-north axis.[117] It would not be surprising if epidemics were conceived in the crowded ports of the south, as the conditions for the spread of the disease existed there with or without the influx of infected migrants. Pagoda festivals were also identified as foci of infection. In 1907, the Shwepaunglaing festival near Pauk was thought to have been the focus of an epidemic in Pakokku district, during which 644 people died. However, an investigation by a local hospital assistant, Maung Aung Pua, found that inadequate vaccination was the underlying cause of the high mortality. His report stated that of 95 villages in the affected locality, 29 had not been visited by a vaccinator for two and a half years, and in six of those villages, no vaccination had ever been performed,[118] although inoculation was said to be widely practised in the district.

Vaccination in Burma

There is no doubt that in the first 20 years of the British administration of Upper Burma, there was a failure to provide and enforce an efficient vaccination policy. Vaccination in Burma was required under the Vaccination Act, India, 1880, but this applied only to municipalities and those towns large enough to have town committees to administer the Act. Rural vaccination was administered and supervised by the district civil surgeons through district superintendents of vaccination and their team of vaccinators. In 1913 for example, there were 278 vaccinators working in the rural and urban areas, all of whom had been trained at the Meiktila Vaccine Depot or had been approved for the work by the superintendent-general of vaccination.[119] Various amendments to the original Act were passed in 1900, 1908 and 1909, regarding the prohibition of inoculation in Burma, the training of vaccinators and the enforcement of the Act. In addition, a series of Port Health Acts amended the regulations governing the vaccination of Indian migrants.

The Vaccination Act though, could be enforced in the rural areas and smaller towns only when a sufficient staff and supply of lymph were available. It was not until 1925 that primary vaccination was made compulsory in the study area of Lower Burma, and even then, an exception was made for Sandoway district.[120] In Upper Burma, the situation was still patchy. In Myingyan district for example, 613 deaths were registered as smallpox in 1926, and neither the Vaccination Act nor the Prohibition of Inoculation Act applied to the rural district.[121]

In the earlier years of the colonial administration, many of the difficulties were associated with the production and transport of reliable vaccine. It was admitted in the health report of 1899 that the most potent cause of the current epidemic was the lack of vaccine.[122] By 1905, the criticism was of "short sighted economy in the matter of the supply of sufficient suitable staffs for the purposes of working compulsory vaccination."[123] This was a familiar situation in Burma: the Acts aimed at health improvement had been passed, but the money to fulfil the aims of the legislation was not available. There was certainly no shortage of legislation — Rangoon was said in 1905 to have greater powers for the enforcement of vaccination than any other city of the British Empire. Any unprotected person could be vaccinated after due notice, and the inhabitants of lodging houses (i.e. Indians) could be operated upon summarily.[124] The 1908 Act extended the summary vaccination to immigrants at the ports, but in 1910, following a year of very low smallpox mortality, this part of the Act was put into abeyance in the port of Rangoon. Instead it became the responsibility of the ships' captains to report infection amongst their passengers and to hoist the quarantine flag.[125] This was probably another example of the conflict between the health authorities and those in charge of trade policies and the budget, but it is also remarkable in view of the official opinion that migrants were responsible for spreading the smallpox infection.

In the rural areas of Burma and the towns of Upper Burma, the problem was the lack of enforcement of the existing laws rather than their suspension. These difficulties were undoubtedly compounded by the basic problem of inadequate numbers of poorly trained staff. As late as 1922, the severe smallpox outbreak in the Upper Burma district of Magwe was attributed to lack of vaccination. The district superintendent of vaccination was said to be incompetent, to have travelled as little as possible, to have faked his diary and provided fictitious figures of vaccinations which were not checked.[126]

The eventual success of the vaccination policy was discussed in Chapters Three and Four. The mortality of infants and children, formerly the chief victims of the disease, declined to insignificance due to the protection of the vaccine. This is further confirmed by the changing mortality pattern, as adults became the chief victims of the disease. As we saw in Chapter Four, smallpox was a childhood disease with 65 to 85 per cent of the total mortality in the 12 years and under age group. But by the late 1920s and 1930s, the balance of mortality had changed, and 68 per cent in 1927 and 78 per cent in 1929 of the deaths were adult. These percentages of the much-reduced total mortality were continued through the 1930s, with approximately 60 to 70 per cent of the deaths occurring in the over-ten years age group.

This brief discussion of smallpox in Burma has concluded that the main significance of the disease was as a killer of children. It was calculated at the beginning of this chapter that the adult population of Burma, that is, 60 to 63 per cent of the total population, was responsible for between 46 and 56 per cent of the total mortality from 1891 to 1931. If adults were not dying in significant numbers from smallpox, and the incidence of cholera and plague was also declining from 1911, then what diseases were the major killers?

Other causes of adult mortality

This chapter has so far examined the mortality from the epidemic diseases of cholera, plague and smallpox, and attempted where possible to quantify the deaths. But this is far from being the full story of adult disease in colonial Burma. The next sections will briefly examine the less specific disease groups as causes of mortality.

Dysentery and diarrhoea

In Burma, the mortality from bowel complaints was recorded from the time registration was introduced, but deaths from respiratory disease were not recorded until 1902. The number of registered deaths from the two categories, and the totals by decade as a percentage of the total mortality are shown in Table 5.8. The figures tell two stories — a decline in the importance of diarrhoeal disease as a cause of mortality, and an increase in the number of deaths from respiratory disease. A decline in the incidence of diarrhoeal disease confirms the evidence presented in the Figure 5.1 histogram series a to f, which showed that the peak periods of mortality had moved from a July/August/September axis to an autumn/winter peak.

One question to be asked is whether the increase in the possible "causes of death" affects the interpretation of Table 5.8 or the histogram series. This would apply only if there was a possibility that, for example,

TABLE 5.8

Registered Deaths from Respiratory Disease and Dysentery and Diarrhoea by Decade, and Expressed as a Percentage of the Total Mortality

Period	Dysentery and Diarrhoea		Respiratory Disease	
	Total Deaths	%	Total Deaths	%
1892–1901	78,399	7.1	*	*
1902–11	100,321	4.6	57,406	2.6
1912–21	99,441	3.7	96,820	3.6
1922–31	78,461	3.5	113,592	5.1
1932–39	47,171	2.2	115,185	5.5

Notes: * This category was introduced on 30 August 1901 as a separate cause of death.

Sources: Annual health reports.

a cause of death formerly registered as "Respiratory" was, by 1930, registered under the "Dysentery and Diarrhoea" group, or was registered as "Respiratory Disease" when formerly grouped under "All Other Causes". In the urban areas of Burma, further "cause of death" categories were added to the registration system in 1922. Additional details were gradually included, and by 1939, the urban data included details of deaths due to malaria, enteric fever, measles, kala-azar, influenza, cerebrospinal fever, typhus fever, blackwater fever, dysentery, diarrhoea, pneumonia, pulmonary tuberculosis, whooping cough, beri-beri, diphtheria, mumps, tuberculosis of joints, other tuberculosis, leprosy and cancer. The first eight categories were listed under "Fevers", dysentery and diarrhoea formed another sub-group and pneumonia, pulmonary tuberculosis and whooping cough were classed under "Respiratory Disease". The last seven diseases listed here were grouped under "All Other Causes".

A disease that could be mis-registered is enteric fever — the disease caused by the bacterium *Salmonella typhi* that was isolated by William Budd of Bristol.[127] It was easily transmitted by contaminated water and was classified in the new urban registration as a "Fever". The disease is usually characterised by a remittent fever, abdominal pain and diarrhoea, but the victim may instead show symptoms of constipation, thus confusing diagnosis. It is likely that a headman in the rural areas could classify a death from enteric fever either under "Fevers" or under "Dysentery and Diarrhoea", but given this possible confusion, did the separate urban category of enteric fever contribute to the decline in the importance of diarrhoeal mortality as a percentage of total mortality? The answer would seem to be no. If the registered enteric deaths between 1932 and 1939 are added to the registered dysentery and diarrhoea deaths for that period, the sum of these is still only 2.7 per cent of the total mortality for those years.

Despite the weaknesses of the Burma registration, there is nothing in the data to refute the premise that dysentery and diarrhoea declined in importance as a cause of death, especially in the 1930s. Table 5.8 shows that the first major drop in the number of deaths from these causes was after 1901. But this drop, from 7.1 per cent of the total mortality up to 1901 to only 4.6 per cent up to 1911, was not very significant. During the first decade of the twentieth century, the new category of deaths from "Respiratory Disease" was introduced, and the registration system extended to Upper Burma, both of which were likely to affect the number of deaths registered in any category.

The importance of bowel disease as a determinant of mortality was described in the first health report of 1867. The surgeon at Toungoo, C. R. S. Parker said that dysentery and bronchitis were the most common causes of death after fevers,[128] while the chief diseases at Tavoy were described as typhoid (enteric fever), dysentery and diarrhoea.[129] Doctor Cowie, the sanitary commissioner, mentioned a typhoid fever in his report on Rangoon in 1868, and this was confirmed by Dr Heffernan, the civil surgeon.[130] Cowie was an unusually enterprising and far-sighted man who advocated, in 1868, that a sewage system with a flushing apparatus should be built in Rangoon.[131] His period as sanitary commissioner was, alas, brief.

The first annual health reports, dated 1867 and 1868, contain the individual surgeons' reports from the towns in British Burma. This makes them uniquely valuable, but also means that the causes of death are subject to individual interpretation. The reports contain many overlapping categories of death, such as bowel complaint, gastritis, dysentery and diarrhoea, but also contain many others that are more difficult to interpret, such as sudden death, thirst with purging, giddiness, sores, drunken, murder, body swelled up and old age. A total of 99 categories were used, but most (with the exception of murder) are descriptions of symptoms rather than the diagnosis of a specific disease. However, the total number of deaths registered under the "bowel" categories listed above was 635, or 8.7 per cent, of the 7,318 deaths listed. These were all urban deaths, and the figure is surprisingly close to the 1922 figure of 7.6 per cent for Rangoon, registered in the first year of the newly detailed urban categories. These figures compare with the 1922 data for the rural areas in Burma, when the dysentery and diarrhoea group were four per cent of the total mortality in Lower Burma and only 1.5 per cent in Upper Burma.

The higher urban mortality throughout the registration period is too consistent to be merely the result of inaccuracies in the Burma registration. High mortality from bowel disease was largely an urban problem, related to contaminated supplies of drinking water and the flies that came with the wet season. The rural population of Burma usually had a regular source of clean drinking water that served the village, and they were only driven to using more easily contaminated sources, such as major rivers, in times of drought. In Lower Burma, especially in the delta, these village supplies could be inundated with flood water during the monsoon, which could contaminate the supplies with human and animal faeces, resulting in a higher mortality figure.

In addition to the Burmese urban population, it is probable that the Indian migrant population also died in disproportionate numbers from dysentery and diarrhoea. In 1882, severe cases of dysentery amongst Indian migrants were attributed to their being given Burmese rice instead of Indian rice.[132] In 1883, however, it was blamed on starvation: D. Sinclair, the sanitary commissioner, stated in the annual health report that "A very common cause of dysentery and diarrhoea amongst Indian immigrants to this province is starvation." He added that coolies employed on public works starved themselves in order to save money to send to India and in consequence, they were found dying by the roadside in the last stages of dysentery although carrying a roll of money.[133]

The delta towns of Burma, with their high concentration of impoverished coolies, had, inevitably, a high death rate from bowel disease. The poor lived in urban areas where overcrowding, poor drainage, lack of clean water supplies and conservancy made them highly vulnerable to diarrhoeal disease. This was acknowledged in the annual health reports with comment in 1900, 1901, 1903 and 1904, when Bassein, in particular, was noted to have markedly insanitary conditions.[134] In 1916, a high rise in the incidence of dysentery amongst the wolfram miners at Tavoy was noted, due no doubt to the usual lack of clean water and sanitary facilities.[135]

The health administrators identified another reason for the high summer incidence of the disease: this was the increased consumption of fruits in season. In 1931, the health officer of Mandalay blamed the high summer mortality from dysentery and diarrhoea on "the indiscriminate consumption of various fruits".[136] It seems probable that the other explanation he put forward for the high death rate was more accurate — the drying up of wells and the consequent increase in water impurities.

Occasionally the health authorities expressed doubts about the accuracy of the urban bias in the death rates for dysentery and diarrhoea. It was suggested that bowel disease was more accurately diagnosed in the urban hospitals, thus raising the urban rate.[137] It is to be hoped and expected that the diagnosis would be more efficiently carried out in a hospital than by a village headman, but it would seem very unlikely that the minority of cases hospitalised could account for the difference between urban and rural rates.

What caused the mortality from bowel disease to decline? The extent of this was greatest in a few urban areas, of which Rangoon is the prime example. The number of registered deaths from dysentery and diarrhoea more than halved between 1927 and 1932. Between 1924 and 1927, more than 1,000 deaths per year were registered as bowel disease, but this dropped to 500 per year by 1932. This was a decline from more than ten per cent of the total registered mortality in Rangoon to just over five per cent, and must be largely attributed to the provision of improved drinking water supplies.

It can be concluded that the mortality from dysentery and diarrhoea fell most heavily on the urban poor. The town dwellers in the wealthier areas with piped water and sanitation facilities were less at risk. In the rural areas, the incidence was much lower, except during the seasons of inundation or severe drought, when contamination of supplies could occur.

Respiratory disease

The new mortality category of "Respiratory Disease" was introduced into the registration system on 30 August 1901. No deaths were notified under this heading in 1901, but 2,439 were registered in 1902. The annual registered total grew steadily until between 10,500 and 14,000 deaths per annum were notified in the last 20 years of registration. In 1922, the category was redefined in the urban area and, as discussed previously, the deaths were registered as pneumonia, pulmonary tuberculosis, whooping cough and other respiratory diseases. Measles was classified as a "Fever" in the urban registration, despite the fact that the disease usually manifests in the respiratory system and is often complicated by broncho-pneumonia.

Table 5.8 shows a sharp increase in the number of deaths registered as "Respiratory Disease" until 1921. Two factors complicate any assessment of this. Firstly, registration under the new disease category was bound to improve as headmen became accustomed to notifying deaths in that way, and secondly, many of the "excess" deaths due to the influenza pandemic were probably notified under respiratory disease. Both these factors would cause the rate to rise, thus obscuring whether there was a true increase in the number of deaths from respiratory disease. From 1922 to 1939, the rate was fairly stable and during that period, the number of deaths recorded in Rangoon from respiratory disease was also constant. In 13 out of the 18 years, the number of deaths in Rangoon was between 2,900 and 3,500.

It is surprising that the registered respiratory death rate shows no greater rise, especially in urban Rangoon. Tuberculosis was known to be important in the towns, and the sanitary commissioners and health officers believed that the incidence was rising steadily. In 1919, the civil surgeon of Myanugmya district described tuberculosis as the commonest of all diseases in Myaungmya and Wakema towns.[138] In 1920, it was stated to be a common disease of urban communities,[139] and in 1923, the civil surgeons of Myaungmya, Pakokku and Myingyan towns commented on the prevalence of tuberculosis.[140] The comments continued with a note in the health report of 1926 that pulmonary tuberculosis was increasing in the towns of Burma,[141] and in 1928, much of the "alarming increase" in the respiratory death rate of Myaungmya town was said to be due to tuberculosis. However, it was also stated that "Tuberculosis is not yet a disease of importance in the rural areas of Burma."[142]

If tuberculosis was increasing sharply in the urban areas, why was there not a greater increase in the total number of deaths from respiratory disease after 1922? There are two possible reasons that may account for this: the urban population was approximately one-tenth of the total population, which limited the impact of an urban disease rate on the province rate, and the accompanying decline in the incidence of plague and smallpox should have lowered the number of deaths registered as respiratory disease.

In the discussion of the major epidemic diseases, it was suggested that the Indian migrant population died of cholera and plague in disproportionate numbers. Could it be said that tuberculosis in Burma also affected one racial group more than another? There is conflicting evidence on this point. In a paper given at a British Medical Association meeting in Burma, W. G. King, a former sanitary commissioner, mentioned the prevalence of tuberculosis amongst the Gurkha battalion of Military Police at Myitkyina.[143] But in the discussion that followed, it was stated that the chief sufferers from tuberculosis in Rangoon were the Burmese and the Chinese.[144]

In 1932, it was noted in the annual health report that tuberculosis was common amongst the Burmese and Chinese at Kyaiklat; the local health officer attributed this to a lowered vitality induced by opium.[145] Two years later, the health officer of Lashio stated that phthisis (an advanced pulmonary tuberculosis) was common in the northern Shan states but not amongst the Shans. Those chiefly affected were Chinese, Gurkhas, Ooriyas and Gharwalis.[146] The evidence is mixed and the assumption should not be made that Indians were the chief sufferers, simply because tuberculosis was an urban disease. If, as mentioned in Chapter Four, tuberculosis was a new disease to Burma, then the lack of natural immunity amongst the Burmese would have made them very vulnerable. Certainly Professor S. Lyle Cummins supported this idea in 1938, when he said that the Burmese were "suffering from a high death rate [from tuberculosis], higher than the Indians residing in Burma". He further suggested that the deaths were due to this susceptibility "and that the disease is a comparatively new one to a great many of the people exposed."[147]

Cummins' theory that the disease was new to Burma supported the opinion of Dr Nisbett, who was the civil surgeon at Bassein in 1868. He stated that the Burmese had a "natural freedom from disease of the tubercular class, the most fatal of all in Europe."[148] This suggests that mid-nineteenth-century Burma was free of tuberculosis, but unfortunately that freedom did not continue.

The balance of the evidence suggests that the heaviest mortality from tuberculosis was amongst adult Burmese, due to lack of immunity. Indians were also victims, but this was probably due to specific circumstances, such as severe overcrowding or the use of infected milk, which was the suggested reason for the prevalence at Myitkyina.[149] There was probably also a sexual, as well as racial, bias in the mortality. The few specific figures that appear in the health records suggest on balance a higher death rate for males than females.[150]

Mortality from tuberculosis was almost certainly increased by complications from other disease factors. Parasite infestations, under-nutrition, poor sanitation or dirty drinking water would pre-dispose the victims to early mortality from tuberculosis, and pneumonia would probably add the finishing blow. This would also complicate the registration of the death, as a high temperature could mean the death was registered under "Fevers" instead of tuberculosis or "Respiratory Disease". The DHO of Myaungmya town suggested that much of the alarming increase in the mortality from respiratory disease was "due to tuberculosis complicated by pneumonia".[151] It is also interesting to note that the sanitary commissioner thought the prevalence of tuberculosis amongst the Gurkha battalion at Myitkyina was due to the men having been weakened by malaria.[152]

Much of the discussion so far has consisted of quotations from the British health administrators about the prevalence of tuberculosis in Burma, but the response of the authorities to the disease has still to be explored. The first enquiry into the disease in Burma was undertaken in 1915, when the Indian Research Fund Association appointed Dr Lankester to report on tuberculosis in the Indian Empire. His enquiry revealed that there had been 545 deaths from tuberculosis in Rangoon in 1915, of which 433 were pulmonary. In one circle of Rangoon, Taroktan, there was a concentration of the disease, resulting in a pulmonary tuberculosis death rate of 2.64 per 1,000. In Mandalay, there were 276 deaths registered from tuberculosis, of which 240 were pulmonary.[153] The disease was reported to be prevalent all over Burma, but with a greater incidence in the wet zone. The investigators found that the heaviest mortality occurred in the 40 to 50 year age group, but child mortality was insignificant.

The second major investigation was that carried out by Professor Cummins in 1938 and 1939. His visit to Burma was the result of a request made by the Central Association for the Prevention of Tuberculosis in Burma to the National Association in England. They asked for the services of an expert in tuberculosis who would study the problem in Burma and suggest ways of controlling and eliminating the disease. The central association and 25 affiliated district associations had been formed following an appeal by the governor of Burma in December 1937 for funds to aid the control of tuberculosis and leprosy. An ad hoc committee was formed to administer the 4,50,681 rupees raised, and from this sum, the committee offered two and a half *lakhs* of rupees to the government of Burma towards the building of a tuberculosis hospital in Rangoon.[154] It should be noted, however, that most of this activity was voluntary, supported by the governor but not part of the sanitary and health services.

The Rangoon Corporation had made a positive effort to tackle the problem in December 1935, when they opened a tuberculosis dispensary in Rangoon. The need was quickly demonstrated by the attendance figures — 24,405 in 1936 and 29,229 in 1937. Presumably not all of these patients were tuberculosis sufferers and many were already under some form of treatment, but 864 new cases of pulmonary tuberculosis were diagnosed at the clinic in 1937, of which 750 were at the third stage. In 1939, the attendance at the clinic had risen to over 38,000, including 5,000 new patients, of whom 1,000 were tubercular.[155]

It would seem that tuberculosis in Burma was a phenomenon of the colonial period. Probably it was introduced by either European or Indian migrants and developed amongst the unprotected Burmese population into a major disease of the urban areas. The number of registered deaths from tuberculosis was not that high, 2,766 in 1939 or a rate of 1.78 per 1,000, but its true incidence was undoubtedly much higher. The introduction of the disease probably had its greatest effect during and immediately after the Second World War. Thein Aung, who wrote a description in 1955 of the "White Plague" in Burma, said that tuberculosis was the chief public health problem of the urban population, aggravated by the influx of people into the towns.[156] This was a colonial legacy that had no benefits.

What other respiratory diseases did adults die of in colonial Burma? The urban registration listed pneumonia amongst others, which is, of course, often a complication of other diseases such as tuberculosis, bronchitis, measles, melioidosis (soil disease), flu, chest infections, and many others. In the towns, more than 40 per cent of the total deaths from respiratory disease were commonly attributed to pneumonia. The rates for all respiratory diseases were much higher in the towns than in the rural districts, but was pneumonia really much more prevalent in the urban areas or was the new registration system the explanation? It was possibly the registration system, as, following a check on the system in the Lower Chindwin district, very high rural death rates for respiratory disease were returned: 3 per 1,000 in 1931, and 3.10 per 1,000 in 1932,[157] compared to province rates of 0.99 in 1931 and 0.98 in 1932.

But these rates pale into insignificance compared to the deaths that occurred from 1918 as the world pandemic hit Burma.

The influenza pandemic

The influenza pandemic is thought to have its origins in the battlefields of the First World War. Probably the virus was carried from the United States of America to Europe, although there may also have been foci in China and Russia.[158] It was a new strain of the influenza virus, and it spread rapidly, reaching Bombay by June 1918. It was recognised in Rangoon in late June and July and had spread to the whole of the study area by September 1918.

It is thought that troop movements were instrumental in introducing influenza to Burma and spreading it within the country. "It was undoubtedly brought to Rangoon by details of troops returning from leave or on transfer from India, and such details probably carried it quickly to cantonments in distant parts of Burma". There were other ways of dissemination: by rail, riverboat, ferries, markets, workplaces and pagoda festivals. The Mahamuni festival at Mandalay was a typical focus; the disease spread rapidly to the villages as the pilgrims returned to their homes.[159]

The influenza appears to have entered Burma in two waves. The first wave peaked in Rangoon in the middle of August and was followed by a second wave of infection that caused 148 deaths in one week of November 1918 alone.[160] The registered death rate for the province was 39.59 per 1,000 in 1918, an increase of 14.31 per 1,000 over the previous five-year mean. During the next two years, a higher than average registered death rate persisted, 31.09 in 1919 and 26.44 in 1920. In subsequent years, the death rate fell below that registered from 1905 to 1917, largely due to the expansion of registration to Upper Burma, as discussed in Chapter Two.

How many people died in Burma as a result of the flu pandemic? Many of the deaths would have been attributed to other causes in the registration, as people died of diseases that were fatal because the victims had been weakened by flu. If the problem of inadequate registration is temporarily ignored, then one of the simplest ways of assessing the excess or flu crisis mortality is to count the additional deaths registered during the three-year period 1918–20. (It should be remembered that 1918 was also a "plague" year, although the 8,840 deaths registered under plague appear almost insignificant compared to the flu mortality.) The mean registered total mortality of the preceding five-year period, 1913–17, was 248,948 per annum. If this mean mortality is subtracted from the gross annual registered mortality for the flu years, then an excess mortality of 139,958 in 1918, 56,513 in

1919, and 10,828 in 1920 is left. The registered crisis mortality therefore totals 207,299.

Of course, this is only part of the actual mortality in Burma, as none of the major hill areas were included in the vital registration, and the registration itself was incomplete in normal times and "completely disorganised for a time" by the pandemic.[161] The sanitary commissioner, C. E. Williams, estimated that the excess mortality in 1918 was not "less than 200,000 up to 31st December 1918",[162] approximately 30 per cent more than the registered figures showed. If the registered figures in the two subsequent years were equally deficient, that is 30 per cent less, then the total mortality for the flu pandemic was approximately 300,000. Given that, by my estimates, the registration under normal circumstances omitted approximately 30 per cent of the mortality, it is probably more accurate to estimate the crisis mortality at 300,000 to 400,000. This is probably a very modest estimate for the whole of Burma, as the infection and mortality rates were known to have been as high in the hill areas as in the study area, but there is no way of arriving at a more accurate estimate. Amartya Kumar Sen quantified the excess mortality due to the Bengal famine from adjusted registration data over a period of four years, but the erratic form of the Burmese data excludes this possibility.[163] The argument, that deaths attributable to a famine are still occurring after the famine is past, is arguable also for an epidemic such as influenza, as the weakening effect of an attack may be the underlying cause of death from malaria or dysentery the following year. The flu mortality in India was approximately 12.5 million, or about four per cent of the population.[164] The Burmese population was approximately 13 million in 1918, and the estimated crisis mortality of 300,000 to 400,000 was therefore 2.3 to 3.1 per cent; a much lower figure, but still a human disaster.

Which age group of the population was most vulnerable to flu? An estimate was made in Chapter Four that childhood mortality (0–15 years) rose by 100 per cent in 1918, the registered deaths of children showing a rise of 50 per cent in the five year and under age group, and nearly 100 per cent in the five to 15 year olds. The registered deaths in the 15 to 50 year age group in 1918 was 107 per cent higher than the average of the two preceding years but, surprisingly, in the over 50 age group, the registered deaths rose by only 24 per cent in that year.

The total picture for the registration data is somewhat unexpected therefore. The mortality fell most heavily on the adult population (the 15 to 50 years) and, less surprisingly, the children. But the supposedly very vulnerable older group appears to have escaped comparatively lightly. This contrasts with the situation in Indonesia, where Brown suggests that the majority of those who died were outside the normal working age, namely the old and the young.[165] More work would be needed on the Burmese data before firm conclusions can be drawn.

How did the infection spread and were there geographical areas in which the mortality was heavier than others? The introduction and spread of infection by troops has already been mentioned, and the sanitary commissioner of the time clearly stated that the rapid dissemination was caused by military movement connected with the war.[166] In effect then, both the origin and spread of the infection were attributable to the war. The troops and military police carried the infection from Rangoon to various military headquarters, and from there to outposts all over Burma, as far as Myitkyina, the Tenasserim district and the Chin Hills by October 1918. It was stated in the annual health report that "All military police posts suffered from one to five deaths".[167]

The Mahamuni festival helped to spread the infection to Mandalay and Sagaing town, districts including Kyaukse and the southern and northern Shan States. In Lower Burma, the pattern of dissemination was mostly the transport network. Infected immigrants from Calcutta arrived in Rangoon and helped to spread the infection over the delta and other parts of Lower Burma. By July 1918, the mortality rates for Hanthawaddy, Insein and Tharrawaddy were rising, and by August, Pegu, Prome, Pyapon, Toungoo, Bassein and Henzada districts were also affected. By September, the infection had spread to all of Lower Burma, and had extended in Upper Burma also. In a few districts, a second wave of infection occurred, the September outbreak being followed by a wave of infection in December. This was noted by the health authorities in Mandalay, Sagaing, Kyaukse and Thayetmyo districts of Upper Burma, but in Lower Burma, this second outbreak was detected only in Akyab and Bassein.

It is probably no coincidence that three out of the four Upper Burma districts where this second outbreak happened were known to be malarial, and the second peak of flu deaths coincided with the month in which the heaviest mortality from malaria normally occurred. Significantly, in Lower Burma, the second wave was noted in districts where the immigrant influx was very high. In 1919, most of Burma continued to show areas of excess mortality, but by 1921, the flu was apparently confined to pockets of less virulent infection with a lower case mortality, although the health authority noted a high mortality from respiratory disease, "which is regarded as a heritage from influenza".[168]

Was there a sexual or racial bias in the mortality of adults? Women aged between 20 and 40 years suffered a far higher registered mortality than men of that age group — 30.88 per 1,000 against 24.70 per 1,000. The sanitary commissioner attributed this to the effect of flu on pregnant and parturient women, but it may also be that women of that age group were more vulnerable to the infection through caring for sick relatives and neighbours.[169]

It is more difficult to assess any racial bias in the flu mortality. The only disease-specific figures available are for Rangoon between July and November 1918. These show a very high proportion of Hindu deaths, more than twice as many as there were for the Buddhist population.[170] The high mortality rate for Hindus is not surprising, given their appalling housing conditions, overcrowding and the absence of effective treatment. The immigrant ships, arriving weekly at Rangoon from Calcutta, carried infected Hindus "scores of whom were ill with influenza", and there were many deaths at sea.[171] The dividing line between those groups with a high or low mortality was financial rather than racial. Europeans, and wealthier Indians or Burmese, were less likely to contract the disease and had a greater probability of surviving if they did. The wealthier "enjoyed a certain amount of immunity" due to "less crowded dwellings, better food and clothes, and willingness to follow western methods of treatment". Despite this neat summary of the advantages that the wealthier enjoyed, the health authorities attributed the higher death rate among the poor to ignorance and lack of precautions, as well as the absence of proper nursing and lack of medical treatment.[172]

This raises the question of the health authorities' response to the epidemic: did they provide a competent service to the populace or were they overwhelmed by the scale and extent of the numbers of sick? To a very great degree, the authorities were simply overwhelmed. This, of course, was partly due to their own vulnerability to the virus. At one point, 50 per cent of the total staff of the Rangoon General Hospital were unable to work due to flu.

In Rangoon, the authorities responded to the outbreak by organising emergency hospitals, temporary dispensaries and transport for the seriously ill, but in the rest of Burma, the response was meagre. There was no central plan for either containment or treatment of the disease, and the "local hospitals were filled to overflowing".[173] Medicine was said to be available to all those who applied for it, but as this consisted mostly of sedatives, gargles, expectorants and cardiac tonics, probably the indigenous medicines were as effective. The authorities produced two initiatives towards the end of 1918 which, if enacted in August, might have had some effect in containing the disease. These measures included the postponing of fairs and festivals and the temporary closure of entertainment areas. The second measure was the distribution of information about the pandemic in pamphlet form, but, by the time these were produced, the disease was already widespread.

Three major criticisms can be levelled at the authorities. Initially, when the case fatality rate in Rangoon was low, the health officials took no measures to prepare the city or the province for the outbreak. This, of course, is a hindsight criticism, but by June 1918, the disease had spread from Europe to India, and surely by July/August, the authorities in Burma must have been aware that this was a medical emergency, not a routine problem. But, by their own admission, the "Province was practically unprepared to cope with it".[174]

The second major criticism is that no attempt was made to stop the immigration of influenza-infected Indians. The port authorities were faced with the huge problem of arriving migrants (1,777 flu cases were dealt with at the ports),[175] many so ill they had to be immediately hospitalised. Indians, who were packed together as deck passengers and highly vulnerable to infection, brought new infections to Burma and further strained the collapsing medical services. Emergency accommodation was found in godowns on the wharves, or in moored flats in which the patients were provided with medical care by the municipal health staff. Many of the migrants left the ships only to collapse in Rangoon. Of the 944 vessels arriving in 1918, less than half were visited by the port authorities, and the masters often failed to report any infectious disease.[176] Those migrants lucky enough to obtain a hospital bed were usually discharged, still infectious and still ill, in order to provide another emergency case with a bed.

As the authorities had very quickly provided themselves with emergency powers when confronted with plague, it seems astonishing that they did not act to suspend immigration. The Sanitary Commission was already short of medical personnel due to war priorities and, for the same reason, there were no additional staff available to help with the emergencies. The commissioner suggested, in the 1918 annual health report, that in the future, a segregation camp for immigrants should be built at the mouth of the Rangoon River to reduce future risks, and that there should be powers to restrict movements of population and large gatherings in *anticipation* (my emphasis) of widespread epidemics.[177]

The third criticism harks back to the original premise on which the sanitary organisations were founded in the 1860s. It was stated in Chapter Two that the over-riding purpose was to protect the lives of European troops, and the wellbeing of the population was pursued only as a secondary condition. In 1918, a policy of segregation was pursued in the barracks of Burma, which, at Maymyo especially, protected the British "rank and file to a very considerable extent from contracting the infections". The health report then continues: "It does not appear to have been possible to protect native units to the same extent."[178] At the military police barracks in Taungyi, there were three successive outbreaks of infection, each one of which coincided with the arrival of police sepoys from other areas.[179] In the suggestions for the future, Williams, the sanitary commissioner, stated that "All movements of troops, in mass or detail, and of Military Police, should as far as possible be postponed until all risk of their transporting infections has ceased."[180] This was a somewhat belated acknowledgement of a previously unjust or medically unjustifiable policy.

The flu pandemic roared through Burma leaving a trail of sickness, death and economic trauma. Agriculture was paralysed as whole village populations suffered.[181] The response of the authorities was belated; they were totally unprepared and unable to cope with the emergency, and outside Rangoon, "little could be done to organise effective relief".[182]

This chapter has considered the major epidemic diseases that affected adults in Burma and also the impact of the diarrhoeal and respiratory diseases. This, of course, is not the whole picture. The major killer identified in the registration from the beginning was "Fevers", and within this blanket term, malaria was the chief cause of mortality. Fevers were responsible for between 30 per cent and 57 per cent of the total registered mortality between 1891 and 1939. Malaria will be discussed in some depth in Chapter Six.

However, there were a number of other conditions that were either direct or underlying causes of adult mortality in Burma. Many of these, such as typhus, blackwater fever, enteric fever, dengue, Malta fever, rabies and venereal disease, have not been fully discussed. But to write even a brief history of all the diseases of colonial Burma would require more space than is available within the main thrust of this study, so the emphasis has had to be on the major causes of death. Some of the diseases, such as syphilis, have already been discussed briefly in terms of their impact on infant mortality, and the debilitating effect of parasites was examined in Chapter Four. This is not to ignore other causes of death, such as accident, snake bite and trampling by wild animals, but such incidents were statistically insignificant compared to those already discussed. Some diseases, such as yaws, goitre and leprosy, caused debility, much misery and made the Burmese more vulnerable to other bacterial or viral conditions. The distribution and treatment of yaws and goitre will be briefly described as examples of the health authority's approach to these chronic diseases.

Yaws and goitre

Yaws has been discussed briefly as a disease of childhood, but what was its distribution and importance as an adult disease in colonial Burma?

If the answer were based solely on the degree of comment in the health reports, then the conclusion would be that, until 1910, yaws was little known in Burma. But suddenly, in 1910, it was reported to be epidemic in south Mergui and the Pakokku hill tracts.[183] Undoubtedly, yaws, like beri beri, goitre, leprosy and parasites, was a disease with a long history in Burma, but had needed both time and medical interest before it arrived on the colonial agenda. In 1910, an assistant surgeon, Maung Shwe Ge, investigated the prevalence of the disease in the Lower Chindwin district as part of a special inquiry into its incidence that year. He identified 344 cases in 74 villages (these numbers included children).[184] A *Spirochete* organism was isolated at the laboratory in Maymyo, but the investigation came to an end with the closure of the laboratory!

From 1910 until the early 1920s, yaws was mentioned intermittently in the health reports, but from 1924 onwards, it was discussed almost every year. In theory, this could be taken to indicate increased incidence, but it is more than possible that the increased reporting was a function of, instead of increased interest by, the administration, as the focus of their attention changed from epidemic disease to chronic disease. It might also reflect the increase in the sanitary personnel.

The distribution of yaws is quite simple to plot. It was a disease of Upper Burma and the coastal districts of Lower Burma, reported occasionally in Sandoway, but described as most prevalent in Tenasserim and Mergui,[185] and endemic at Victoria Point.[186] In Upper Burma, the disease was repeatedly reported in the Upper and Lower Chindwin, Mandalay, Kyaukse, Katha and Pakokku districts. The 1926 health report stated that knowledge of the distribution of the disease was still incomplete,[187] but the continuing medical surveys from that date and the treatment campaigns identified the affected districts.

Yaws is a disease of poverty and overcrowding leading to unhygienic living conditions. It is therefore not surprising to find that it was common in the malarial districts of Burma, where the population of many villages were described by the health report of 1912 as being "extremely dirty in their persons and clothing, which condition was probably the result of long continued ill-health of all members of the family".[188]

The importance of the disease in terms of the numbers affected can only be guessed at from some of the reports. During the 1920s and 1930s, regular campaigns were run in the infected districts to establish the distribution of the disease, and occasionally, to offer treatment. The number of cases reported were sometimes astonishingly high. In 1928, epidemic conditions were found in 36 out of 50 villages visited in Katha,[189] and during a campaign in the Upper Chindwin district in 1939, more than 10,000 cases were treated.[190] It is impossible to establish from the health records whether these high levels of incidence were new to Burma, or, as has already been suggested, reflect instead the activities and interests of the health officers, and Sanitary Commission.

The response of the colonial administration, therefore, could be described as somewhat belated. It took the form of the campaigns described above, but all too often, there was no money available to treat the victims of yaws. Time and again in the health records, the report states that no treatment was available because there were no funds.[191] Money, when it was raised, came from a variety of sources — from district councils, from the government, from the deputy commissioner's fund, and in 1936, application was also made to the Red Cross for grants.[192]

Another chronic and debilitating disease was goitre, again a disease of very specific localities. It is caused by iodine deficiency and appears in areas where the diet is deficient in iodine. In Burma, it was prevalent in the watersheds of the major rivers — the Irrawaddy, Chindwin, Salween and Sittang. From 1913, it was described as endemic in these hill areas,[193] but the Pakokku hill tracts were undoubtedly the district most often identified in the health records and in 1924, some parts were described as having an 80 per cent incidence in the population.

The approach of the medical authorities in Burma to the investigation, recording and treatment of goitre was very similar to that already described for yaws. Until 1924, the disease received only occasional comment in the health reports, but from that date, it was reported almost every year. Treatment, however, was haphazard. In 1924, medication, in the form of potassium iodide, was given to schoolchildren in the Pakokku hill tracts and Bhamo,[194] but in 1927 and 1930, treatment was offered only to those who sought it.[195] This somewhat half-hearted approach continued until 1937, when a detailed study was conducted in Salin township, and over 8,000 cases were treated in the upper Shan states.[196] In the two subsequent years, further surveys were carried out, culminating in a request, in 1939, from the Inspector General of Civil Hospitals that all schoolchildren in nine affected districts should be treated, and that there should be a census of the children to determine the disease's incidence.[197]

This has a sad and familiar ring to it. The colonial medical authorities were coming to grips with an eminently treatable deficiency disease just before the Second World War put a temporary stop to all progress.

It is perhaps salutary to remember at this point that human beings have to die of something; therefore any discussion of adult mortality must be sensitive to the necessary nature of adult deaths. However, mortality from major epidemic diseases such as cholera, plague, smallpox and malaria were no longer seen as inevitable by the end of the nineteenth century. Medical and sanitary knowledge was advanced enough to prevent most of the excess mortality from these diseases, given the will and the money to employ the necessary measures. The same argument could be advanced about that other great cause of catastrophe mortality — famine. But despite this, there was a huge loss of life due to famine in the Indian sub-continent during the late nineteenth and early twentieth centuries. Was hunger also a potent determinant of mortality in British Burma?

Famine and scarcity

This section will briefly examine the role of famine and food scarcity in the mortality and morbidity rates of colonial Burma. Did many people die of hunger? Was the mortality from the diseases often associated with food scarcity, such as cholera and typhoid, exacerbated by want?

Famine was a familiar occurrence in Burma. Scott and Hardiman described a three-year famine in Magwe district in the late 1770s, during which "Half the population is said to have died."[198] The demographic consequences of the famine that affected most of the country between 1805 and 1814 were discussed in Chapter One. In 1824/25, "The *Mahathayayawgyi*, or great famine … is said to have occurred …. While it was raging the *indaing* tracts were deserted and lapsed into jungle, and a number of people died of starvation."[199] In 1842, outbreaks of cholera in Insein and Syriam were so severe that the fields were not planted and "for two months rice was very scarce and so famine prevailed."[200]

These four periods — 1778, 1805–14, 1824/25 and 1842 — show clearly that more than crop failure or adverse weather was involved in Burma's famines. Each period is complicated by other factors: warfare with the Thais and social upheaval between 1778 and 1814; war with the British in 1824/25, and disease in 1842. No evidence of a direct connection between the British invasion and the famine has been found, but it is probable that a food shortage was exacerbated, firstly by the Burmese attempts to raise a defending army, and then by the movement of armies and disturbance of agriculture as the British occupied Prome, just south of Magwe district.[201]

This pattern was continued in the nineteenth century, as the two succeeding Britain–Burma wars brought food shortages and famine to parts of Burma. In 1852/53, the Burmese army was said to have passed through Magwe district, devastating the country as it went.[202] In 1853, during the struggle for Tharrawaddy and Henzada districts, the price of rice soared to eight rupees a basket, 16 times the normal levels. Destitute people moved into Henzada town, and parts of the rural district were deserted.[203] Prices also reached eight rupees a basket in Hanthawaddy district.

The third war brought similar disasters. In Tharrawaddy district, the natural disasters of a cholera outbreak and crop failures in 1888 were aggravated by the uprising against the British. The resulting distress and poverty caused many families to offer their children for adoption.[204] These parents were not selling their children into slavery, but were instead seeking adoptive parents who were wealthy enough to feed them, usually in return for a small sum of money. This should be interpreted, therefore, as an indication of great distress and hunger, not venality. This practice was also recorded in Shwebo district during the famine of 1891/92. Children were given away at Mandalay and Sagaing in exchange for a few *pyis* of rice for the parents, and for the children the hope that they would be fed.[205]

It is difficult to judge the severity of the food shortages and famines that occurred in Upper Burma between 1891 and 1894, and it is also difficult to judge how much of the shortage was due to natural disaster and how much to guerrilla warfare. The districts affected were Lower Chindwin, Pakokku, Thayetmyo, Yamethin, Meiktila, Minbu, Myingyan and Shwebo. It is impossible to ascertain whether mortality increased in these districts during the famine period, as the registration of deaths had not been introduced into the rural areas, but there is no doubt that there was severe distress. This is illustrated by the degree of depopulation that occurred as families or whole villages emigrated to Lower Burma. In Shwebo district, the "majority of the jungle population are said to have left the district. Whole families moved away, and in some villages not a soul was left behind."[206] This migration was encouraged by the British authorities, as land was available in Lower Burma and the movement relieved them from the responsibility of providing famine relief in the affected villages.

The duration of this type of migration (a response to the "push" of famine) varied in its extent from one season to permanent settlement. Sometimes the move was a temporary expedient, involving a larger proportion of the adult male population seeking seasonal work than was necessary in a good agricultural year, but even when whole families moved, a rapid return to Upper Burma was quite common. In 1891, more than 6,000 families emigrated from Meiktila district to Lower Burma, but "a large number of these returned" to their villages in the good agricultural years of 1893 and 1894. However, famines in the following two years led to another large migration.[207] In Shwebo district, the interval between the out-migration and return was, for some of the people, 30 years. "A few village sites which were deserted at that time (1891/1892) have been re-occupied thirty years later on the opening of the Yeu Canal by the former occupiers or their descendants who in the interval had been residing in Toungoo District."[208]

The British response to famine and food shortages in Upper Burma was governed largely by their experience in India. In some years, relief works were opened, which provided either food or the money to buy food, in return for labour on, for example, road construction. This approach to famine relief was used in Minbu, Yamethin, Pakokku and the Lower Chindwin districts in the 1890s. The alternative, used when material distress was the problem rather than outright famine, was to relieve or remit the *thathameda*, or poll tax. The 1890/91 growing season in the Lower Chindwin was so poor that the *thathameda* tax was reduced from ten rupees to four or five rupees, and remittance of the tax was also necessary in 1891/92, 1895/96 and 1896/97.[209]

In 1897, cholera added to the existing distress in Meiktila district. The death rate in Meiktila town rose to 42 per 1,000 from a previous average of 25 to 30 per 1,000. The *thathameda* tax was remitted on 3,863 households, and reduced for the rest of the district population.[210]

Other bad years followed. Many of the dry zone districts suffered food shortages or famines between 1895 and 1898, and between 1904 and 1908. The season of 1896/97 was remarkable in that the word "famine" was used to describe the situation in Upper Burma, a phrase of admission that was very seldom used in British India.[211]

Charles Keeton argued in *King Thebaw and the Ecological Rape of Burma* that the wet-rice agriculture of Upper Burma was severely damaged by deforestation during the reigns of Mindon and Thebaw.[212] There is no doubt that deforestation causes loss of water through flash flooding, but was this exacerbated in Upper Burma during Thebaw's reign? Keeton attributed the famine of 1883–85 to new deforestation, and this would perhaps partly account for the continuous problems experienced by districts such as the Lower Chindwin, where, he argued, new dry crops such as sesamum and millet were by necessity replacing upland rice.[213] Crop changes were also necessary in Myingyan district following the 1856/57 famine. New cultivation patterns were developed; more sesamum and jowar were grown and less of the more water-dependent rice.[214]

It is probable that deforestation was a contributing factor to famine, but in many dry zone districts, forest clearance predated Mindon's reign and other factors were therefore involved. When the government or local authority was weak or the country disturbed, the maintenance of the irrigation canals was neglected. In Kyaukse district, the canals were said to be in "a bad state" following disorder under Thebaw and guerrilla fighting against the British.[215] The Burmese people had an additional explanation for the bad harvests following the British invasion which was noted by the settlement officer of Mandalay district: it is "impossible not to notice the fact that the succession of dry years since 1887 is more or less associated with and attributed to the entrance of a non-Buddhist power."[216]

There were few years of outright famine between 1920 and 1940, although economically, there were some years of "unrelieved gloom for the agriculturalist" in the 1930s.[217] The 1920 and 1921 seasons were remarkable for soaring rice prices, but these were probably a product of the flu pandemic which must have disturbed the planting and harvesting. The 1932 season was notable for the failure of the middle rains in the dry zone. Relief works were opened in Myingyan, Yamethin, Meiktila, Kyaukse and Magwe districts due to the "wholesale failure of early sesamum and cotton."[218]

The sanitary commissioners used their annual reports to debate a possible connection between scarcity, high food prices and fluctuations in the mortality rate. However, due to the erratic nature of the mortality rates recorded by the registration system, they were unable to draw any firm conclusions and, even with the benefit of hindsight, the connections are complicated by other factors. For example, in 1938, the registered mortality rate was 25.73 per 1,000, the highest since the flu pandemic, and the annual health report described a disastrous agricultural season. The sanitary commissioner commented that December 1937 "will long be remembered for the unusual and abnormal wetness of the first and the last weeks and the consequent damage to crops in many parts of the country."[219] But simplistic assumptions should not be made: the "Fever" death rate rose steadily throughout the 1930s, and from 1936 to 1939, "Fever" deaths were between 38 and 40 per cent of the total registered mortality. The erratic and unseasonable rainfall that destroyed crops in December 1937 may have raised the death rate from malaria by the provision of more breeding places for anophelines. Therefore the high death rate in 1938 may well have been due to the combination of food scarcity and increased malarial parasitaemia.

The low annual rainfall of many dry zone districts made them vulnerable to scarcity and crop failure. Such scarcity or famine could be very local, severely affecting only one or two districts, whereas other dry zone districts would receive normal rainfall. Unfortunately the British administration altered the locality of the weather recording stations many times, making it almost impossible to plot these local fluctuations. Also, the rainfall was often described in the annual health reports as being in "excess", or "normal", or in "slight defect" instead of a directly comparable measurement. Despite these defects in the records, it is apparent that a variation of ten inches in the measured annual rainfall of dry zone districts was common, and as this was up to 30 per cent of the total rainfall, it could be critical. The seasonal distribution was also important, because in the fragile agricultural ecology of the dry zone the timing and duration of the rains could be as important as their quantity. In 1926, the total rainfall was above average but the monsoon was late, causing scarcity of water in April and May, and then flooding from the excess water in June and July. Forty-four inches of rain were recorded in Minbu district in that year, which compares to a ten-year average of 34 inches; and in Yamethin district, 47 inches were recorded, compared to a ten-year average of 38 inches.[220]

This brief examination of famine and food scarcity in Burma has not revealed the extent of the mortality attributable to hunger. The agricultural ecology of Upper Burma was unstable due to the low and uncertain rainfall, and this situation was probably exacerbated over time by deforestation. But the evidence suggests that real famine was usually local, unless accompanied by social catastrophe of some kind. If there were no exceptional circumstances creating a general famine, then the effects of local famine were usually relieved by the availability of food and work in adjacent districts. The British relief works therefore, in many ways, fitted into a pattern that already existed, that of emigration to obtain work and the ability to buy food. On some occasions, the Burmese preferred their traditional safety nets to those provided by the British. In 1897 and 1907, test famine relief works were opened in Thayetmyo district, but "not a single volunteer" was found as the cultivators refused to accept work at such low rates of pay.[221]

If the registration statistics had been more reliable, it would have been possible to analyse the data on a district-by-district basis for the famine-related diseases where the excess mortality is normally found. Sen noticed that the excess mortality in the Bengal famine of 1943 followed the normal seasonal pattern, "just linearly displaced severely upwards". He also described the main causes of this excess mortality as the endemic diseases of the region.[222] But the Burma registration data is so erratic that it would be very easy to "prove" both excess mortality and a decline in mortality following scarcity or famine. It can only be concluded therefore that the mortality from endemic disease was almost certainly increased by periods of famine and food scarcity, but that quantification of this is not possible.

Conclusion

In summary, this chapter has attempted to discuss the levels, causes and seasonality of adult mortality in the colonial period. The estimates from the life tables suggest that this adult mortality, as a percentage of the total mortality, fell in the 1920s and 1930s, although the overall CDR levels rose from 32.5 in 1901 to over 37 per 1,000 from 1921 onwards. Also, the registration data strongly suggests a seasonality shift in the total mortality from summer to winter (Figure 5.1a to f), which is a very significant indicator of changing disease patterns.

The role of the major epidemic diseases, cholera, plague, and smallpox in the history and pattern of mortality has been discussed. It was found that, statistically, the decline in these epidemic diseases could not explain the changing percentages of adult and child mortality, despite their accounting for the decline from a total of 7.6 per cent of registered mortality from 1902 to 1911 to two per cent between 1932 and 1939. An attempt was made within the discussion of these epidemic diseases to assess two other factors, the role of the Indian migrant in the dissemination of infection and the response of the colonial authorities to public health needs. Two ideas emerged from these discussions: firstly that the migrants from India became both victims and "whipping boys", in that their social and economic circumstances made them vulnerable to disease and they were then accused of disseminating it. The second fact to emerge was the formative role that the epidemic diseases, especially plague, took in the development of a public health service in Burma.

What also emerges from the colonial health records is the, perhaps astonishing, number of improvements that were planned by the commissioners, but which "died" or were "stillborn" due to scarcity of money and resources. A clear change can be seen between the laissez-faire policies of the closing decade of the nineteenth century and the more interventionist years of the 1930s, as views of governmental responsibilities changed across the world.

An attempt was also made to assess the significance and the mortality from other diseases such as bowel and respiratory infections. It was found that bowel disease affected the urban poor and Indian migrants disproportionately, but declined sharply as a percentage of the overall mortality. Deaths from respiratory diseases rose, but as this overall category was not introduced into the registration system until 1901, the numbers would be expected to rise as familiarity with the classification improved. Complicating the respiratory registration was the rise in urban tuberculosis, which all the evidence suggests was imported with the British annexation. A major factor influencing the number of deaths from 1918 to 1921 was of course the flu pandemic. A very rough estimate was made that the total "excess" deaths due to the pandemic in the whole of Burma was 400,000, though this may well be too modest a figure.

Another factor that this chapter attempted to assess was the role of food scarcity in the overall mortality. The registration and health records are too erratic to enable firm conclusions to be drawn, but food scarcity probably exacerbated disease levels. During the colonial period, the scarcities were usually localised and relieved by the seeking of work in adjoining districts.

Ironically, as will be discussed in Chapter Six, in the areas of malnutrition and malaria the initiatives were half-hearted, belated and ineffective. This was despite the huge erosion of life through "Fever" deaths and the morbidity caused by nutritional diseases.

6 The determinants of mortality: Nutrition and malaria in colonial Burma

The object of this chapter is to examine and expand the argument, already put forward in the earlier chapters, that the population of Burma grew more slowly from 1911 onwards. Two underlying reasons have been suggested for this: a chronic state of under- or malnutrition in much of the population, and a high and increasing number of deaths that were malaria-related.

In this chapter, both nutrition and malaria will be discussed in relation to the whole population, and not for their effects on specific sectors (such as infant mortality) as has already been examined. An attempt will be made to discover how these changes (if they were changes) arose, their results as determinants of demographic change, and the reaction of the British administration to the problems.

Nutrition

Jacques May, author of *The Ecology of Malnutrition in the Far and Near East*, wrote in September 1960 that diets in the Far and Near East "are usually sufficient to sustain a miserable life for a short duration".[1] Certainly the average Burmese life under British rule had a short duration, but was it also nutritionally a "miserable life"? Rice is and was the staple food of Burma, but was it an inadequate food, and did the diet change for better or for worse in the colonial period?

How ancient is the cultivation of rice in Burma and the rest of Southeast Asia? At the present time the answer is not proven, although Anthony Reid suggested that "rice is probably indigenous to Southeast Asia and has been for millennia the basic staple of the great majority of its people."[2] George Coedès wrote of "the rich rice-producing plain of Kyaukse" in connection with the existence of groups of Pyus in

Burma prior to the sixth century AD.[3] Victor Lieberman mentions that sixteenth-century European visitors to Burma commented on the prosperous rice-growing districts of the Mon country, and the Burmese Land Rolls of 1784 and 1802 record paddy areas in Hanthawaddy, Martaban, Kyaukse, Minbu and the Mu valley, as well as dry-rice cultivation in many areas.[4] It will probably be the sophisticated testing of rice seeds by archaeologists that will confirm the very early existence of the crop in Southeast Asia, but what must be remembered is that the long history of rice consumption in the region has contributed to the great cultural and religious significance of rice in Burma.

During the colonial period, both change and continuity are apparent. Agriculture and, therefore, the choice of food crops are dependent on soil and climate, and there is no evidence of substantial climatic change. Wet- and dry-rice cultivation had traditionally dominated Burmese agriculture, with the additional dry zone crops of pulses, sesamum and millet.[5] In areas of lower population density, for example in the delta prior to the 1850s, and in the hill districts, shifting cultivation was practised. In 1940, rice was still the most important crop in Burma. Pulses, sesamum and millet were grown in addition to rice in the dry zone, and shifting cultivation was still practised in the hills.

These are obvious and simplistic statements of continuity but one major change is equally manifest — the enormous expansion of rice cultivation in the delta. This extension of the cultivated rice acreage, from around 1.3 million acres in 1860 to 9.9 million acres in 1940,[6] produced a huge surplus of rice, and turned the country into a major food exporter. In the next section, the effect of this development on the Burmese diet will be discussed.

Effect of the expansion of rice milling on the Burmese diet

The new rice export industry was responsible for producing another major change — the development of a large rice-milling industry. The history of the rice industry and the European, Chinese and Indian involvement in its development has been well documented by Cheng Siok-Hwa and M. S. I. Diokno among others,[7] and will not be discussed here, but the consequences for the Burmese diet of the introduction of power mills has not been fully explored.

According to Cheng, until about 1900, "the bulk of the mills were situated in the four main ports",[8] but from that date there was a very rapid development of small, upcountry mills owned and/or operated by Burmans.[9] The problem is that the exact number of these mills is not known, as only the larger mills that employed ten or more people were required to be registered under the Factories Act or the List of Industrial

Establishments, and "many escaped enumeration and inspection by employing less than ten workers each".[10]

Some guidance to the probable growth rate in the number of the small mills can be taken from the very rapid expansion of the larger, registered mills. These grew in number from a total of 83 in 1900 to 353 in 1920 and 683 in 1940,[11] and of these large mills, two were owned by Burmans in 1898 and 334 in 1936.[12] (There is no evidence to suggest that the number of small mills did not expand as rapidly as these larger units, especially as cheap and efficient milling units were imported from Germany.[13]) Both Diokno and Cheng have ably documented the growth of the industry and the imbalance of economic power that existed between the very large European mills and the small Burmese mills; but the significant factor for dietary analysis is that, especially in Upper Burma, much of this milling was done "for home consumption".[14]

These indigenous mills were established in paddy-growing areas "where knowledge of local conditions was an advantage"[15] and where small lots of paddy could be economically machine-milled for home consumption without incurring heavy transport costs. The Burmese ate by preference a milled rice known as "Small Mills Specials", or one of a slightly better quality known as "Bazaar Quality".[16] The Small Mills Specials was milled from "poor to medium qualities of paddy", and up to 42 per cent of broken grains were allowed in the finished product.[17] The name and the quality of the product therefore indicate that it was the produce of small, local mills and that it was essentially a poor product containing many broken grains.

The change from the habitual consumption of hand-milled rice to machine-milled rice was rapid. An *Agricultural Bulletin Report* in 1913 stated that "In a survey carried out by Government officials it was found that even the very poor Burmese considered unpolished rice unfit for consumption and that according to Burmese consumers the more perfect the polish the better in taste, flavour and appearance was the cooked rice".[18]

Comparing the nutritive values of home-pounded rice to machine-milled rice
The discussion so far has examined the history of rice consumption in Burma and the expansion from 1900 of the rice milling industry, especially the small mills that produced rice for home consumption. But to understand why a change from eating home-pounded rice to eating highly milled rice was important, it is necessary to understand the structure of the rice grain.

In the following discussion the terms used are those defined by the United Nations Food and Agriculture Organisation. "Paddy" is rice that is still in the husk, while "husked" or "brown rice" is paddy minus its husk but with the germ, pericarp and aleurone layers intact. "Home (-pounded)" or "hand-pounded" rice has had the husk and aleurone layer removed without the use of power machinery. "Milled", "highly milled" or "white" rice has had the germ, pericarp and aleurone layers removed by power machinery, while "under-milled" or "lightly milled" rice retains a degree of the germ, pericarp and aleurone layers.[19]

It can be seen that the effect of milling is to remove the outer layers of the rice grain, but unfortunately, "protein, fat, vitamins and minerals are present in greater quantities in the germ and the outer layers than in the starchy endosperm".[20] Thus the degree of milling determines the degree of lost nutrients, and also the percentage of water-soluble nutrients lost when the grain is washed.

The percentage of nutrients lost is not insignificant. The FAO Nutritional Survey of 1948 reported that 76 per cent, 56 per cent and 63 per cent respectively of the thiamine, riboflavine and niacin contents of husked rice were lost during the processing that turned paddy into milled rice.[21] But home or hand-pounded rice, due to the retention of the germ and parts of the aleurone layer, retained 2.4µg per gram of thiamine compared to only 1µg per gram in milled rice — or more than twice as much.[22]

In 1967, Pe Kyin, the director of Health Services, published tables showing the nutritive values of five different types of rice grown in Burma. The amounts of thiamine, or Vitamin B1, in the dehusked rice was between 0.37mg and 0.48mg per 100g of edible portion of rice. The loss of thiamine through milling was progressive, until in the final product of polished white rice, the content was between 0.07mg and 0.10mg per 100g of edible portion. This represents a loss of approximately 80 per cent.[23]

An alternative method of preparing paddy found little favour with Burmese consumers. This was the technique of parboiling, widely used in India, which involved the soaking and then the steaming of the unhusked grain. The paddy was then dried and milled in the usual way, either by machine or by hand. Large quantities of parboiled rice were exported from Burma, a million tons a year by the late 1930s, but the small amounts retained in the country were bought by Indians.[24] Both the process and the product were unpopular with the Burmese. Complaints about the odours from parboiling were common, although in 1923, the agricultural chemist in Burma was said to have devised a process that mitigated the nuisance.[25]

Nutritionally, parboiled rice is far superior to machine-milled rice. During the steaming process, thiamine and other water-soluble nutrients from the germ and aleurone layers diffuse through the grain.[26] The result is that the final product, the parboiled milled rice, contains more than twice the amount of thiamine and niacin and one and a half times the amount of riboflavine of the milled, raw rice.[27] The other advantage that parboiled rice has over milled rice is that the vitamin content of the rice is affected far less by washing. For example, while between six and 15 per cent of the thiamine in parboiled rice is lost during washing, more than 40 per cent of the thiamine is lost from milled rice.[28]

All the evidence suggests that the consequence of changing from hand-pounded rice to machine-milled rice entailed a damaging loss of vitamins and protein from the Burmese diet. Machine-milled rice after cooking contains only 0.7 to 0.9µg per gram of thiamine, whereas hand-pounded rice contains 1.6 to 2.8µg per gram of thiamine. Deficiency of this vitamin in the diet causes the disease beri beri. "The loss of thiamine due to machine milling is the main cause of beri beri in rice eaters."[29] Is there evidence to show that beri beri existed in Burma and that it was extensive enough to be considered an important determinant of mortality? Did the incidence of the disease increase after 1900 with the rise in the availability of milled rice?

The history of beri beri in colonial Burma

Confirmation of the existence of beri beri in Burma appears in the first health report of 1867, when several deaths were reported amongst the population in Bassein gaol. The treatment given to the other affected prisoners was a "nourishing diet with a free use of Gin Punch combined with Calomel"[30]; the treatment was said to have had satisfactory results. In the same year, outbreaks were also reported in the Irrawaddy division.

This theme of beri beri in gaols was to prove a constant one in British Burma,[31] and 52 years later, in 1919, the sanitary commissioner, C. E. Williams, stated that "The frequently recurring outbreaks of beri beri among under-trials and others confined in lock-ups undeniably constitute a stigma upon Police Administration in this Province, and call for close investigation and remedial measures."[32] Unfortunately, it was not only in the gaols that investigation and action were required.

Beri beri in gaols, lighthouses and timber camps could be defined as "industrial or contract" beri beri, and appeared with depressing and shameful persistence. It was associated with both large and small groups of workers who, for reasons of economy and or isolation, were fed on rations usually supplied by contractors.[33] A common practice of the contractors was to purchase three or six months' supply of milled rice for their workers or gaol inmates, which was then stored (often under damp conditions) until it was required. This process was frequently followed in the timber camps, lighthouses and mining camps.

Industrial beri beri

The first reference to beri beri in lighthouses appeared in 1908[34] when, in response to reports of the disease in several light-stations, a special enquiry was initiated. As a result of this enquiry, and information gained from experiments undertaken in the Federated Malay States,[35] it was decided to issue only parboiled rice to lighthouse keepers. This change, which increased the vitamin content of the diet, was put into effect in May 1911 and was presumably effective as little further reference is made in the health reports to beri beri in lighthouses or lightships.[36]

The swift moves to protect the efficient manning of the lighthouses appear in stark contrast to the inaction in other fields. Despite the acknowledgement that "The prevention, the prophylaxis of beri beri is the avoidance of stale, uncured rice",[37] no regulations were passed to protect the health of the general population or those on diets supplied by the contractors.

The mission schools and training schools cannot be exempt from criticism. The occurrence of beri beri at mission schools (discussed in Chapter Four) was not confined to any particular denomination, but occurred wherever rations were inadequate in thiamine. The recruits at the Police Training School at Mandalay suffered an outbreak in 1913; with further cases reported amongst Karen recruits at Shwebo in 1918.[38] In 1923, there were outbreaks at Myingyan amongst students at the Police Training School, and also at the Teachers Elementary Training School.[39]

Probably most shameful, because it was the most persistently recurring, were the beri beri outbreaks in timber camps. References to this appeared in the annual health reports in 1909, 1918, 1919, 1930, 1932, 1933, 1934, 1935 and 1936. J. H. Williams, who worked at the timber camps of the Bombay Trading Corporation from 1920, described women in forestry camps with their breasts split like ripe tomatoes from beri beri swelling.[40] In addition, John Taylor, C. de C. Martin and U Thant, who published their "Preliminary Enquiry into Beri Beri in Burma" in 1928, reported outbreaks in forest camps in Pegu, Toungoo, Tharrawaddy, Upper Chindwin and Myingyan districts and recorded "serious" outbreaks with many deaths each year from 1921 to 1924. An example of these outbreaks was the 41 deaths recorded in the two reserves of Kadat and south Zamayi between October 1923 and March 1924.[41]

An outbreak of beri beri on Cheduba island (Arakan district) cost 188 lives in 1929. The disease was found to be endemic in the rainy seasons but was particularly severe that year, affecting 1,650 people. Most of the victims were men between the ages of 18 and 30 years and engaged in strenuous work in the fields. Despite a population of 32,500, there were no medical staff on the island, no dispensaries, no hospitals and, perhaps even more importantly, no roads. During the rainy season, when food was at its shortest and the work hardest, communications between the inland and coastal villages became impossible. During the other seasons, fish from the coast was exchanged for pulses, peas and beans from inland villages. But during the wet season, there was no fishing and the coastal villagers lived on rice and a little *gnapi* (fish paste). The rice was stale by then and, although hand pounded, "was exceptionally thoroughly decorticated for hand pounded rice".[42]

Two important omissions should be noted at this point in the discussion. The first is that the evidence from the British records, with few exceptions, concerns mission students, prisoners, and industrial workers only, while very little attention is paid to the possibility of beri beri amongst the mass of the Burmese population living in the rural areas. The second omission is the authorities' lack of effective response to the repeated outbreaks of the disease in gaols and camps. It should be remembered that the Sanitary Commissioner had taken action to prevent beri beri in lighthouses from May 1911, and that enough was known about the disease to make this prevention relatively simple, but despite this, regular outbreaks in the timber camps were still being reported as late as 1936.

Taylor, Martin and U Thant had found that the occurrence of beri beri in timber camps was always linked to one of two factors: either the buying in bulk of milled rice and its storage in the forest through the monsoon period, or the bulk buying of hand-pounded rice and its prolonged storage. In the forests of the Taungdwin Circle (Upper Chindwin district), hand-pounded rice was stored for nine months in a godown by the Bombay Trading Corporation for their Burmese workmen. Samples of the rice from different levels in the heap "were all found to be friable and dirty and the outer layers of the grain powdered off easily. At the bottom and sides white ants had tunnelled into the grain which was caked with the earthy matter of which the tunnels are constructed."[43]

The poor condition of this rice was not exceptional. Samples from a contractor's camp in Pegu district were found to be "composed of opaque yellowish grains, dirty, mouldy and friable".[44] At this camp, of 19 men employed, 12 contracted beri beri and some died.[45]

The reserves in Pegu district were worked by Messrs Foucar and Company, and it was their practice to import milled rice from Pegu for their employees and contractors, and to store it during the monsoon period. However, in 1925, "Owing to their previous experience of the *serious interruption of their work* which had been caused by beri beri over the past four years" (my emphasis), they arranged to purchase local paddy and to send a month's supply of freshly hand-pounded rice to each camp as needed.[46] No beri beri cases occurred amongst those who ate this rice.

Part of the problem for those who worked in the forests (and the military police) was that their isolation made it difficult to obtain the variants of green vegetables, fruits and some fish proteins used in the Burmese diet. In one outbreak of beri beri at a military police outpost in Shwebo in 1918, 25 out of 129 recruits contracted the disease. Their issued rations consisted of rice and salt only; it was milled rice and stored under damp conditions.[47] Chin and Karen military police received only this very meagre ration, but Indian recruits were given the full official rations, which included *atta*,[48] and they did not succumb to beri beri. It is notable that this outbreak was dealt with in the same way that many forestry outbreaks were dealt with, that is by sending the sick Karens back to their own hill villages where they could obtain hand-pounded rice and vegetables. Although it is not explicitly stated in the report, it is quite clear that the police authorities and forestry officials were aware that the diets in the villages would probably effect a cure. This type of outbreak, whether it was at a school, a military police outpost, a forest or a mining camp, resulted from dependence on issued rations, where the location made it difficult to supplement a nutritionally inadequate diet.

Poverty-induced beri beri
Most of the other recorded beri beri deaths in colonial Burma were associated with a poverty-induced poor diet. Inevitably Hindu coolies were noted to be amongst the greatest sufferers. Between 1909 and 1938, 19 separate references appear in the annual health reports to the prevalence of beri beri amongst Indian coolies. In 1909, it was described as "endemic in many places in the Irrawaddy Delta", mainly amongst Indian coolies eating inferior rice.[49] Bassein town and Rangoon figured largely in these reports due to their high proportion of temporary migrant labour, identified in Taylor, Martin and U Thant's beri beri enquiry as having the poorest diet in Burma. The comments were continuous, the mortality inexcusable. In 1913 at Bassein, 61 deaths occurred, "mainly Indian coolies",[50] and in the same year at Mandalay town, there were many cases "mostly among the poverty stricken classes".[51]

The Hindu coolies in the mining populations of Tavoy and Mergui were noted as prone to beri beri outbreaks, which were reported in 1916, 1917, 1919 and 1920. The vulnerability of Hindu coolies was emphasised by the disproportion in the number of deaths. For example, in Rangoon in 1922, 86 out of 183 beri beri deaths were Hindu. In

Bassein town in the same year, there were 18 deaths of which 11 were Hindu.[52] In 1923, the proportion was much higher. Of 116 deaths in Rangoon, 75 per cent were coolies,[53] and in 1929, 97 out of 128 deaths were Hindu.[54] In Bassein, the reports note that the deaths are all "from the poorest Indian classes"[55] or, in another year, "in the poorer quarters of the town where people of the coolie class reside."[56]

Some recognition of the responsibilities of the employers of this labour was shown by the sanitary commissioner in 1922, who suggested in his report that employers of labour on rice diets should see that these men were supplied with more lightly milled rice, or an addition to the diet of items such as germinated beans.[57] However, the continuing mortality suggested that these remarks had little effect, and no legislation to protect these men was put into place.

The evidence of the Royal Commission on Labour, whose report was published in 1931, shows all too clearly that the problems of poverty, unemployment and malnutrition amongst Indian coolies were still not considered by employers to be worthy of action.[58] The mortality in towns continued to show high proportions of Hindu deaths: in Rangoon in 1931, 55 out of 74 deaths from beri beri were Hindu,[59] in 1932 in Rangoon, the proportion was 81 of 97 deaths.[60] In 1935, 72 per cent of those affected in Rangoon were Bengali,[61] and it was noted that in Pyapon district the disease was confined to Indian coolies, who had an ill-balanced diet due to their low standard of living and their consumption of damp and deteriorated rice.[62] It must be emphasised again that these are registered deaths, and the deaths in the rural areas probably went unrecorded.

The vulnerability of this group of migrant workers to beri beri is clear. Taylor, Martin and U Thant published tables of diets (in their 1928 report on beri beri) that show variations between the poorest industrial workers, such as Rangoon dock labourers or workers in the rice mills, and the non-coolie class Hindus and Muslims with more stable employment. The main difference is in the quantity of rice each consumed daily; the poorer labourers ate about 2.25 to 2.75 pounds (1 to 1.2 kg) of rice, compared to average urban Burmese, Muslim, or better off Hindus who consumed 1.25 to 1.5 pounds (0.55 to 0.7 kg) per day.[63]

Taylor, Martin and U Thant found that the poorest labourers not only ate an unbalanced diet with excessive rice carbohydrate, but that the rice purchased by these coolies was often mixed, broken and remilled.[64] Due to the paucity of vegetables and meat, there was no compensation in the diet for the vitamin deficiency of this rice.

The recorded incidence of beri beri in British Burma was severe enough by 1925 to warrant the investigation by Taylor, Martin and U Thant (this will be examined in the next section). Although the diets of four sample villages were looked at, little or no attempt was made to discover the extent of the disease in the rural population. This was despite the inconclusive investigation of a village outbreak in Maubin district, about which a civil surgeon notified the investigators. The surgeon made no visit to examine the 18 cases, no dispensary or hospital treatment was sought and, as the report noted, the outbreak did not appear in any statistical record, "and it seems quite possible that similar instances occur and beri-beri of a mild form may be considerably more common in Burma than the records suggest."[65] This lack of interest in the mass of the population can only lead to the conclusion that the survey was instigated for economic reasons, because the ill health amongst coolies and forestry workers was causing financial damage.

This discussion has established sufficient evidence to confirm a widespread incidence of recorded beri beri outbreaks, usually amongst the poorer coolies or labourers subject to feeding by "rations". But to this point it has been mainly a disease history of Hindus, Chins and Karens, with little evidence as to whether or not the health of the Burmese rural population was being affected by the introduction of milled rice.

Evidence of nutritional deficiencies in the Burmese population

On occasion, references appeared in the records to suggest that beri beri was more widespread than was commonly admitted. The health report of 1910 stated that the chief centres for beri beri in Burma were the districts of Bassein, Toungoo, Henzada, Pyapon, Insein, Maubin and Thayetmyo, as well as Rangoon and Thonze, with cases also appearing in Shwebo, Kindat and Mandalay.[66] It seems unlikely, given the number of districts named, that the authorities were referring to "industrial" beri beri only.

An isolated comment in 1919 by C. E. Williams, the sanitary commissioner, reveals a remarkable early assessment of the problem, and his analysis predates the comments of the Union of Burma survey, which was conducted 42 years later on the nutrition of the security forces and their dependants: "There is constantly a very narrow margin in their [the Burmese] diets of the quantity of nerve food in excess of the minimum supply necessary to prevent actual nerve starvation, resulting in beri beri."[67] Williams saw this equilibrium as being easily upset by changed conditions. The 1963 report of the Union of Burma survey, which was conducted in 1961, also assessed the situation: "the thiamine problem is a borderline one ... beri beri does exist in Burma and in particular is an ever present danger given the proper stressful situations."[68] These situations were suggested as pregnancy, diarrhoea, strenuous military operations, or a partial famine from an environmental catastrophe.[69]

By 1927/28, the discussion had widened slightly and included mention of the increase in registered deaths from beri beri, which were recorded in urban areas only. But the health reports also contained reports from district health officers (DHOs) of deaths in rural areas. It is significant and indicative of the developing official interest in beri beri and deficiencies that in 1931, the sanitary commissioner noted that the Burmese people were known to use fresh country liquor, or "rice beer", as a beri beri cure; a local response to a local problem.[70]

It is possible to say that by the mid-1930s, beri beri was recognised as a problem in rural Burma by the health authorities. But significantly, by that date, interest in the disease more broadly had risen and the district authorities were looking for incidence in the rural areas. When the medical staff looked for beri beri they found it, but previously the DHOs had, on the whole, not looked.

In 1935, the director of public health expressed concern because no figures of beri beri incidence were available for the rural areas,[71] and two years later, there was more criticism of the lack of information on the disease in the countryside.[72] These remarks in the health reports indicated, for the first time since 1919, official unease that a common and widespread disease might exist in the rural areas of which very little was known. In 1938, J. T. Davidson, the director of public health, wrote that beri beri was now appearing among Burman and Karen field labourers. "It appears at a time when this class is engaged in strenuous labour and subsides at harvest season when more food is available."[73]

This description by Davidson defines exactly the condition of "sub-clinical" beri beri noted by Williams in 1919 and the Union of Burma survey report in 1963. This was a state of deficiency, not yet overt beri beri until the stress of lactation, pregnancy, hunger or heavy physical exertion precipitated the disease.

Taylor, Martin and U Thant did not believe that beri beri was a problem in the rural areas of Burma, despite their comment that mild beri beri may be considerably more common in Burma than the records suggest. They concluded in their report that "Such information as has been obtained very strongly suggests that over the greater part of the populous agricultural areas of Burma beri beri is not endemic or epidemic to any extent and although cases do occur their total number is very small."[74] They reached this conclusion despite admitting that the "statistical evidence is weak"[75] and that the records "are very incomplete as regards the Districts".[76]

Their inquiry was based on an investigation of reported cases, which were either urban hospital returns or reported incidents from employers of labour. In addition, the investigating team visited eight selected districts, but again the case figures were drawn from the headquarters town, the civil hospital, the gaol and military police lines, not from the mass of the rural population that lived in the smaller towns and villages. An attempt was made to assess the rural figures for the selected districts, but the only cases reported were deaths in timber camps. No sampling of rural populations was undertaken, and the absence of reported cases was taken as negative evidence, despite the information from the village in Maubin district confirming that villagers did not seek western medical help.

The enquiry team based this opinion partly on their examination of the diets of four villages near Pegu, Prome, Thayetmyo and Mektila. They reported that "as a rule" the rice used was hand pounded, but in the case of the Pegu village, "75 per cent of the inhabitants take their paddy to Pegu for machine milling and store when returned milled [*sic*]."[77] The report adds: "This practice is increasing in regard to villages in the vicinity of milling centres."[78]

It is in this part of the report that the weakness of the enquiry would seem to lie. Only four village diets were sampled to provide a picture of village Burma from which the generalised conclusions were drawn. In contrast, the diets of eight district towns were examined. In four of them — Bassein, Myingyan, Pegu, and Mandalay — the poorer Burmese were found to eat milled rice, though seldom highly polished. In Thayetmyo and Prome, either milled or hand-pounded rice was used, and in Toungoo and Meiktila, the rice was hand pounded.

This means that of the four villages selected for dietary examination, three were close to headquarters towns where hand-pounded rice or a mixture of machine-milled and hand-pounded rice was commonly used. This led to the conclusion that Burmese villagers had a diet that was "not of a type to favour the occurrence of beri beri",[79] but it is clear that the choice of villages caused considerable bias. If the investigators had examined the diet of villages near Bassein, Mandalay, Myingyan and Pegu, they might well have concluded that most Burmese villagers ate machine-milled rice, a diet that was likely to cause beri beri.

Perhaps it is too easy to criticise past investigations, as all enquiries have to work within a brief and a budget. But the conclusion of the report into beri beri was also contrary to the *Agricultural Bulletin Report* of 1913 (mentioned previously), which stated that even poor Burmese considered unpolished rice unfit for consumption and had a marked preference for the highly polished finish.[80]

At this point we may assess the argument so far. The suggestion has been made that the introduction of machine mills into Burma caused damaging changes to the Burmese diet. The evidence for this was the rapid spread of small mills specialising in milling for local consumption, the wide incidence of reported beri beri cases of the "industrial" type, and the evidence from the health records, especially in the 1920s and 1930s, of clinical and sub-clinical beri beri amongst the rural population. Against this must be weighed the conclusion of Taylor, Martin and U Thant's report that beri beri was not endemic or epidemic to any great extent in the rural areas. However, the hypothesis of nutritional deficiency and the critically low levels of thiamine are supported by the first nutrition survey ever undertaken in Burma, which started in 1939. (This has already been discussed with reference to the diets of children in Chapter Four.)

Nutrition survey 1939–41

Doctor U Maung Gale, DHO of Myaungmya district, was appointed Special Nutrition Officer for Burma following a training period at Coonor. The survey that he undertook was a five-year project (curtailed by the Second World War), which included the examination of village children between the ages of four and 12 years, as well as diet surveys. This survey, therefore, entailed actively looking for signs of deficiency diseases; checking the heights and weights of children, and making chemical analyses of the foodstuffs. The survey was conducted between 1939 and 1941 in Bassein, Insein, Thaton, Mergui, Yamethin and Minbu districts, and the findings contrast remarkably with those of Taylor, Martin and U Thant's enquiry into beri beri.

U Maung Gale found a deficiency of calcium and Vitamins A and B "in all classes irrespective of the economic status of the bread winner".[81] There was also a shortage of animal proteins in the diets of the poorer class. This survey, thus, underlines the hypothesis that a high percentage of the Burmese population was suffering from dietary deficiency, especially the critical thiamine deficiency.

Having already examined children's diets, what needs to be discussed in this chapter are the major findings of U Maung Gale's report concerning adult diets and the evidence for the argument that a majority of the Burmese population were eating machine-milled rice by the end of the 1930s.

Before discussing the survey, it is perhaps worth asking why it was conducted? Why, after largely ignoring the health and certainly the diet of the Burmese population for so long, did the colonial administration train a medical officer in nutrition and organise such a survey? It is notable that in contrast to the malaria surveys undertaken, this nutrition survey concentrated on those involved in agriculture, petty trading, crafts and clerical work, and not the minority of the population working in industries such as mining or the military. The answer seems to lie in a complex ideological change that occurred in the scientific, administrative and economic polices of the empire.

A number of developments were associated with this change. The League of Nations was founded, and sponsored, as part of its work, meetings such as the Conference of Far Eastern Countries on Rural Hygiene in 1937. The 1930s was also the time when the idea of "welfare" in the colonies was accepted and was, of course, a period of great economic depression, when governments were looking for innovative ways of improving trade and reviving colonial markets. Michael Warboys has identified these economic factors as one of the major reasons for the sudden, and formerly atypical, anxiety about the health of rural people in the colonies. His analysis (made on the situation in the African colonies but seemingly equally applicable to Burma) was that the administrators saw an attack on colonial malnutrition, when combined with a more balanced agrarian development, as necessary to "aid colonial revenues and trade balance".[82]

When the developments in Burma are viewed through this analysis, they appear quite logical. The Royal Commission on Agriculture visited Burma in the 1930s, and its report was followed promptly by the formation of the Nutrition Advisory Committee of the Indian Research Fund Association in 1936.[83] The committee recommended that a representative from each Indian province should be trained in nutrition; this led directly to the appointment of Dr U Maung Gale as Burma's nutritionist, and the beginning of what was planned as a five-year programme of research.

It may seem harsh to suggest that the British investigated rural diets in Burma only when larger economic reasons made this imperative, but the idea is substantiated by the history of beri beri treatment in Burma. The point has already been made earlier in this chapter that the authorities moved quickly to adjust the diets of military policemen and lighthouse keepers when this was thought necessary in 1911. The scientific knowledge existed early in the twentieth century, but the will to apply it to the general population of Burma was lacking until the late 1930s.

The survey began in January 1939 and was continued in different districts of the country until March 1941. As this was the only authoritative and detailed nutritional survey of Burma in the colonial period, the findings and methodology of the survey will be considered in some detail.

The dietary survey was intended to be thorough and informative. The objective was to establish the nature and amount of the food consumed by families, and the method was to examine, record and weigh family food twice daily for seven days. This work was done by trained volunteers, usually known to the family, who visited the house twice daily at the time of meal preparation. As far as was possible, only the edible portion of the food was weighed, and as any food that was surplus at one meal was consumed at the next, there was very little waste to account for. The analysis covered the calculation of total calories, per cent calories from cereals, total protein and animal protein, total fat, and carbohydrates. The quantities of minerals, calcium, phosphorous, and iron were calculated, and also the values in the diets of Vitamins A, B and C. The foodstuffs that were peculiar to Burma and for which no standard analyses were available were sent to the Harcourt Butler Institute of Public Health in Rangoon.[84]

In each of the districts selected for survey, villages were chosen which represented the different communities within the area, such as rice-growing villages, urban villages or craft villages. The first survey was undertaken in Insein district, where the presence of the Rural Health Unit at Hlegu would be of assistance to the survey team. The methodology and the results of this first survey will be explained in some detail as it set the pattern for the following district surveys, and demonstrates the validity of the findings.

The villages chosen for the survey in Insein district were Hlegu town, Yemun village, Laydaunggan village, Taikkyigon village, Tantabin town and Insein town. Hlegu and Tantabin, although headquarters of townships, were more accurately described as urbanised villages in paddy-growing areas with, in addition, a fishery at Tantabin. Yemun was a Karen village where paddy was the chief crop, but where fruit gardening was also carried out. Laydaunggan and Taikkyigon were paddy-growing villages, although in the latter, market vegetables were also grown and a few cows were kept by Indians. Insein town was a municipality and the headquarters of the district.

The diets of 158 families were examined from these towns and villages in Insein district. A wide range of occupations and social strata was covered, including traders and petty traders, clerks, school teachers, subordinate government servants, cultivators, agricultural labourers, landowners and salary owners.[85]

The results of the survey showed, not surprisingly, that the diet tended to improve with the economic status of the family. This, Dr U Maung Gale warned, was not always a simple equation, as the size of the family, its indebtedness and a natural reluctance to reveal information about the family income also needed consideration. The

TABLE 6.1
Mean Intake of Calories per Head in Insein District

Town/Village	Calories
Hlegu	2,143
Tantabin	2,228
Insein town	2,418
Taikkyigon	2,527
Laydaunggan	2,559
Yemun	2,986

Sources: U Maung Gale, *Reports on the Dietary and Nutritional Surveys.*

survey showed that the mean intake of calories consumed varied between villages, and this is shown in Table 6.1. The number of calories per head per day varied between the low of 2,143 at Hlegu and the high of 2,986 eaten at Yemun. Dr U Maung Gale attributed the high calorie intake at Yemun to the increased consumption of rice by agricultural labourers during the harvest.

Dr U Maung Gale's report judged the calorie intake at Hlegu and Tantabin to be slightly inadequate. He based this on a recommendation from the Health Bulletin that 2,600 calories per day were needed by an Indian in "easy-going agricultural or coolie work".[86]

The survey in Insein district found that the families' diet was nutritionally inadequate in several ways. The consumption of animal proteins and total proteins was too low in Taikkyigon and Laydaunggan, and the total protein intake was also too low at Hlegu and Tantabin. The consumption of fat was inadequate and the calcium intake was unsatisfactory in all the villages. Milk and milk products were absent from nearly all diets, but a higher intake of calcium was found amongst those families using leafy vegetables. *Ngapi*, the fish paste that early European travellers to Burma found so offensive, was found to be rich in calcium due to the shells of small shrimps, and the families who ate *ngapi* with their rice had the highest intake of calcium.

The intake of Vitamin B in the diets was measured by the survey team in international units, and the consumption range was found to be 128 to 266 IU. The report suggested that 300 IU was the desired level, and this level was only approached at Yemun (266 IU) "where home pounded rice is more largely used".[87]

The above discussion has referred to the findings of the survey team and Dr U Maung Gale's assessment of the nutritional adequacy of the diets in Insein district; no attempt has been made to judge the findings by modern nutritional standards. It is a very complex and technical matter to decide whether a diet is sufficient or contains the recommended intake of all the necessary components. The FAO standards are "designed for a well-developed, healthy human being, usually called Reference Man".[88] But not only is Reference Man not necessarily the "average" rural Asian, but his protein requirements depend on the level of the other essential nutrients in his diet. The intricate physiological interactions between the fats, vitamins and proteins make it very difficult to judge dietary requirements in different countries, where lifestyles vary and the available foods differ. There have also been many developments in the science of nutrition since the 1930s, including changes in the terminology employed. These factors complicate direct comparisons between Dr U Maung Gale's findings and a modern assessment of recommended food intakes. A simple example of this is the measurement of the amount of Vitamin B in the Burmese diet. Dr U Maung Gale calculated a daily intake of between 128 and 266 IU in Insein district, and suggested that 300 IU was the daily requirement. Modern surveys measure the B group vitamins separately as thiamine, riboflavine and niacin in mgs or μgs per day. This is very difficult to compare to international units, which are a measurement of response to treatment or of bodily activity.

Despite these problems, some conclusions can be drawn. Dr U Maung Gale calculated that the diets were deficient in Vitamin B and that only 43 to 89 per cent of the daily requirements were available. (The percentage varied from village to village depending largely on the method of rice milling.) Doctor S. Postmus, surveying diets in Burma on behalf of the WHO in 1957, reported that only 65 per cent of the daily requirement of thiamine and 26 per cent of the requirement of riboflavine were present in the diets of the districts of Burma, excluding Rangoon.[89] These measurements are average; adult daily requirements and the daily needs of groups under physiological stress, such as pregnancy or lactation, are much higher. Postmus calculated that pregnant and lactating women in Burma were receiving only 30 to 32 per cent of their daily requirement of thiamine, and 11 to 12 per cent of their requirement of riboflavine.[90]

During the next two years (1939–41) surveys were carried out in Bassein, Yamethin, Minbu, Thaton and Mergui districts. The population surveyed in the Mergui district has not been included in the calculations or the discussion about the survey because the district lies outside the study area, and the population examined was atypical, in that the families surveyed were mine workers, plantation workers or town dwellers. Dr U Maung Gale also examined the diets of various schools, and the results of these were discussed in Chapter Four (see Table 4.7, which summarises his findings on malnutrition in children). In addition a special survey was done in Taungdwingyi town, Magwe district, to investigate the possibility of links between nutrition and the high registered IMR.

All the districts showed a very similar nutritional pattern to that of Insein district. With the exception of Bassein, the intake of proteins was inadequate, and in all districts, except Yamethin, the consumption of Vitamins B and C was well below what was necessary. The consumption of pulses, beans and fruit was too inadequate to compensate for these deficiencies. Dr U Maung Gale stated that the survey team did not find the high consumption of pulses that was reputed to exist in Upper Burma. In Yamethin district, for example, he found that the consumption was half of one ounce per day,[91] and Taylor, Martin and U Thant reported an average intake of less than two ounces per week.[92] All the district diets were deficient in calcium due to the lack of milk, and most diets were also deficient in phosphorus. Dr U Maung Gale described quite wide fluctuations in the standards of the diet, which were not only dependent on the economic standing of individual families but sometimes on the economy of the whole village. This was particularly true of villages in the dry zone. The people of Shwezanthi village in a hilly part of Minbu district were described as very poor and their crops barely sufficient for subsistence.[93] There was no fresh fish in their diet; beef was eaten once a week and vegetables had to be obtained from other villages. Another poor village in Minbu district was Ywathya, again very dry, where only a little sesamum and groundnut could be grown, and the main occupation of the village was the making of earthenware pots.[94] The children in both these villages were much lighter in weight than the average for the district.[95]

In Yamethin district, the vitamin content of the diet was up to standard, due to the high proportion of families eating home-pounded rice. It was notable that in most of the districts surveyed, one or perhaps two villages were found to have adequate or near adequate intakes of Vitamin B due to the consumption of home-pounded rice, but overall, 73 per cent of the families surveyed ate machine-milled rice.

This is a major finding. In Minbu, Thaton, Insein, Magwe and Bassein districts, 60 to 100 per cent of the population surveyed ate machine-milled rice. Yamethin was the only district surveyed in which the majority of the population ate home-pounded rice. Table 6.2 shows the numbers of families surveyed in each district and the percentage of those families that ate machine-milled rice.

TABLE 6.2
Surveyed Families Eating Machine-milled Rice

District	Area	No. of Families	Percentage Eating Machine-milled Rice
Minbu	Dry Zone	131	60
Yamethin	Mid Burma	182	21
Insein	Mid Delta	158	100
Bassein	Delta	211	87
Thaton	Coastal	129	95
Magwe*	Dry Zone	33	70

Notes: *Taungdwingyi town only.

Sources: U Maung Gale, *Reports on the Dietary and Nutritional Surveys.*

Of the populations surveyed, the highest percentage eating milled rice, between 87 and 100 per cent, were in the south of Burma. This is not surprising; in the ten districts of Bassein, Myaungmya, Pyapon, Maubin, Hanthawaddy, Thaton, Insein, Henzada, Tharrawaddy and Pegu, there were 469 registered mills in 1940 and, no doubt, many smaller ones. The population of these ten districts, the most densely settled in Burma, was approximately half that of the study area in 1940. If a conservative estimate is taken, that approximately 80 per cent of the population of Lower Burma and 50 per cent of the population of Upper Burma was eating milled rice by 1940, then this represents a major and damaging change to the Burmese diet.

Nutritional effect of eating machine-milled rice

The loss of vitamins and protein from the rice grain during the milling process has already been discussed in general terms, but in this section an attempt will be made to apply that information more specifically to the Burmese diet. How much rice did the Burmese eat? In 1928, Taylor, Martin and U Thant estimated that the consumption was between 1 pound and 1.5 pounds (470 to 624 grams) a day of uncooked rice, the larger amount being eaten by poorer Burmese.[96] In the immediate post-Second World War period, B.O. Binns estimated in his calculations of the pre-war diet that the average rice consumption was 425 grams a day,[97] and Postmus estimated 441 grams daily in the 1950s.[98] The quantities of rice suggested by Taylor, Martin and U Thant look high, as do their suggested daily meat consumption figures for Burmese, on average seven ounces per day. It is possible that these figures are distorted by being urban only, but they are certainly wildly different to Binns' estimate of half an ounce of meat per day including poultry, although both reports estimate the fish consumption at approximately three ounces per day. Dr U Maung Gale stated that the Burmese diet was deficient in animal proteins, so it is probably safe to regard Taylor, Martin and U Thant's figures for meat and rice consumption as too high.

The estimates of thiamine consumption will be based therefore on the estimated rice figure from Postmus, slightly more generous than Binns, at 441 grams per day, but not as high as Taylor, Martin and U Thant's figures. The FAO estimated that home-pounded rice contained 2.4µg per gram of thiamine, and that milled rice contained 1µg or less per gram.[99] At an estimated rice consumption per day of 441 grams, if home-pounded rice was eaten, the thiamine intake was 1.05mg. If milled rice was eaten, then the intake was only 0.4mg. In 1957, R. G. Chitre and Tin Tin Oo calculated that the daily thiamine requirement per adult per day in Burma was 1.2mg, but found intakes per day of between 0.57 and 0.86mg.[100] Alternative food sources of thiamine are some vegetables and liver, and it is probable that the Burmese obtained some of the daily requirement from leafy vegetables, although the intake of these was often inadequate.

If the diet of the poorer Burmese had contained more pulses, beans and germinated beans, then compensation for some of these protein and vitamin deficiencies might have been achieved. However, Dr U Maung Gale found that the consumption of pulses was low, and this was confirmed by Binns (just under one ounce per day),[101] and Taylor, Martin and U Thant, who reported that on average less than two ounces was eaten per week.[102] The director of public health, G. G. Jolly commented in 1923 that germinated beans were freely available in most Burmese markets, but Taylor, Martin and U Thant had measured the consumption of these beans at less than one ounce per week, and Binns made no mention of them as an item of diet.[103]

These figures can only be taken as an approximate indication of what was happening during the colonial period. But there is sufficient evidence to say that the change to machine-milled rice reduced the thiamine in the Burmese diet to an inadequate level. Beri beri was not new to the Burmese people, but probably previously occurred only when turmoil and distress forced the population to eat stale, damaged or mouldy rice. The difference brought about by the habitual eating of milled rice was that a permanent deficiency state was created, with subclinical or frank beri beri a constant danger.

The population most at risk from this deficiency were undoubtedly pregnant or lactating women, infants, those engaged in strenuous labour and children or adults attacked by infections.[104] The earlier chapters have discussed beri beri amongst these various groups, but undoubtedly the mortality would have weighed most heavily on the infants, children and mothers. It is amongst those groups that the thiamine deficiency must be seen as a determinant of mortality.

The post-war picture

Several post-Second World War surveys support this picture of a population suffering sub-clinical nutritional deficiencies, especially thiamine. Reports and papers written in 1953, 1957, 1961, 1967 and the 1970s have a consistent theme, which includes sub-clinical beri beri.[105]

The WHO surveys, conducted in the 1950s, found a beri beri incidence of 43.7 per cent amongst adults in Burma.[106] The Union of Burma nutrition survey of the military forces and their dependants, conducted between October and December 1961, found clinical signs of thiamine deficiency in two to four per cent of those examined, but biochemical analysis revealed thiamine deficiency in 43 per cent of defence personnel, in 55 to 65 per cent of military dependants, and 30 per cent of the civilian population.[107] The report stated: "The consumption of polished rice as the major food staple … is responsible for the prevailing inadequacy of thiamine and riboflavine nutritive. This problem is further compounded by the practice of discarding the water in which rice is cooked and insufficient diversification of the diet."[108]

Ba Tin, for his 1969 dissertation, studied 4,320 workers from factories, government departments and rural areas. He found that 31 per cent of the total group were deficient in Vitamin B complex, and that thiamine deficiency was most frequently found amongst those doing heavy work, especially in the rural areas.[109]

The situation appeared to be unchanged in the 1970s. Dr Daw Sein May Chit in her paper "Nutritional Problems in Burma", stated that "clinical signs of overt (thiamine) deficiency were uncommon, but low urinary excretion rates and suboptimal dietary intakes are prevalent throughout the country. Thiamine problem is a border line one but beri beri has been shown to be an ever present danger given the proper stressful conditions like pregnancy, diarrhoea or natural catastrophes."[110]

It is also interesting to note that the prestige value of white or machine-milled rice has remained high. It was noted in the *Agricultural Bulletin Report* of 1913, and was commented on in the 1970s by Sein May Chit: "White rice also is considered high prestige value and it is thought shameful to admit eating under-milled rice."[111]

A post-war report indicated that the change was not confined to Burma. The FAO's 1957 report of the fourth session of the Nutrition Committee for South and East Asia commented on the "recent rapid extension of small mills into rural rice producing areas where much rice was previously home pounded, a tendency which seems to be particularly prominent in Burma, Thailand and Vietnam."[112] Unfortunately the committee did not define "recent" in this context, but the FAO nutritional survey of 1948, *Rice and Rice Diets*, criticised the spread of mechanical rice mills in rural areas on nutritional grounds, and said that in practice "few governments have attempted to check the spread of rice milling or to reduce the number of existing mills."[113]

Beri beri was certainly experienced in Malaya. The report of this country's delegation to the League of Nations Conference in 1937 stated that protein and Vitamin B deficiency were "commonly prevalent" in Malaya.[114] A more detailed examination of beri beri in Malaya was published by C. E. Cobb in 1924. He suggested that the problem was largely confined to the Chinese in Malaya, and was almost unknown amongst the Indians, who ate parboiled rice, and rare among the Malays, who ate hand-pounded rice. Cobb, who was a medical officer in Kuala Pilah, noted that "the more wealthy Chinaman, however, is able to afford a more varied diet together with his white rice, and therefore does not suffer to the same extent as the labourer".[115]

Cobb described a two-year period, August 1919 to August 1921, when beri beri admissions first declined and then became negligible from December 1919. The explanation was a shortage of rice in Malaya from early 1919, which caused the government to institute profiteering controls and distribution orders.[116] Wheat flour was used as a rice substitute, and Chinese rice purchasers found that many dealers would sell rice only when an equal quantity of flour was also bought, and much of the available rice was lightly milled or hand-pounded Malay rice instead of the highly milled variety to which they were accustomed. There was also an increase in the consumption of sweet potatoes, Indian corn and other vegetables. The result of this enforced dietary change was "the disappearance of beri beri in Kuala Pilah in about four months", although the beri beri apparently returned when the former diets were resumed.[117]

Was the situation in Thailand and Vietnam similar to that in Burma? A large milling industry, 90 per cent Chinese-owned, developed in Thailand,[118] and this may well have caused a substantial proportion to change to white rice consumption. Certainly the Vietnamese experience has parallels with Burma's history. Charles Robequain described the development of a large rice milling industry at Saigon–Cholon, which used German or American machinery and was French or Chinese in ownership. But in addition to the development of major milling centres, Robequain described the growth of small, Annamite-owned factories in Cochin China which milled rice for home consumption.[119]

Malaria

"Malaria kills more people and does more damage to physical, social and economic welfare ... than any other disease .... Yet malaria is insidious, and except in epidemic form, it does not manifest itself with dramatic power sufficient to attract attention and funds commensurate with its ability to destroy health and prosperity."[120] This quotation from a 1937 report by the League of Nations Health Organisation summarises neatly the situation in colonial Burma: the people were suffering morbidity from malaria; that the costs in deaths and to the economy of the country were huge, and yet it persisted comparatively without attention and funding for far too long. This section will examine malaria in Burma, its causes and its impact.

Malaria is one of the oldest diseases known to man. It is characterised by periodic fevers, followed by chills and heavy sweating. Certainly there are references to periodic fevers in early Chinese, Chaldean and Hindu writings. The Greeks described an association between swamps and the development of periodic fevers and splenomegaly in the fourth century BC.[121] It would seem very unlikely that Burma escaped a widespread disease that was well established in neighbouring countries and for which her terrain was environmentally suitable. Lieberman refers to the existence of malaria in the delta in the fifteenth and early sixteenth centuries,[122] and Michael Adas described it as an obstacle to agricultural development there in the mid-nineteenth century.[123] It is highly probable that malaria was known to the earliest inhabitants of Burma.

The author of *Hunter's Tropical Medicine*, G. T. Strickland, describes malaria as "stable endemic ... when natural transmission occurs over many successive years and there is a predictably constant incident of cases", and "unstable ... where the amount of transmission varies from year to year, collective immunity is low, and epidemics are therefore likely". He classifies the degree of endemic malaria by the spleen or parasite rate in children of two to nine years old. His four classes of endemic malaria are "hypoendemic" (spleen rate of zero to ten per cent), "mesoendemic" (11 to 50 per cent), "hyperendemic" (over 50 per cent) and "holoendemic" (over 75 per cent). The adult spleen rate is low, and the parasite rate in infants is high.[124] These terms will be used in this section.

What are the symptoms of malaria? It is usually described as giving "periodic" and "intermittent" fevers[125] with anaemia as a common complication and, sometimes, pulmonary edema, renal failure and cerebral dysfunction.[126] The spleen may rupture and the fever itself result in tachycardia, nausea, vomiting, delirium, etc. The very wide range of symptoms helps, of course, to explain the difficulties of diagnosis, even when medical help was available, and the further difficulties headmen in Burma had in classifying deaths for registration. If a headman was confronted with a death, and reported symptoms included fevers, coughing and diarrhoea, was the death registered under "Fevers", "Respiratory Disease" or "Bowel Disease"?

These symptoms are caused by a tiny organism (protozoa) of the *Plasmodium* genus, of which there are four species that infect man — *falciparum, ovale, vivax* and *malariae.* Part of the life cycle of the plasmodium takes place in the female anopheline mosquito and part in man or other host.[127] A bite from the infected mosquito will initially infect the bloodstream of the human host, and after going through various changes and arriving at the form of a gametocyte, it can in turn infect a non-carrying female mosquito as she feeds from her human host.[128] This is a vital factor to remember in the transmission of malaria — an area previously free of the disease can be infected by the immigration of human carriers, as well as infected anophelines. As this is not a medical study, a further description of the complex changes in the life cycle of the plasmodium in the human body and its effect on the symptomatic process of the disease will not be attempted.

Who and how many were affected by malaria?

It would be sensible to pose the same questions about malaria in Burma as were posed about the other major diseases. A description of the disease itself and how long it may have existed in Burma has already been attempted; but how many died of the disease in colonial Burma, and how efficient (or otherwise) was the recording of these deaths? Also, was there a racial, sexual or age bias to the morbidity and mortality of malaria? Some of these questions have already been addressed in earlier chapters, but a reminder of those findings, before the causes of the disease are considered, would be timely. The other factors to be considered are the significance of the child/woman ratio and the seasonality of deaths.

There have already been discussions of the registration of "Fever", and therefore malaria deaths, in earlier chapters, particularly Chapter Five where the reclassification of urban data and the sub-division of fever categories were discussed. Did the new category of "Respiratory Diseases", which first appeared in 1902 records, absorb some of the fever deaths? It was concluded in Chapter Five that there was

TABLE 6.3

Registered Fever Deaths, Estimates of Malaria Deaths and Comparisons
with Registered Deaths from Epidemic Diseases

Ten-year Period	Registered Fever Deaths Over Total Registered Mortality (%)	Registered Fever Deaths p.a., Averaged (1,000s)	Estimate of Registered Malaria Deaths p.a.* (1,000s)	Estimate of Malaria Deaths p.a., Averaged (1,000s)	Total Reg. Cholera, Smallpox and Plague Deaths p.a., Averaged (1,000s)
1892–1901	39–51	53.9	27.0	40.0	–
1902–11	32–57	76.0	38.0	50.7	14.7
1912–21	30–33	98.1	49.1	66.7	13.7
1922–31	30–37	76.8	38.4	51.2	10.3
1932–39	36–40	101.0	50.5	67.4	5.4

Notes: * Assumed to be 50% of registered Fever deaths, see *RSABB*, 1880, p. 7; *RSAB*, 1939, p. 19.

Sources: Annual health reports.

undoubtedly an initial tendency, although in the early 1920s there was a reverse effect as later deaths from the 1918 pandemic were registered as fevers.

Table 6.3 is an attempt to illustrate the importance of malaria deaths in colonial Burma, as shown by the registration data. Its inaccuracy has been extensively discussed, but the core of truth, that on average more than 50,000 people a year died from malaria, is there. So also is another truth that, while the combined total of deaths from cholera, plague and smallpox declined to an average of less than 5,000 a year, estimated malaria deaths climbed to over 67,000 a year in 1932 to 1939.

A sexual bias in registered fever deaths can be seen very clearly from the registration figures. On average, between 1914 and 1939, the number of male deaths exceeded the number of female deaths per year by 5,743.[129] This is only to be anticipated and is largely due (where these are malarial deaths) to division of labour. Men made up the greater part of the casual labour force employed on civil engineering projects, such as canal building, railway embanking and new road development. Groups of labourers, some infected with the malarial parasite, moving into areas previously free of malaria, could rapidly infect the local anophelines and, hence, their fellow labourers and the local population. Also, men are more likely to go to woodland areas looking for fuel and timber for items such as house repairs.

Was there a racial bias in the mortality? It could be argued that there was, at times. But the pattern of the mortality depended on geographical locality. The deaths could be shown to be Chinese and Indian labourers, who were brought into an area for a specific project. For example, R. C. Robertson, author of *A Malaria Survey on the China–Burman Highway*,[130] could be said to have shown the susceptibility of Chinese labourers, but in actual fact admitted that the survey was carried out mainly on Chinese, as the Shans and local tribesmen were difficult to approach.[131] However, when the stimulation of the malaria is by irrigation, the high mortality is found amongst the local villagers as well as construction workers and it may well continue at hyper- or holo-levels. An unhappy example of this can be seen in Minbu district where, after the opening of the new canals in 1911/12, the death rates soared in some administrative circles (from 725 in Legaing and Konsaung in 1922, to 1,363 in 1924), and the births fell in Sinbyugyun (from 1,327 in 1922, to 862 in 1924).[132] The post-canal construction condition of this valley is discussed later in this section.

The disastrous effect of malaria on the Infant Mortality Rate (IMR) and the morbidity and mortality of children in colonial Burma was discussed in Chapters Three (Table 3.6 and Figure 3.2) and Four (Table 4.8). Although it was not possible in Chapter Three to precisely quantify the percentage of the IMR attributable to malaria, it was noted that the difference in the IMR between the Tatkon and Hlegu health centres was nearly 140 per 1,000. Tatkon Centre, in the malarial district of Yamethin, had an IMR of 300 in 1938, and Hlegu (less malarious) only 162. In both health centres, the IMR was believed to be under-recorded and, of course, excluded stillbirths and abortions. These figures would suggest that approximately 50 per cent of infant and *in-utero* deaths were malaria related.

The mortality and morbidity of children due to malaria were discussed in Chapter Four and it was suggested that the major evidence for this lay in the child/woman ratios. These were found to have declined overall from approximately 2.2, up to and including 1911, to approximately 2.1 from 1921 onwards. More significantly, the district variations were much greater and a strong correlation was drawn between the irrigated districts and persistently low child/woman ratios.

Were there other geographical links between malaria and the deaths of children? Did other areas show significant variations? Table 4.8 indeed showed that there were three distinct regions of Burma in the 1920s and 1930s. In the majority of the districts of Lower Burma, the child/woman ratio had remained "healthy", and in the three out of ten districts in which it had fallen below 1.0 in 1921, it had recovered by 1931. However, in the mid-Burma districts of Prome, Toungoo and Thayetmyo there was only a marginal recovery in 1931, and in Upper Burma, the ratio was still below 1.0 in four of the nine districts.

The seasonality of mortality and its significance in proving the high number of malarial deaths has already been discussed in the preceeding three chapters. Figure 5.1 is particularly significant as the histograms show how the total registered mortality swung from a July/August/September axis to an autumn/winter peak. It is not intended to reiterate here all the points that have already been made, but merely to refresh the previous ideas. It was noted for example that in Kyaukse district, the IMR was at its highest from December to January, and that in Minbu district, following the opening of the canal, the spleen rate in one circle was very little short of 100 per cent, even as late as the end of January.[133] However, Figure 5.1 achieves new significance in the light of the discussions so far, and particularly the discussions of irrigation technology and irrigation to come, where it will be argued that the experiences in Kyaukse and Minbu districts were experienced elsewhere, and for the rest of the colonial period.

This section has so far examined malaria in the same context as other major diseases. An attempt was made to estimate the number of deaths per annum in the colonial period, whether there was sexual, racial or age bias within that mortality and what was indicated by the child/woman ratios.

Why did mortality from malaria rise and remain high?

What is needed now is an examination of the determinants of the disease. Why did malaria persist during the colonial period and why, as has already been suggested in earlier chapters, did the mortality from the disease apparently rise and stay persistently high? To understand the probable causes, it is necessary to look back briefly through the irrigation history of the area.

Irrigation works in Burma

Most of the material wealth of the Burmese kingdoms lay in their agriculture, particularly the wet-rice lands that provided the staple food for the population. These *ledwins*, or rice bowls, depended on extensive irrigation systems that were fed by perennial rivers and streams. Many of the canals, weirs and tanks predated the Burmese kings in both construction and design,[134] but their maintenance and improvement of the irrigation was a matter of royal prestige, due to its economic importance to the state. A strong king who was also an effective administrator would ensure that the canals were well maintained and the allocation of water supervised, but lack of control at the centre resulted in the silting of canals, water wastage and therefore, an impaired tax base for the kingdom. King Mindon Min (1853–78) had the irrigation tanks in Shwebo district, including the famous Mahananda Tank, repaired in 1853, and in 1866, ordered the repair of the Old Mu Canal, which ran from north of the Mahananda Tank to the Yemyetgyi Lake in Sagaing district. During Thebaw's reign (1878–85), however, many of the canal systems were thought to have suffered from silting and poor maintenance, and in the vital Kyaukse district, the population was reduced and the canals fell into disrepair.[135]

The rice-growing regions lay within Kyaukse, Magwe, Minbu, Mandalay and the Lower Chindwin districts, but of these Kyaukse, in particular, was of vital and strategic importance to the Burmese kings. The long period of insurgency and guerrilla warfare that followed the British struggle to establish control of Burma resulted in further neglect of the irrigation systems, as villagers either fled the fighting or joined the resistance forces. It was 1889 before the last resistance was quelled in Kyaukse district, and 1890 before peace was finally established in Shwebo district.

Despite these difficulties, the British lost no time in surveying the irrigation works, where it was possible and safe to do so. Initial approval for work on the Mandalay Canal was given by the Secretary of State for India on 12 November 1896, and a first report on Kyaukse district by D. J. Grant, special irrigation engineer, was dated 12 May 1887.[136] The British sanctioned canal improvements as "Productive Public Works" on which the outlay and interest charges were to be recovered by an increase in revenue from the improved land.

The senior irrigation officers who were appointed to Burma were experienced men who had worked on major projects in India. They were confident that their modern scientific skills would effect radical improvements on the existing irrigation works, and could also be deployed to build efficient and modern new systems Unfortunately, some engineers applied this Indian experience to Burma without due regard to the very different physical relief, geology or local epidemiology of disease. For example, the irrigation engineers calculated the desired critical velocity of the canal waters by reference to their India experiences, using a formula known as Kennedy's Vo with insufficient regard for local conditions.[137] The original survey and estimate for the Ye-u Canal in Shwebo district had to be discarded and a re-survey and new estimates were put in hand in 1905. The first survey was said to have assumed a heavy silt, characteristic of an Indian river rather than the Mu River, and the canal was therefore designed with excessive grading to carry this away (see further discussion below).[138]

The list of irrigation works that were newly built or renovated and repaired by the British is long, and only a brief summary is given here. A more detailed discussion of some of the works follows later in the section on technology and epidemiology, but a brief account of the British engineering work gives some idea of its scope.

One of the first works to be sanctioned by the Government of India was the Mandalay Canal, running nearly 40 miles south from the Madaya River through Madaya township to the Myitnge River. Three estimates were prepared for the work, ranging from 32,95,000 rupees in 1896 to 51,04,225 rupees in 1906. Two hundred and eighty miles of watercourses were constructed by the engineers at a cost of 4.8 rupees per irrigated acre, more than twice the price originally quoted to the cultivators. It was hoped that 65,000 acres would be irrigated in total, with double cropping on 15,000 acres. However, it was found that the soil was not fertile enough for double cropping, and the areas irrigated did not reach the target until extensive distributaries were developed.[139]

There is nothing unusual, of course, in civil engineering projects outrunning their original estimates, but it seems probable that at least part of the cause in Burma was the over-hasty estimates made in the light of Indian and not Burmese experience. The over-optimistic estimates of double cropping are one example, and the problem of the rising estimate for shoddy mis-forecasts in the Ye-u Canal is another. The latter was a new work, with a 42-mile-long main canal drawing water from the Mu River near Kabo. The Ye-u Canal had its own head-works on the Mu River, but shared a common head weir with the Shwebo Canal, which was situated just to the south of the Ye-u.

The Shwebo Canal was first sanctioned in 1900 at an estimate of 48,04,093 rupees, which was raised in 1908, to 53,70,532 rupees, and which had necessitated a total capital of 61,13,549 rupees by 1921. The main canal ran for 28 miles before dividing into two branches of 25 miles and nearly 22 miles in length. The Shwebo and Ye-u canals shared more than a common head weir, however, as miscalculations of the critical velocity required led to the canal bed having too steep a slope, thus producing a scouring action.

There were other difficulties associated with these canal systems. The Old Mu Canal (repaired by Mindon Min) was also supplied by the Mu River, but, except at times of flood, the river could not adequately supply the three canals, and water shortages could occur in the irrigation systems. In 1917, the settlement officer, R. B. Smart, described several of the problems faced by the cultivators.[140] The Irrigation Department would not supply until 1 June, although the water was usually needed prior to that date for the nursery rice beds. Also the revenue assessment for the area took insufficient account of the lower rice prices prevailing locally, and the problems of water rationing that often occurred because of the three canals that were draining the Mu River.

The other major new canals that the British built were in Minbu district. They comprised two canals taken from the left and right sides of the Mon River at Mezali. The canals were designed to irrigate the Mon valley, which in some years received only 15 inches of rainfall. Substantial head-works were constructed for the canals as the river was periodically subjected to massive flooding, destroying crops in a valley otherwise subject to drought. The canals were first opened for irrigation in the season 1911/12, and as discussed later, turned the valley into an epidemiological disaster area!

The ancient Kyaukse canal systems, which drew water from the Panlaung and Zawgyi rivers, were described by the irrigation engineer in 1887 as being "unexpectedly good", a somewhat barbed compliment.[141] The canals irrigated 203,000 acres, nearly two-thirds of the cultivable land in the Kyaukse district. Despite them being "unexpectedly good", the British engineers put in hand many changes to the canals, and particular emphasis was placed on straightening the channels. This reduced the length of many canals by up to one-third or half, and necessitated the building of falls along their course. Also, regulators were constructed at the heads to control the admission of water, as under Burmese management, the canals had open heads. However, Gibson, the settlement officer in 1903, reported that the water supply in some canals had deteriorated, and that the new British practice of withholding the water when the rivers were low was resulting in the loss of nursery rice crops.[142]

The British also carried out repairs and remodelling on other irrigation works, such as the Meiktila Lake, which supplied drinking water to Meiktila town and, in addition, irrigated nearly 46,000 acres. The bunds or banks of the lake were raised, the sluices repaired and regulators built at the head of the irrigation channels. Work was begun in 1892 and continued intermittently until 1911, with additional alterations to the sluices planned in 1914.

Other tanks and minor canals were altered in Minbu, Magwe, Myingyan, Yamethin and Meiktila districts. Works consisted of re-bunding and building new distributaries or falls, weirs and sluices. In some cases, such as the Kanna Tank in Myingyan district or the Nyaungyan-Minhla Tank in Meiktila district, the alterations were originally approved as "Famine Relief Work" in the drought years of 1891/92 and 1896 respectively, but were later sanctioned as "Public Works".

This brief outline of the irrigation canal engineering work in Upper Burma has suggested that these engineering changes had adverse epidemiological consequences for the rural Burmese. But, before this idea can be discussed, it is necessary to examine the other factors in this hypothesis — malaria and mosquitoes.

Significance of the anopheline mosquito

Malaria was not new to Burma in the British occupation, but was well known in regions such as the foothills and forests, and also the irrigated districts. The Burmese were well aware of the link between irrigation and malaria in their land, so much so that there is a cynical proverb about a village near Nga Pyawn weir, Kyaukse district, reputedly built by King Anawrahta in the eleventh century. The saying goes: "If you like to die, don't take arsenic, go to Than Ywa village".[143]

However, acknowledging the prior existence of malaria does not invalidate the central notion that the British system of water management exacerbated the problem, resulting in hyperendemic or even holoendemic malaria in the canal areas. The prior existence of the disease as stable endemic malaria, with occasional instability, strengthens the probability, because it was the alterations to the canals that increased the breeding sites for the existing anopheline mosquitoes, thus interrupting the stable transmission pattern of the disease.

How did this happen? The explanation rests on an understanding of the vector's habits and how its effectiveness or success can be increased in Darwinian terms. This depends on the physical environment that the individual mosquito and its larvae require. For example, all mosquito larvae live in water, but some species require sun, others shade; some require moving water, yet others, still water.

The larvae of *Anopheles balabacensis*, for example, require still water, though this mosquito was not a very important vector of lowland Burma, as it was usually found in areas of forest. The only irrigated district in which it was important was in the forested part of Madaya township. The larvae require shaded water and they thrive happily in small stagnant pools, such as cattle hoof prints, stagnant ditches and paddy fields, but never breed in moving water, whether shaded or not. This mosquito is a monsoon breeder, highly anthropophilic (likes to feed on humans) but is only important in thickly forested areas.[144]

Another mosquito that breeds in stagnant water is *A. barbirostis*, one of the most widespread anophelines in Burma. But despite this prevalence, it is primarily a cattle feeder and is not important in malaria transmission in Burma.[145] *Anopheles annularis* has a similarly wide distribution in Burma, breeding in stagnant ponds, borrow pits and rice fields, but it is only important as a malaria vector in the Arakan region, as its feeding habits are largely zoophilic, that is, it shows a preference for cattle.[146]

All adult mosquitoes need to feed, and therefore the proximity of humans or cattle is important. Some species, such as *A. culicifacies* (another minor vector in Burma), are primarily zoophilic, and their local importance as a vector of malaria depends on the ratio of man to cattle in the vicinity.[147] An outbreak of cattle disease can, by lowering the cattle population, result in a local epidemic of malaria as the mosquitoes are forced to turn from cattle to man for food.

Another important requirement of mosquitoes is a rest area, which may be limited by the proximity of water as many mosquitoes have only a short flight range. Bush and scrub are important as resting places, but some species will be found resting in houses or sheds, even the mainly zoophilic *A. culicifacies*.[148]

The primary vector of malaria in Burma and the mosquito whose breeding requirements were unwittingly provided by the British, was a tiny anopheline called *Anopheles minimus*. This mosquito's larvae need lightly shaded, slowly moving, clean water. It is often found in the "hilly regions, either low rolling foothills or narrow river valleys in mountain ranges. When found on the plains, it is always in association with extensive irrigation systems".[149] The larvae prefer the grassy edges of the irrigation canals or the light shade and protection provided by tree roots or backwaters in clear perennial streams.

Several malariologists have described the characteristics of *A. minimus* in Burma, and have found that, most importantly, the mosquito is highly anthropophilic.[150] One malariologist, on a single evening, collected 846 *A. minimus* from houses in one village, but could find only 51 in cowsheds.[151] Some of these mosquitoes would have been looking for food, others resting after feeding, but both groups were staying in close proximity to humans, their preferred host.

Anopheles minimus reaches its maximum prevalence in the post-monsoon period from October to December, although in areas where perennial water is available, the mosquito may breed from April to December.[152] During the monsoon, the larvae tend to be flushed out by the pulsing velocity of the water in the hill streams, but post-monsoon the larvae experience the conditions they need to thrive. In the irrigation canals, the water was kept (as far as possible) at a constant, low velocity by the British engineers.

Probably the simplest way to describe the suitability of the canal environment for *A. minimus* is to compare the description of a "natural", that is, hill breeding site to the man-made canal zones in Kyaukse district. In 1941, a survey by a malariologist of 40 villages in Amherst district, south Burma, found hyperendemic malaria in those villages that had perennial hill streams. *Anopheles minimus* was found to be breeding amongst the fallen leaves, grassy edges or tree roots in these otherwise swift-flowing streams. All of the villages were next to, or within a furlong of their stream, thus putting them well within the flight range of the mosquito. The survey area was forested, with scrub and trees surrounding the villages and lining the banks of the streams, providing small bays and backwaters for the anopheline larvae.

Maung Tin, a malariologist and the author of the report, examined 2,372 children in the villages and found that 828, or one in three, were infected with malaria.[153] He attributed this to the high number of breeding places for *A. minimus* adjacent to the villages. He also found that the malaria was seasonal and that the highest incidence of the disease was in November and December.

The report showed that the villagers were chronically impoverished, a state that Maung Tin attributed to the prevalence of malaria. He described the disease as "hindering greatly the economic and social development of the villagers" and "checking the natural increase of the population".[154]

There are many similarities between this natural breeding area for *A. minimus* and the man-made area of the canal zones of Kyaukse district. The description of the district in the *Gazetteer* of 1925 makes this very clear: "The banks of the canals themselves are in many cases planted with fine trees, ... which have grown to a great size and spread a cool shade over the water and the bridle paths. Behind these trees the meandering depression, which marks the course followed by the canal before its straightening, is often filled with a dense and luxuriant mass of bushes, ... broken only by the villages and monasteries which occur at frequent intervals along the banks. But the wealth of trees is not limited to the main canal alone; they are scattered along the larger distributaries ...."[155]

Therefore the basic and vital requirements for *A. minimus* to breed successfully existed in both Kyaukse and Amherst districts. The slowly moving, clean and shaded water, the dense scrub for resting places and the close proximity of the human food were available in both districts; but one was a man-made environment and the other was natural.

The other irrigated areas such as Shwebo district and the Mon valley also provided the environmental factors necessary for *A. minimus*, although not all were as rich in trees as Kyaukse district. However, the grassy edges of the canals and adjacent scrub made up any possible shade deficiency.

Perhaps this is the point at which the importance of *A. minimus* as a vector should be discussed. It was stated earlier that the anopheline was the most important vector of malaria in Burma, but this was not understood at the time of British rule and acknowledgement of its importance in the irrigated areas of Burma is largely a post-Second World War development.

The reasons why the British malariologists underestimated the importance of *A. minimus* can be divided into two main groups. Firstly, there was the problem of preconceptions: malariologists investigating the disease in Burma had either worked or trained in India. Many of them assumed that the vectors that had been important in India would also be important in Burma and were satisfied that they had identified the culprit when they found the breeding sites of anophelines familiar to them. However, a mosquito that was involved in malaria transmission in India might well be, and often was, free of the parasite in Burma.

The other reason why the importance of *A. minimus* was not recognised lies in the criteria governing malarial investigation in pre-war Burma. Surveys fell into three categories: those protecting economic investments, such as the railways or mines; those protecting the troops or military police, and those protecting the towns and thus Europeans. Therefore no attempt was made to establish a countrywide catching and dissection programme to establish which anophelines were the main carriers of the parasite in the widely differing areas of Burma.

These pre-war malarial surveys were scattered and haphazard, and many made no attempt at dissection as this was time-consuming and required some laboratory facilities. But in the last few years of the British administration, a new awareness of the health problems of the rural areas developed, and this is shown in three malarial surveys. One of these was the 1941 survey, carried out by Maung Tin, of 40 Karen villages in Amherst district, in which *A. minimus* was identified as the major vector. Unfortunately there was no dissection, as the villagers had a "superstitious objection" to allowing the mosquito catchers to enter their huts.[156]

A 1940 survey of Kengtung town in the Shan states positively identified *A. minimus* and *A. maculatus* by dissection as the vectors responsible for the endemic malaria of the town and surrounding countryside.[157] The other survey in which *A. minimus* was identified was referred to in the health report of 1939.[158] This mentioned a new survey of Yamethin township in Upper Burma, in which both *A. minimus* and *A. culcifacies* were identified but, unfortunately, the report did not make clear whether or not this was confirmed by dissection.

These three reports show that the administration was aware of the importance of *A. minimus* as a major vector in Burma by the end of the 1930s. But were the British also aware that the anopheline was the cause of the hyper- and holoendemic malaria in the irrigated zones? There is little sign in the records of any awareness, although by the early 1930s there was little excuse for this ignorance as world knowledge had advanced rapidly. This was illustrated at the Intergovernmental Conference of Far-Eastern Countries on Rural Hygiene, organised by the League of Nations Health Organisation in 1937. The reports make it very clear that *A. minimus* had been recognised as a major vector associated with irrigated rice cultivation in other Southeast Asian countries. The Preparatory Report mentioned the hyperendemic malaria in northern Siam, "with its usual corollary: economic distress".[159] This was attributed to *A. minimus*, as was malaria in the Philippines.[160]

There was also extensive discussion in the conference report on the appalling amount of engineer-induced malaria in some Far Eastern countries.[161] The recommendations of the report reveal that knowledge of the breeding requirements of anophelines was far advanced. The suggestions for remedying the problems, which were particularly relevant to the situation in the irrigated areas of Burma, were the periodic sluicing of small streams, the automatic sluicing of large streams, the removal of sheltering vegetation, changing the water levels and agitating the surface water.[162] Instead the British engineers were discussing in 1929 the reduction of the scouring (and therefore the sluicing) of the Shwebo Canal in Volume A Kyaukse *Gazetteer*, and the *Gazetteer* (admittedly a few years previously in 1925) was eulogising the shady canal areas.

Early malarial investigations in colonial Burma

Why were the British apparently unaware of the importance of *A. minimus* in the irrigated areas? To understand this, it is necessary to go back to some of the early malarial investigations in Burma, and to appreciate the narrowness of their brief and the lack of attention given to those rural areas that did not include the protected categories of Europeans, military forces or economic investment. The narrow interpretation of the instructions and the preconceptions that anticipated finding Indian problems in Burma can be seen from the following examples.

There was an explicit and understandable preoccupation with the health of the military police and troops. The investigation of malaria in Katha district in 1912 was almost undoubtedly to protect the military forces stationed there, as more than one in three of the military police at Wuntho town in Katha district were admitted to hospital with malaria in June and July of 1908 and 1909.[163] The total population of the town was less than 2,000, but it was chosen for survey and subjected to intensive investigation by the Malarial Committee in Burma presumably because of its strategic importance, although the official reason given was that it was an example of a typically diseased sub-montane tract.

The investigating officer, Major O'Gorman Lalor, concluded that the "essential element" in malarial prevalence at Wuntho was the presence of stagnant water all the year round, and it would appear that he concentrated his search for anophelines on these areas.[164] Later research has shown that *A. minimus* was the dominant vector of the region, breeding all the year round in the local streams.[165]

A more extreme example of the British preoccupation with the military police, to the disadvantage of the local population, can be found in the unpublished records of the administration. In January 1911, a military police unit was permanently withdrawn from a village on the salt fields of Myaungmya district following severe outbreaks of malaria. The Home Medical Department Proceedings record that "The Commissioner added that the Deputy Commissioner, Myaungmya, had been instructed to encourage the villagers at Sagyin to take [anti-malarial] action on the lines suggested, but that the matter was obviously now of but little importance."[166] The lack of concern for the rural population could hardly be stated more clearly.

O'Gorman Lalor, as malarial officer, carried out a series of investigations in 1911 and 1912, which included a study of the mosquitoes prevalent in Rangoon, particularly with regard to yellow fever, and a detailed investigation of the malaria at Kyaukpyu. The latter town is situated on Ramree island and was an administrative and, periodically, a military centre, for the oil-rich island. O'Gorman Lalor made extensive recommendations for the control of malaria at Kyaukpyu, which included engineering work to reduce the sub-soil water.

These activities were described in the *Annual Report of the Provincial Malarial Committee, Burma*, for the year ending 31 March 1912. But there was an extraordinary omission from this report, and from the malarial officer's activities. During the year 1911/12, there had been a disastrous outbreak of malaria in the Mon valley, following the opening of the Mon Canal in July 1911. By December 1911, death rates of over 200 per 1,000 were being recorded in some of the administrative circles near the canal, and in the Legaing Circle, the registered death rate climbed to over 300 per 1,000.[167] This epidemic was investigated by the local health officials only, and no attempt was made to identify the anophelines involved in the transmission of the disease or to investigate the causes. The outbreak, of course, involved no Europeans, military aspects or private investment. There had admittedly been government investment in the new canal; but that was nearly completed and, presumably, it was considered at the time that the disease would not interfere with the eventual recovery of the capital from the cultivators.

In fact, the British were still obsessed with the danger from rising sub-soil water, and the problem of irrigation canals as breeding areas was still not recognised. The sanitary commissioner for Burma in 1905 and 1906, W. G. King believed that if there was "unfit surface drainage and obstructed sub-soil drainage, evil will result."[168] This had probably been true in Madras, where King had formerly been the sanitary commissioner, and was true of certain areas of Burma but sub-soil waters did not provide the most important anopheline breeding areas in Burma.

The scale and funding of these first investigations are also worthy of comment. The appointment of a special malarial officer with the rank of major, the recruitment of his staff including a laboratory assistant, and the detailed work undertaken (which included the catching and dissection of adult anophelines) indicates a pre-First World War lavishness that was not repeated. The appointments were the result of the decisions taken at the 1909 Simla Conference on malaria, which emphasised the necessity of systematic investigation into the distribution and epidemiology of malaria.[169]

One more malarial survey of this early period should be mentioned. This was a spleen census of the principal towns and selected villages of Burma conducted by O'Gorman Lalor in 1911/12. A spleen census required an external examination, or palpation of the spleen of a child between the age of two and nine years. The purpose of the examination was to assess the size of the organ, as an enlarged spleen is considered diagnostic of malarial infection, and is also a measurement of endemicity. As noted earlier a spleen rate of zero to ten per cent is classified as hypoendemic malaria, 11 to 50 per cent is mesoendemic, over 50 per cent is hyperendemic, and over 75 per cent holoendemic.[170]

In the spleen census, O'Gorman Lalor recorded rates of 100 per cent in the Ye-u Canal area, the Lower Chindwin district and parts of Akyab, but there was no malarial investigation of the rates in the Ye-u or Lower Chindwin areas, and only a recommendation for a yellow fever survey at Akyab.[171] The only measurements taken in Kyaukse district for the spleen census were in the headquarters town and in Myittha, a railway town. In both cases the results were negligible. The lack of response by both the sanitary commissioner and the malarial officer to the 100 per cent rates in Ye-u and the Lower Chindwin illustrates all too clearly the policy of putting the resources where the military forces or Europeans were threatened by malaria. There can be no excuse on the grounds of contrived ignorance (which perhaps could be claimed for Kyaukse district) because the data was there for all to see. Two of the most respected malariologists in India, Samuel R. Christophers and C. A. Bentley wrote in 1909 that "It often happens that the effect upon the actual labourers and native populations in the neighbourhood may pass unrecorded and unnoticed, the outbreaks of [malarial] disease and death among Europeans alone attracting attention".[172] However, it is all too clear that, even when the extent of the disease was measured in the "native populations", there was not always a response from the health authorities.

If the canal areas were largely ignored by the administration, then how can it be shown that the malaria incidence in those regions was high? What sources are available?

The answer lies in a number of sources, of which perhaps the most important are the calculations that the health authorities made on child / woman ratios in Burma using the data from the 1911 census. These calculations revealed that the proportion of children was much lower in the irrigated districts of Upper Burma than in other areas of the country. It was also reported that the population of Kyaukse district, despite a slight net gain from migration, had grown by less than one per cent in the decade 1901 to 1911, whereas the average growth rate in Burma was 1.2 per cent per annum.[173] The reason for this stagnation seemed to be the high registered mortality under "Fevers" and "All Other Causes".

This was followed in 1917 by a spleen census of villages in Mandalay district. The authorities found that 47 per cent of the villages in the survey showed spleen indexes of between 50 and 100 per cent, indicating hyper- or holoendemic malaria. In addition, the authorities reported that a comparison by age group of the population of the district to other similar Buddhist groups in Burma showed a 25 to 30 per cent "deficit" of children.[174]

Plates 1 and 2 (taken in 1987) show what are commonly known as one-season dams. These were, and have been during recorded history, built by the local cultivators for the control of agricultural water supplies. The British administrators, however, considered their use in Burma to be inefficient and ineffective because they were frequently washed away during periods of rain or slight flooding. However, the epidemiology of *A. minimus* required the slow-moving, controlled water preferred by the British to the spasmodically flooding or checked water provided by the Burmese, and this anopheline therefore thrived. There was another simple practical advantage to one-season dams: they were cheap and easily replaced.

Effects of other civil engineering projects

Hyperendemic conditions were also caused by other civil engineering projects in Burma. The building of railways, roads, drinking water storage, etc. could all create hyperendemic outbreaks of malaria through the disturbance of the epidemiological balance. It was common for labour to be drafted into areas free or relatively free of malaria, and

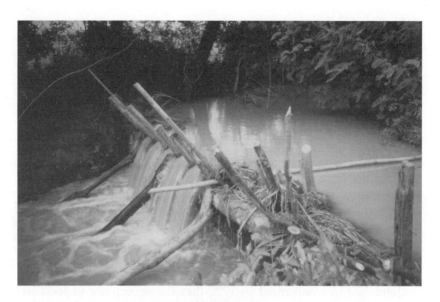

PLATE 1

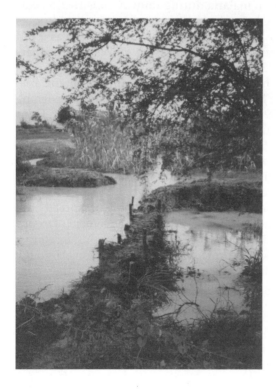

PLATE 2

through the parasitaemia of some of the workers, the local anophelines could be infected and epidemics started.

The situation, of course, was not unique to Burma, but was noted earlier in India. Christophers and Bentley described, in 1909, how the aggregation of labour, exposure of the workers to anepholines through poor housing and poverty led to sickness and higher malarial rates. This in turn would ensure a greater turnover of labour (as often there were no medical facilities available), so infected labourers would return to their own villages, thus spreading the cycle of infection.[175] Ronald Ross, in 1911, was clearly still trapped in the Darwinian view evident in the health records of the 1860s, as his comment on the problem was: "Stupid, poor, lazy people, living in badly made huts ... bitten much more easily than more civilised races".[176] Remarkably, but unfortunately without effect, Patrick Hehir suggested in 1910 that coolies should be given a minimum wage to ensure that they had a sufficient quantity of wholesome food to protect them against malaria,[177] a proposition that was both humanitarian and economically sensible.

John Sinton commented in 1928 that the occurrence of localised epidemics was associated with the aggregation of labour and economic stress. It is in this report that the phrase "a life a sleeper" can be found.[178] The mortality from malaria during railway construction was so high that the lives were being lost at the same rate as the sleepers were laid, though this fact hardly received the same publicity as it did when equal losses were sustained by Caucasian POWs on the Thai–Burma border during the Second World War.

The construction of railways in Burma was catastrophic in malarial terms. The building of the Mu valley railway (347 miles) from Sagaing to Myitkyina between 1889 and 1898 resulted in what O'Gorman Lalor called an "exaltation of malaria". The population in the area was previously low, but the entry into the district of first Indian, and then Chinese, labourers, followed by 1,400 military police, meant that "a great influx of people susceptible to malaria and unprotected by immunity" was now vulnerable.[179]

This was, of course, another common method of spread and transmission to previous (non-epidemic) areas; the movement of troops had been noted to spread infection since the early part of the century, although action was not taken to protect the local population. Although in 1909, in a discussion about "malaria bearing police",[180] there was some talk about removing persistently infected individuals from the area, little, if any, action was taken, and the problem persisted throughout the colonial era. It was noted that when Mingaladon Cantonment, built in a previously malaria-free area, was occupied from December 1928, it took just over two years for the new cases amongst the troops to rise to 37 and the relapses to rise to 109.[181]

This section set out to examine two questions: why did malaria persist during the colonial period, and why did the mortality from the disease apparently rise and stay persistently high? The increase in malaria was shown to be related to canal design and exacerbated, until the end of the 1930s, by an apparent unawareness of the full causes by the health authorities, who were understandably reluctant to provide resources to alleviate the problem in areas other than those where military forces or Europeans were threatened. Another contributory factor in the spread of malaria was the movement of large groups of personnel, such as troops, around the country. The various engineering projects undertaken by the colonial government, too, entailed moving large gangs of cheap labour, who carried the disease with them.

The malaria lesson – learnt or lost?

Was it apparent that the British administration before and after World War Two or the new Burmese administration learnt anything from the history of malaria in Burma? Was there any obvious awareness in the management of irrigated districts, movements of police, or control of other civil engineering projects, etc., that knowledge acquired in the prevention of malaria was being put into effect? It would appear that the answer is no. Modern transmission was discussed in 1975,[182] and reference was made to hyperendemic conditions in connection with dams and irrigation water; similarly, references were made to movements of the army and smuggling groups causing malaria. In 1947, a malaria commission was recorded as discussing the importance of construction works, such as roads, to malaria transmission, but great emphasis was laid on the lack of importance in Burma, unlike India, of borrow pits.[183]

A report covering the period from 1981 to 1986 was given to the author. It was on the Sedawgyi Dam Hospital Project and shows that in many cases little or nothing had been learnt. The dam, which was being funded by the World Bank and other international organisations, was being built in Medaya township to provide additional water for irrigation. Shortly after the beginning of the civil engineering work, workers were falling prey in large numbers to disease, mostly malaria, and it became necessary to build a hospital urgently to cope with the need. During the first year (1981), over 53,000 patients attended hospital. By 1985, this had increased to over 93,000 but declined quite dramatically to 68,000 in 1986. During the period from 1981 to 1985, the highest proportion of those patients treated (50 per cent) were suspected of suffering from malaria. This seems to show an amazing unawareness on the part of not only the Burmese administration but also the international organisations that nearly 50,000 people per year were contracting malaria when forward planning and historical knowledge should have prevented most of this.[184] It would seem that the historical knowledge of prevention and treatment was there, but the will to apply it (with the necessary application of funds) was not. Perhaps, after all, nothing had changed: the knowledge existed but the funds did not.

The determinants of mortality

This chapter was titled "The Determinants of Mortality" because it aimed to show how nutrition and malaria were the real, underlying causes of the slow population growth experienced by Burma during the colonial period.

Throughout the book, mention was made of the typical Burmese diet, which was often lacking in first-class proteins and sufficient variety. The poverty of the ordinary Burman (and Indian migrant) meant that under-nutrition was a way of life. The development of the rice-growing industry led, ironically, to a worsening of the food problem. Machine-milled rice, as opposed to the traditional hand-pounded rice, became the favoured staple of the diet. It was shown how machine-milled rice meant that much of the nutritious outer covering of the grain was removed. This loss of vitamins (B1, in particular) manifested itself in the form of beri beri. A malnourished person is weakened and unable to fight off infection or survive a sudden trauma.

The mortality figures show that "Fevers" were the biggest killers in Burma. Malaria falls under this category and was estimated to make up about 50 per cent of the "Fevers" death. That, alone, is enough to make malaria deadly. The problem was exacerbated by the civil engineering works undertaken by the colonial authorities to improve the agriculture of the country. Not only did the irrigation works provide breeding places for the malaria vector, but their construction involved the intro-duction of sources of infection, in the form of the labourers contracted to do the work, to previously malaria-free areas.

Sad to say, both these "determinants of mortality" were capable of solution, and in both cases, the health authorities were slow or reluctant to take the necessary measures to address and alleviate the problem.

Conclusion

This book forms part of the social and economic history of the colonial era in Burma and has attempted to identify and explain the determinants of demographic change in that country during the study period. The period in question includes the nineteenth century, but places the main emphasis on the years 1891 to 1941. A demographic framework was developed for Burma in Chapters One and Two, by using sophisticated methods to calculate the numbers of its population and the rate of increase. In the subsequent chapters, an examination was carried out on infant, child and adult mortality, and disease; the Burmese family; and the economic and social developments that caused the demographic changes in Burmese society.

The number of the Burmese population during the British colonial administration from 1850 to 1941 was established and the methods used were reported in Chapter One. The most reliable estimates of the Burmese population were identified by inspection and analysis of all the available data, and adjustments were made for variations in the area covered compared to the study area. Thus it was established that the population of the study area remained relatively stable from 1783 to 1826, and then, between 1826 and 1891, the population rose at approximately one per cent per annum. This latter estimation can be described as an attainable figure when compared to the population growth rates of India, the Malay Peninsula, Thailand and other neighbouring states. Then, to establish the size of the population from 1891 onwards, some general adjustments to the raw data had to be made. The decennial censuses were examined, but it was found that changes in the study area and the flawed nature of the figures made the data unusable without a great deal of adjustment. Some reconstruction of district boundaries in Upper Burma had to be made to provide a consistent baseline for the figures, due to the increasing area covered by successive censuses. In Lower Burma, more drastic reconstruction was required to subtract the number of Indian migrants who, by 1931, numbered over one million. Using this adjusted data, estimates of the growth rate were made for the period 1891 onwards. The growth rates calculated for each inter-censal decade from 1891 to 1941 were

0.96 per cent, 1.25 per cent, 0.82 per cent, 1.04 per cent and 1.32 per cent. These figures show an increasing growth rate, interrupted by a sharp decrease caused by the flu pandemic, and then followed by a further period of increasing growth. This showed that Burma achieved a population growth rate of, on average, approximately 1.0 per cent per annum between 1891 and 1941. An attempt was made to establish whether the population growth rate achieved during the study period in Burma was indeed lower than that achieved in neighbouring countries. From 1911 onwards, India, Malaya, the Philippines and Thailand boasted an average population growth rate of approximately 1.8 per cent; but most of these figures were based on untreated census data, and hence may not be reliable. However, Peter Boomgaard and A. J. Gooszen provided data for Indonesia, based on treated census data, which show a growth rate rising from 1.0 per cent (1900–30) to 1.5 per cent (1930–40). Since these figures were obtained from treated data, they are believed to be more reliable, particularly the 1930 ones.[1] These figures are not dissimilar to the Burma figures, but do indicate that Indonesia's growth rate was higher than Burma's from 1930.

The immediate reason for this relatively slow population growth was established in the birth and death rate figures presented in Chapter Two. Again, accurate calculation was not easy. The obvious source was the vital registration records of Burma. However, even the local sanitary commissioners admitted that these records registered only an estimated one in three vital events, and hence they were discarded here as a source. The other option was to use the census data to estimate the vital rates through the use of life tables. Due to the peculiarities of the census data, a large amount of "smoothing" of the figures was required. Even so, it was felt that the resulting figures were more reliable than those obtained from vital registration. The resulting figures showed that the increase in the birth rate in Burma lagged behind the increase in the death rate. An estimated crude birth rate of 45 in 1901 rose to 48 in 1921; meanwhile, the crude death rate rose more sharply from 32.5 in 1901 to over 37 in 1921.

In particular, Burma suffered from a comparatively high infant mortality rate, as detailed in Chapter Three. Once again, the inaccuracy of the vital registration data made it necessary to find an alternative method of establishing the IMR. This was done by use of the life tables to provide estimated data. By the 1930s, of every 1,000 infant births registered, 200 babies died before their first birthday. The estimated figures, from the life tables, showed an even higher rate. The estimated IMR for females rose from 250 per 1,000 in 1891 to 295 in 1931. The figures for males are even more telling, rising from 295 in 1891 to 335 in 1931. When compared to the IMR data of neighbouring countries, the

Burmese data were not only relatively high but were increasing at a time when those for the other countries were decreasing. This high IMR was found to be largely due to malnutrition, the debilitating effects of which worsened the effects of infectious childhood diseases. The response of the colonial administration to the rise in infant mortality was inadequate, at best.

The study of the family and childhood in Burma (Chapter Four) focused on childbirth, the age of marriage, birth control practices, levels of fertility, the size of the family unit, and disease among, and mortality of, children. The most important finding was of a similar pattern of malnutrition and disease among one- to 15-year-old children as that found among infants (Chapter Three). Studies revealed that approximately 50 per cent of this age group were malnourished. Nutritional deficiencies, dysentery, measles, respiratory diseases and intestinal parasites were shown to be the main and synergistic causes of childhood death. Malaria was also found to be a major cause of death; but once again, the action taken by the colonial health administration had little effect. The high mortality rates among babies and infants during the study period, due to a combination of malnutrition and disease, caused a shortage of children in Burma, particularly in some Upper Burma districts.

The investigation of adult morbidity and the development of a public health system in Burma, detailed in Chapter Five, further follow this pattern. It showed that the seasonality of mortality shifted from a summer to an autumn/winter peak, indicating a change in the pattern of disease, and evidence was given of a steady decline, from 1911, in deaths caused by cholera, plague and smallpox. Although the mortality due to hunger was not quantified, death due to dysentery and diarrhoea fell over the study period, believed to be largely attributable to improved drinking water supplies. Mortality from bowel disease mainly affected the urban poor, as the wealthier urban areas had piped water and sanitation facilities, and the incidence of these diseases was generally lower in the rural areas.

The effect of respiratory diseases was investigated but, despite increases shown in the registered data, no trend could be confirmed, due to the newness of the registration system (introduced in 1901) and the huge increase in mortality that came in the wake of the flu pandemic between 1918 and 1921. What was apparent was that the authorities did little to prepare for the effect of the pandemic, and were unable to cope with the emergency except in Rangoon. The mortality rates were significantly affected by the flu pandemic, and a modest estimate was made that flu caused 400,000 additional deaths between 1918 and 1921.

There were three significant facts that emerged in the chapter. The use of life tables showed that, although the overall crude death rate rose during the study period, the increase in childhood mortality was greater than that of adults. Indian immigrants became both victims of the major epidemic diseases and 'whipping boys' because their social and economic circumstances led them to be blamed for disseminating these diseases. Another significant fact to emerge was the formative role that the epidemic diseases played in the development of a public health service in Burma.

Nutrition and malaria in Burma during the study period were examined in Chapter Six. It was found that malnutrition, which was rife in all ages of the Burmese population during the years under British rule, was exacerbated by a dietary shift from hand-pounded to machine-milled rice. A big expansion in rice production in Burma, with a more than seven-fold increase in rice crop acreage between 1860 and 1940, changed the country into a major rice exporter. This led to a rapid expansion in the number of rice mills, the majority of which were machine powered. Machine-milled rice contained less vitamins and protein than home-pounded rice and, in particular, thiamine levels were reduced by a very significant amount. A deficiency of thiamine in the diet causes beri beri. Although little quantitative evidence has been found, there is considerable circumstantial evidence that the change to machine-milled rice reduced thiamine in the Burmese diet to an inadequate level, and hence resulted in an increase in the incidence of beri beri. The evidence was primarily from health reports, which showed an increasing realisation of the problem, almost certainly indicating an increasing prevalence. Further weight is added to this argument by the nutritional survey, carried out between 1939 and 1941, which found nutritional deficiencies in a sample of six districts. Unfortunately the effect on the death rate is not quantifiable from the health reports, as mortality from beri beri was not listed separately but was included in the category of "All other causes" until the latter part of the study period, when more detailed data was recorded for the urban areas of Burma. The effect on the death rate must be expected to be most significant among infants, children and mothers. There was also evidence from the reports that beri beri was not recognised as a problem in rural Burma until the early 1930s, despite reports of its effect on industrial labour, and measures taken to reduce it from 1908, when the problem arose in lighthouses, and in later years in police training schools, teacher training schools, and timber camps.

While the ability of the population to repel diseases undoubtedly lessened with worsening nutrition, other factors meant that malaria was also becoming more prevalent. It was shown that colonial civil engineering projects, such as new irrigation works, gave malaria the means to travel further afield and to reach new victims. A detailed analysis of the mosquito in Burma was also carried out in Chapter Six, in particular covering its breeding locations, and confirming that *A. minimus* was the most important vector of malaria in Burma. It was pointed out that improvements and extensions to existing canals and the building of new ones contributed to an increase in malaria deaths, due to the resultant increase in the breeding locations of *A. minimus*. Evidence was given of the increasing prevalence of malaria at a time when there was a steady decline in the other major diseases, namely cholera, plague and smallpox. It is almost inevitable, therefore, that the increases in the incidence of beri beri and malaria were significant contributors to the increased death rate that occurred during the study period.

In order to provide comparative data, mortality rates from Indonesia were investigated. However, Boomgaard stated that the data available was not sufficiently reliable to establish an accurate level of mortality.[2]

It is worthwhile summarising the data on diseases affecting mortality rates in colonial Indonesia during the nineteenth and twentieth centuries. Boomgaard stated that reliable information is only available for a few epidemics, and that data on endemic diseases are much scarcer, making it virtually impossible to identify any changes in endemic disease patterns. He also wrote that it is almost certain that endemic malaria became more significant after 1850, but it is possible that the increasing availability of quinine reduced the effect of the spread of malaria, either wholly or partly.[3] Between 1889 and 1892, reports of cholera outbreaks became more numerous, and malaria claimed large numbers of victims, especially in 1891. Flu was also widespread in 1890 and 1891. Various actions initiated by the authorities, and their effect, are summarised here: "It can be established that preventive and curative measures — although very modest in terms of scope and effectiveness — would have led to a situation where the mortality rate no longer lay completely outside the control of the authorities. In this context reference has already been made to the introduction of smallpox vaccination and the establishment of schools for native doctors and midwives earlier in the 19th century. A first step towards the prevention of disease was also made by the sinking of artesian wells in an effort to improve drinking water supplies. The foundations were also laid in some areas for a greater public awareness of the importance of hygiene."[4]

In the period 1895 to 1911, "there is no evidence of any significant improvements in preventive and curative medical care. As for the main causes of death, the Medical Service reports suggest that, as in the preceding period, swamp-fever, i.e. malaria, was seen as a significant cause of death."[5] Smallpox continued to recur sporadically, and cholera recurred in epidemic form in 1897, 1901, and 1910. Plague broke out in 1910 and "The slow official response was all the more remarkable considering that this particular epidemic had already spread from 1894 onwards via China and Japan to India and thence to the Far East."[6]

During the period from 1912 to 1929, the mortality peak of 1918 was, according to the system of registration, to be attributed to the effects of a flu epidemic. Plague broke out in 1910 to 1915 and again in 1919, 1921 to 1925, and in the 1930s. Other diseases were also prevalent. The Medical Service's registers show that "smallpox occurred throughout the entire period; it was however a less significant cause of death than bacillary dysentery and typhoid; cholera was still fairly prevalent — mainly in the 1912–1920 period — but was being fought with increasing success by vaccination programmes and had virtually died out in the course of the 1920s."[7] Malaria, although still very common, was no longer so frequently regarded as the direct cause of death. Between 1910 and 1929, research was carried out to identify the most dangerous species of mosquito and to establish the location of their breeding grounds. This led to anti-malaria measures such as the draining of marshlands and swamps, and the cleansing of saltwater fishponds. The idea also gained acceptance in the 1920s that improvements in hygiene were, in themselves, vitally important preventive measures in the fight against disease.[8] During the period 1930 to 1942, a severe outbreak of plague may have been responsible for an apparent rise in mortality between 1930 and 1933.[9]

Unfortunately, as no quantitative data is available from Indonesia for the mortality caused by each of the major diseases, no direct comparison can be made with the Burma figures. However, it is apparent that, as in Burma, malaria was one of the major killers. Studies were carried out in Indonesia to establish which mosquito type was the main carrier and to identify its main breeding grounds. The Dutch authorities then took steps to reduce these breeding areas. In Burma, however, the irrigation systems were altered and extended on the incorrect assumption that the anopheline identified by the malariologists as the major cause of malaria in India would be the same in Burma. This led to an increase in the breeding grounds of the mosquito species that was primarily responsible for the spread of malaria in Burma. Malaria surveys carried out in Burma were inadequate until the last few years of the British administration, and hence *A. minimus* was not identified as the major vector until the problem had worsened considerably.

It is interesting to note that, in both Burma and Indonesia, the official response to many health problems is believed to have been slow or inadequate. As has always been the case, the authorities would have had to divide the available resources across many areas, and decisions were undoubtedly made that, particularly with the benefit of hindsight, can be considered to have been mistaken or inappropriate. However, in Burma, there appears to have been a consistent pattern of slow or inadequate response to major disease crises.

There are several topics, highlighted by this book, on which further research would be very useful for our understanding of the causes of demographic change in Southeast Asia. One of these is the infant mortality rate, which is believed to have been high in Burma compared to neighbouring countries. Why was malnutrition, believed to be the cause of the high IMR in Burma, less serious in the other countries of the region? Another topic is the increase in the incidence of beri beri witnessed in Burma. As this is believed to have been the result of thiamine deficiency in the Burmese diet caused by the change to machine-milled rice, were there similar effects in other Southeast Asian countries, or did particular conditions prevail in Burma which made the situation worse? It is interesting to note that beri beri was not listed as a significant disease by Boomgaard in his discussion of disease patterns in Indonesia, although this may simply be due to a lack of specific data from the available health records.

In summary, this book has sought to establish the best estimates of population numbers for colonial Burma that are achievable from the available raw data. This treated data was used to establish best estimates of birth rates, death rates and overall growth rates. The determinants of these vital rates have been established and some comparisons made with neighbouring countries, which indicate that the population growth rate of Burma was relatively low. It was further shown that an increase in mortality from beri beri was caused by the change from hand-milled to machine-milled rice. It was argued that the colonial powers were partly responsible for this low growth rate by assisting the spread of malaria through irrigation improvements and other civil engineering projects, and by their slow and inadequate responses to numerous health crises.

Appendix 1

Burma: Chinese Population by District (Including Yunnan Chinese)

District	1901			1911			1921			1931		
	M	F	Total	M	F	Total	M	F	Total	M	F	Total
Sandoway	270	240	510	90	2	92	65	9	74	123	26	149
Rangoon town	8,872	2,146	11,018	12,941	3,114	16,055	15,928	7,891	23,819	19,917	10,707	30,624
Bassein	1,700	278	1,978	2,504	254	2,758	3,146	812	3,958	4,511	1,769	6,280
Prome	1,507	1,130	2,637	1,216	229	1,445	1,125	325	1,450	1,661	710	2,371
Toungoo	838	344	1,182	2,154	346	2,500	2,107	653	2,760	2,460	1,122	3,582
Hanthawaddy	3,507	535	4,042	505	777	1,282	3,272	941	4,213	3,717	1,635	5,352
Tharawaddy	1,381	224	1,605	1,902	231	2,133	1,888	508	2,396	1,895	792	2,687
Henzada	780	200	980	1,719	282	2,001	1,594	409	2,003	1,900	724	2,624
Pegu	2,269	543	2,812	4,464	1,045	5,509	4,467	153	5,980	5,031	2,521	7,552
Myaungmya	1,514	196	1,710	3,075	256	3,331	3,657	834	4,491	5,384	1,946	7,330
Thaton	2,212	826	3,038	3,089	870	3,959	3,002	1,423	4,425	3,141	1,841	4,982
Thongwa	2,951	451	3,402	–	–	–	–	–	–	–	–	–
Maubin	–	–	–	1,950	182	2,132	2,015	372	2,387	2,685	925	3,610
Pyapon	–	–	–	2,982	431	3,413	3,479	1,042	4,521	4,493	1,613	6,106

Region												
Insein	–	–	–	–	–	–	2,614	709	3,323	3,572	1,841	5,413
Thayetmyo	818	718	1,536	220	17	237	280	81	361	497	201	698
Mandalay	1,365	211	1,576	1,461	251	1,712	1,846	420	2,266	2,215	938	3,153
Katha	232	25	257	379	63	442	1,952	719	2,671	1,870	845	2,715
Ruby Mines	938	146	1,084	2,465	1,625	4,090	–	–	–	–	–	–
Shwebo	106	15	121	192	27	219	358	83	441	581	230	811
Sagaing	52	12	64	141	15	156	118	19	137	176	53	229
L. Chindwin	65	–	65	146	22	168	188	61	249	315	160	475
Myingyan	220	28	248	274	53	327	299	97	396	504	223	727
Pakokku	405	325	730	–	–	–	230	36	266	352	150	502
Minbu	249	76	325	408	40	448	417	90	507	488	139	627
Magwe	69	5	74	355	24	379	522	102	624	969	320	1,289
Kyaukse	69	19	88	124	1	125	172	64	236	237	110	347
Meiktila	145	48	193	498	18	516	346	41	387	294	90	384
Yamethin	368	131	499	863	58	921	705	195	900	1,027	412	1,439

Sources: *Census of Burma*.

Appendix 2

Upper Burma: Hindu Population by District, Including Jain and Brahmanic

District	1891	1901	1911	1921	1931
Mandalay	9,613	13,427	16,071	22,103	28,396
Katha	1,116	1,237	1,429	3,990	5,653
Ruby Mines	775	1,982	2,505*		
Shwebo	2,093	1,586	2,305	2,548	3,463
Ye-u	425*				
Sagaing	1,319	930	1,772	1,958	2,690
L. Chindwin	374	911	784	1,299	1,338
Myingyan	1,386	686	1,787	1,748	2,284
Pakokku	1,798	965	1,170	891	1,358
Minbu	975	817	2,651	1,995	2,016
Magwe	711	634	2,632	7,315	10,314
Kyaukse	528	684	815	1,028	1,419
Meiktila	1,109	1,647	2,931	2,650	3,381
Yamethin	1,213	2,126	3,766	6,304	7,323
Pyinmana	1,054*				
Thayetmyo	2,524	2,352	2,186	1,946	2,276

Notes: *This district was amalgamated with the district above it from that date.

Sources: *Census of Burma*.

Appendix 3

Upper Burma: Muslim Population by District

District	1891	1901	1911	1921	1931
Mandalay	18,493	20,342	20,845	23,209	24,456
Katha	893	941	1,156	2,478	2,256
Ruby Mines	302	767	1,205*		
Shwebo	3,391	4,335	6,326	7,610	9,112
Ye-u	394*				
Sagaing	1,541	1,803	2,815	2,811	3,044
L. Chindwin	426	786	876	1,025	1,156
Myingyan	1,213	670	1,529	1,156	1,345
Pakokku	1,311	702	894	1,022	1,166
Minbu	698	922	1,061	1,223	1,446
Magwe	725	641	1,617	3,521	5,286
Kyaukse	3,133	3,431	4,954	5,740	7,300
Meiktila	1,274	2,631	4,253	4,283	4,931
Yamethin	5,289	7,804	11,057	12,908	15,343
Pyinmana	1,876*				
Thayetmyo	2,149	2,431	2,164	1,994	1,995

Notes: * This district was amalgamated with the district above it from that date.
Sources: *Census of Burma*.

Appendix 4

Lower Burma: Hindu and Muslim Populations by District

District		1872	1881	1891	1901	1911	1921	1931
Sandoway	Hindu	86	124	175	558	386	376	696
	Muslim	2,121	2,509	3,128	3,906	4,257	5,251	6,286
	Total	2,207	2,633	3,303	4,464	4,643	5,608	6,982
Rangoon	Hindu	934						
	Muslim	518	*	*	*	*	*	*
	Total	1,452						
Rangoon town	Hindu	14,108	35,871	57,845	82,994	108,350	125,002	141,344
	Muslim	12,067	21,169	28,836	43,012	54,634	61,954	70,791
	Total	26,175	57,040	86,681	126,006	162,984	186,956	212,135
Bassein	Hindu	721	4,851	6,577	12,562	11,822	14,947	15,648
	Muslim	2,671	4,925	5,795	6,378	8,107	9,994	11,393
	Total	3,392	9,776	12,372	18,940	19,929	24,941	27,041
Prome	Hindu	791	978	2,382	2,612	5,152	5,509	7,886
	Muslim	1,112	1,795	2,276	2,629	3,536	4,174	4,958
	Total	1,903	2,773	4,658	5,241	8,688	9,683	12,844
Thayetmyo	Hindu	2,029	2,620					
	Muslim	1,174	1,861	**	**	**	**	**
	Total	3,203	4,481					
Moulmein town	Hindu	11,040	12,853					
	Muslim	7,810	9,307	*	*	*	*	*
	Total	18,850	22,160					
Shwegyin	Hindu	291	958	3,927				
	Muslim	423	855	1,673	*	*	*	*
	Total	714	1,813	5,600				
Toungoo	Hindu	1,535	2,086	3,056	5,385	14,220	19,575	23,859
	Muslim	1,001	1,962	2,551	4,227	6,369	8,163	9,644
	Total	2,536	4,048	5,607	9,612	20,589	27,738	33,503
Hanthawaddy	Hindu	7,908	8,534	39,529	57,137	47,326	52,248	
	Muslim	*	4,085	4,682	11,979	16,307	12,811	13,535
	Total	11,993	13,216	51,508	73,444	60,137	65,783	
Tharrawaddy	Hindu	2,029	1,985	2,845	8,454	7,406	9,179	9,086
	Muslim	1,174	1,110	1,681	3,132	3,857	5,421	5,511
	Total	3,203	3,095	4,526	11,586	11,263	14,600	14,597

continued

Appendix 4

continued

District		1872	1881	1891	1901	1911	1921	1931
Henzada/	Hindu	378	703	2,701	4,298	6,600	6,703	7,279
Myanaung	Muslim	977	1,192	2,171	3,028	4,657	5,211	5,826
	Total	1,355	1,895	4,872	7,326	11,257	11,914	13,105
Pegu	Hindu			11,904	18,602	34,350	40,856	41,060
	Muslim	*	*	3,353	4,782	7,384	9,745	11,038
	Total			15,257	23,384	41,734	50,601	52,098
Myaungmya	Hindu				2,405	6,128	9,533	13,803
	Muslim	*	*	*	4,008	7,103	11,361	15,150
	Total				6,413	13,231	20,894	28,953
Thaton	Hindu				13,166	16,805	21,112	22,612
	Muslim	*	*	*	6,867	10,221	13,405	16,047
	Total				20,033	27,026	34,517	38,659
Maubin/	Hindu	723	3,895	11,374	6,392	6,833	8,537	
Thongwa	Muslim	*	1,650	3,695	5,530	4,864	6,001	6,266
	Total	2,373	7,590	16,904	11,256	12,834	14,803	
Pyapon	Hindu					12,164	16,431	22,569
	Muslim	*	*	*	*	3,540	5,640	7,162
	Total					15,704	22,071	29,731
Insein	Hindu						24,640	31,318
	Muslim	*	*	*	*	*	7,990	10,249
	Total						32,630	41,567
Amherst	Hindu	1,441	6,690	24,383	25,348	23,864	25,415	24,706
	Muslim	3,681	7,599	18,890	18,012	22,893	26,678	31,865
	Total	5,122	14,289	43,273	43,360	46,757	52,093	566

Notes
*District was not in existence at that date.
**District was part of Upper Burma at that date.

Sources: *Census of Burma.*

Appendix 5

Lower Burma: Hindus and Muslims as a Percentage of the District Population, from Contemporaneous Census Records

District	1872	1881	1891	1901	1911	1921	1931
Sandoway	4.03	4.11	4.28	4.90	4.51	5.00	5.40
Rangoon	0.43						
Rangoon town	26.50	42.51	48.06	53.64	55.56	54.67	52.97
Bassein	1.05	2.51	2.60	4.83	4.51	5.09	4.73
Myanaung	0.28						
Prome	0.69	0.86	1.29	1.43	2.29	2.60	3.12
Thayetmyo	–	2.64					
Moulmein town	40.56	41.72	–	–	–	–	–
Shwegyin	0.55	1.05	2.82				
Toungoo	2.94	3.14	3.45	3.44	5.86	7.26	7.81
Hanthawaddy	–	2.80	4.94	10.62	13.62	19.74	16.00
Tharrawaddy	–	1.11	1.30	2.92	2.59	2.96	2.87
Thongwa	–	0.83	1.70	3.48			
Henzada	–	0.59	1.27	1.51	2.11	2.16	2.13
Pegu	–	–	5.06	6.88	9.72	11.35	10.65
Myaungmya	–	–	–	2.11	3.95	5.63	6.50
Thaton	–	–	–	5.83	6.48	7.32	7.25
Maubin	–	–	–	–	3.68	3.88	3.98
Pyapon	–	–	–	–	6.12	7.61	8.89
Insein	–	–	–	–	–	11.13	12.54

Sources: *Census of Burma.*

Notes

INTRODUCTION

1   For dissertation papers on contemporary Burmese demography, see Tin Tin Nyunt, "Estimation of Vital Rates for Burma and Their Effects on the Future Size of the Population", MA thesis, Australian National University, Department of Demography, Research School of Social Sciences (Canberra: ANU, September 1978); Aung Myint Thein, "Estimation of Infant and Childhood Mortality from Burma's First Stage Census: 1953", MSc Demography project paper, London School of Economics and Political Science (July 1975); and Lay Maung, "Methods of Obtaining Vital Statistics from Rural Areas with Particular Reference to Burma", project report for Board of Examiners of the MSc Medical Demography examination, London School of Hygiene and Tropical Medicine, University of London (August 1971).

2   Michael Adas, *The Burma Delta: Economic Development and Social Change on an Asian Rice Frontier 1852–1941* (Madison: University of Wisconsin Press, 1974).

3   James R. Andrus, *Burmese Economic Life* (Stanford: Stanford University Press, 1948).

4   John S. Furnivall, *Colonial Policy and Practice: A Comparative Study of Burma and Netherlands India* (Cambridge: Cambridge University Press, 1948).

5   Charles A. Fisher, "Some Comments on Population Growth in South-East Asia with Special Reference to the Period since 1830", in *The Economic Development of South-East Asia*, ed. Charles D. Cowan (London: George Allen and Unwin, 1964)

6   Irene B. Taeuber, *Population Growth and Development in Southeast Asia*, SEADAG report, Population Panels Seminar, New York, 1972.

7   Kingsley Davis, *The Population of India and Pakistan* (Princeton: Princeton University Press, 1951).

8   A. R. Vyatkin, *The Population of Burma: Historio Demographic Outline* (Moscow: Chief Publishing House of Oriental Literature, 1979).

9   R. M. Sundrum, "Population Statistics of Burma", economics research project, Statistical Paper No. 3, (Rangoon: University of Rangoon, December 1957).

10 June Nash and Manning Nash, "Marriage, Family and Population Growth in Upper Burma", *Southwestern Journal of Anthropology* 19, no. 3 (1963): 251–66.

11 Maung Ba Aung, "Why Burma Is Sparsely Populated, a Suggestion", *Journal of the Burma Research Society* IV, part 2 (1914); J. Stuart, "Why Is Burma Sparsely Peopled?", *Journal of the Burma Research Society* IV, part I (1914) and part V (1915).
12 Nash and Nash, "Marriage, Family and Population Growth in Upper Burma", p. 265.
13 Ibid., p. 260.
14 Edward A. Wrigley, *Population and History* (London: Weidenfield and Nicolson, 1969), p. 13.
15 Carlo M. Cipolla, *The Economic History of World Population* (London: Penguin, 1974), p. 85; Kingsley Davis "Population Policy and the Theory of Reproductive Motivation", in *Essays of Economic Development and Cultural Change in Honour of Bert E. Hoselitz*, ed. M. Nash (Chicago: University of Chicago Press, 1977), p. 160; Wrigley, *Population and History*.

CHAPTER 1

1 J. A. Stewart, "Kyaukse Irrigation — A Side-light on Burmese History", *Journal of the Burma Research Society* 11, part 1 (1921): 4.
2 *Burma Gazetteer, Vol. A, Thayetmyo District* (Rangoon: 1911), p. 11.
3 *Burma Gazetteer, Vol. A, Toungoo District* (Rangoon: 1914), p. 6.
4 Ernest Henry George Dobby, *Southeast Asia* (London: University of London Press, 1950), p. 152.
5 Daniel George Edward Hall, *A History of South-East Asia*, 4th edition (Basingstoke: Macmillan, 1981), p. 158.
6 Ibid., p. 155.
7 Ibid., p. 156.
8 Ibid., p. 157. It is interesting to note here that the Burmese, at least, were distinguished by what Hall describes as "a desire for independence which has been such a strong feature of their mentality through history".
9 Edmund Ronald Leach, *Political Systems of Highland Burma: A Study of Kachin Social Structure* (London: Athlone Press, 1977), p. 235.
10 For a more detailed discussion of the pitfalls of this broad-brush approach to the divisions between the races, see Leach, *Political Systems of Highland Burma*, chapters 1–3.
11 Leach, *Political Systems of Highland Burma*, p. 2.
12 Moshe Yegar, "The Panthay (Chinese Muslims) of Burma and Yunnan", *Journal of Southeast Asian History* 7, no. 1 (Mar. 1966): 81.
13 See J. Baxter, *Report on Indian Immigration* (Rangoon: Superintendent, Government Printing and Stationery, 1941); Usha Mahajani, *The Role of Indian Minorities in Burma and Malaya* (Bombay: Vora and Co., 1960); and Michael Adas, *The Burma Delta: Economic Development and Social Change on an Asian Rice Frontier 1852–1941* (Madison: University of Wisconsin Press, 1974).
14 *Report on the Public Health Administration of Burma* 1931 (Rangoon: 1932), p. 2.
15 Mahajani, *Role of Indian Minorities in Burma*, p. 3.
16 Michael Symes, *An Account of an Embassy to the Kingdom of Ava* (London: W. Bulmer and Co., 1800), p. 314.

17 Father Sangermano, *A Description of the Burmese Empire*, translated by William Tandy. Originally published in Rome by Oriental Translation Fund of Great Britain and Ireland in 1833 (New York: Augustus M. Kelley, 1969), p. 97.

18 Henry Burney, Godfrey Eric Harvey, ed. "On the Population of the Burman Empire", *The Journal of the Burma Research Society* 31, pt. 1 (Apr. 1941): 27.

19 Sangermano, *Description of the Burmese Empire*, p. 97.

20 Ibid., pp. 42–3.

21 Henry Yule, *A Narrative of the Mission Sent by the Governor-General of India to the Court of Ava in 1855*. Originally published in 1858 (Kuala Lumpur and New York: Oxford University Press, 1968), p. 288.

22 Economic and Social Board, *A Study of the Economic and Social History of Burma*, Pt. 3, Administration Report (Rangoon: Office of the Prime Minister, 1957), pp. 4–6. See also Adas, *The Burma Delta*, p. 20.

23 William J. Koenig, "The Early Konbaung Polity 1752–1819: A Study of Politics, Administration and Social Organisation in Burma" (PhD dissertation, University of London, 1978), p. 84. In a footnote Koenig says that there is no evidence that systematic resettlement resulted in Upper Burma, but there are references in Vol. A of the various Burma district *Gazetteers* to possible descendants of the Assamese.

24 Frank N. Trager and William J. Koenig, *Burmese Sit-tans 1764–1826* (Tucson: University of Arizona Press, 1979), p. 30.

25 Ibid., p. 30. Any judgement of the numbers involved is hazardous, but Trager and Koenig say "tens of thousands starved to death".

26 Accounts of the epidemic in Siam were evaluated by Barend Jan Terwiel, "Asiatic Cholera in Siam: Its First Occurrence and the 1820 Epidemic" in *Death and Disease in Southeast Asia*, ed. Norman G. Owen (Singapore: Oxford University Press, 1987), p. 148.

27 Sangermano, *Description of the Burmese Empire*, p. 168.

28 For more general discussion of demographic loss from crown control see Victor B. Lieberman, *Burmese Administrative Cycles: Anarchy and Conquest c 1580–1760* (Princeton: Princeton University Press, 1984).

29 Koenig, "The Early Konbaung Polity", p. 88. See also Sigfrid Henry Steinberg, *The Thirty Years War and the Conflict for European Hegemony 1600–1660* (London: Edward Arnold, 1977). Although it is hazardous to make comparisons between Europe and Southeast Asia, it is worth noting that Steinberg argued effectively that displacement of communities, not wholesale death, was the reason for the decline of 60 or 80 per cent in the population of some areas of Germany during the Thirty Years War. This study showed that a decade after the end of the war, these populations had returned.

30 Koenig, "The Early Konbaung Polity", p. 96.

31 Ibid., p. 98.

32 Adas, *The Burma Delta*, pp. 20, 21.

33 Ibid. See also Widjojo Nitisastro, *Population Trends in Indonesia* (Ithaca: Cornell University Press, 1970), pp. 21, 22. There is a similar discussion here of the under-enumeration in Raffles' assessment of the population of Java. Village heads were forced into the dual role of representatives of the people and tax collectors for the government. The collector had to obtain population

information from these headmen, which, as the headmen and villagers were both aware, was directly related to taxation.

34 Kingsley Davis, *The Population of India and Pakistan* (Princeton: Princeton University Press, 1951), p. 26.

35 Economic and Social Board, *Economic and Social History of Burma*, p. 5.

36 My own suggestion would be to roughly double the figures, which would then bring them into alignment with the totals estimated for Upper Burma, to form, between them, an "acceptable" figure for Burma Proper.

37 Hall, *History of South-East Asia*, p. 772.

38 See Bernard Benjamin, *The Population Census* (London: Heinemann, 1970), p. 158. In the post-enumeration survey taken three weeks after the 1961 Census of Great Britain, it was found that of the sample of 146,692 people, 209 were counted twice and 240 missed at the census. These are described as "small errors", due to a census held "with a high degree of simultaneity in such a highly urbanised and densely populated country". Therefore the margin for error in a disturbed rural, non-bureaucratic, potentially hostile Upper Burma must be high. For discussion of the estimated under-enumeration in the Indian post-war census, in particular the under-counts of six per cent in 1951 and 1971, see Tim Dyson, "Preliminary Demography of 1981 Census", *Economic and Political Weekly* 16, no. 3 (1981): 1349–56, and Pravin M Visaria, "Provisional Population Totals of the 1971 Census", *Economic and Political Weekly* 6, no. 29 (1971), p. 1459.

39 Albert Fytche, *Burma Past and Present,* Vol. II (London: Kegan Paul & Co., 1878), p. 222.

40 Adas, *The Burma Delta*, p. 22.

41 Norman G. Owen, "Southeast Asia — The Paradox of Nineteenth Century Population Growth" (Unpublished paper, Mar. 1985), p. 8.

42 *Census of India 1901, Vol. 1-A, India, Pt. 2, Tables* (Calcutta: Government Printing, 1903), p. 5.

43 *Imperial Gazetteer of India, Burma*, Vol. 1 (Calcutta: 1908), p. 336.

44 *Burma Gazetteer, Vol. B, Maubin District No. 14* (Rangoon: 1912).

45 *Burma Gazetteer, Vol. B, Myaungmya District No. 13* (Rangoon: 1912).

46 *Census of India 1911*, Vol. 9, *Burma, Part 2, Tables* (Rangoon: Superintendent, Government Printing, 1912).

47 *Census of India 1901*, Vol. 12-C. *Burma, Part 4, Upper Burma Provincial Tables* (Rangoon: Superintendent, Government Printing, 1905). See comment on p. 656: "The area synchronously and non-synchronously enumerated at the 1891 census, was far smaller than that so dealt with at the 1901 enumeration and the area estimated was far larger, thus no comparison can be instituted between the two sets of figures."

48 *Census of British Burma 1872*, Report (Rangoon: Government Press, 1875), p. 3.

49 Benjamin, *The Population Census*, pp. 157, 158.

50 *Burma Gazetteer, Vol. A, Mandalay District* (Rangoon: 1928), p. 163.

51 Ibid., p. 79.

52 Hall, *History of South-East Asia*, p. 771.

53 *Burma Gazetteer, Vol. A, Lower Chindwin District* (Rangoon: 1912), p. 149.

54 *Census of British Burma, 1872*, p. 2.
55 Ibid., pp. 4, 5.
56 For a full discussion of the development of agriculture in the delta see: Adas, *The Burma Delta*.
57 Baxter, *Report on Indian Immigration*, p. 5.
58 Hall, *History of South-East Asia*, p. 626.
59 *Census of India 1891*, General Tables for the British Provinces and Feudatory States, Vol. 2, Statistics (London: Eyre and Spottiswoode, 1892).
60 *Census of India 1901*, Vol. 12-C. Burma Part 4, Upper Burma Provincial Tables (Rangoon: Superintendent of Government Printing, 1905).
61 *Burma Gazetteer, Vol. A, Shwebo District* (Rangoon: 1929, reprinted 1963), p. 46.
62 *Census of India 1891*, General Tables ... Vol. 2.
63 J. G. Scott and J. P. Hardiman, *Gazetteer of Upper Burma and the Shan States*, Pt. 2, Vol. 1 (Rangoon: Superintendent of Government Printing, 1901), p. 326.
64 *Census of India 1931*, Vol. 11, Burma Part 2, Tables (Rangoon: Superintendent of Government Printing, 1933).
65 *Burma Gazetteer, Vol. B, Yamethin District No. 39* (Rangoon: 1924).
66 *Burma Gazetteer, Vol. B, Myingyan District No. 38* (Rangoon: 1913).
67 *Census of India 1911*, Vol. 9, p. 4.
68 *Burma Gazetteer, Vol. B, Myingyan District No. 40* (Rangoon: 1924).
69 Ibid.
70 *Census of India 1931*, Vol. 11.
71 *Burma Gazetteer, Vol. A, Kyaukse District* (Rangoon: 1925), p. 106.
72 For an example of the complexity of these adjustments see *Burma Gazetteer, Vol. B, Tharrawaddy District No. 8* (Rangoon: 1912), and *Burma Gazetteer, Vol. B, Myaungmya District No. 13* (Rangoon: 1912), where it is stated that "No township as at present coincides with the township area of 1901".
73 *Census of India 1911*, Vol. 9, p. 4.

CHAPTER 2

1 Henry S. Shryock and Jacob S. Siegal, *The Methods and Materials of Demography*, condensed and edited by Edward G. Stockwell (New York: Academic Press, 1976), p. 1.
2 HMSO, *Memorandum on Measures Adopted for Sanitary Improvements in India up to the end of 1867* (London: Eyre and Spottiswoode for HMSO, 1868), p. 1.
3 Ibid., p. 2.
4 Ibid., p. 2.
5 Daniel George Edward Hall, *A History of South-East Asia*, 4th edition (Basingstoke: Macmillan, 1981), p. 664.
6 *Report on the Sanitary Administration of British Burma*, 1870, Resolution, p. 1. These reports are generally referred to in the text as annual health reports, and they were issued yearly by the Government Press of Rangoon. From 1870 to 1889, their title was as above and they will be referred to as *RSABB* and the designating year. From 1890 to 1920, their title was *Report on the Sanitary Administration of Burma*, and they will be referred to as *RSAB* and

the designating year. From 1921 to 1936, the report was titled *Report on the Public Health Administration of Burma* and will be referred to as *RPHAB* and the designating year. Finally in 1937, the title was changed to *Report on the State of Public Health in Burma* and will be referred to as *RSPHB* and the designating year.

7 *RSABB*, 1883, Resolution accompanying the Report, p. 1.
8 *RSABB*, 1876, pp. 29, 30.
9 *RSAB*, 1898, p. 1.
10 Ibid., Appendix, p. V.
11 *RSABB*, 1870, p. 99.
12 *RSABB*, 1875, p. 20.
13 *RSABB*, 1870, p. 100
14 *RSABB*, 1883, Resolution, p. 1.
15 *Proceedings of the Chief Commissioner, Burma. In the General Department. No. 44.S. (Sanitary)*, (26/8/1891).
16 *RSABB*, 1882, p. 2.
17 *RSAB*, 1895, p. 2.
18 *RSAB*, 1897, p. 1.
19 *RSAB*, 1904, Resolution, p. 1.
20 *RSABB*, 1885, p. 4.
21 *RSAB*, 1901, p. 3.
22 *RSAB*, 1905, p. 2.
23 *RPHAB*, 1921, p. 4.
24 *RSABB*, 1883, p. 4.
25 *RSAB*, 1894, p. 6.
26 *RSABB*, 1870, pp. 108, 109.
27 *RSABB*, 1877, p. 25, and *RSABB*, 1878 Table VI respectivelty.
28 *RSAB*, 1911, pp. 1, 3.
29 Ibid., p. 3.
30 J. I. Clarke, *Population Geography and the Developing Countries* (Oxford: Pergamon Press, 1971), p. 259.
31 *RSAB*, 1906, p. 2.
32 *RSAB*, 1894, p. 3.
33 *RSABB*, 1879, p. 2.
34 *RSABB*, 1883, p. 3.
35 *RSAB*, 1892, p. 1.
36 *RSABB*, 1871, p. 4.
37 *RSAB*, 1896, p. 5.
38 Ibid., p. 4.
39 *RSABB*, 1882, p. 2.
40 *RSAB*, 1907, p. 3.
41 *RSAB*, 1892, p. 29; *RSAB*, 1894, p. 7; *RSAB*, 1910, p. 2.
42 *RPHAB*, 1923, p. 3.
43 Patricia Herbert, *The Hsaya San Rebellion (1930–1932) Reappraised*, Working Paper No. 27 (Melbourne: Monash University, Centre of Southeast Asian Studies, 1982), p. 1.
44 *RSAB*, 1912, p. 4.

[45] *RPHAB*, 1930, p. 50.

[46] *RPHAB*, 1934, p. 29.

[47] *RSPHB*, 1939, p. 36.

[48] *RSPHB*, 1937, p. 41; *RSPHB*, 1938, p. 41; *RSPHB*, 1939, p. 38.

[49] Ansley Johnson Coale and Paul Demeny, "Methods of Estimating Basic Demographic Measures from Incomplete Data", *Population Studies* no. 42 (New York: UN Department of Economic and Social Affairs, 1967), pp. 57–61. Hereafter referred to as UN Manual 4.

[50] This detailed breakdown into religions was not constant in all districts, and those that had only small populations of Animists, Hindus, Mohammedans or Christians gave these religious populations in totals only with no age groupings detailed. Districts which had large populations of Hindus and Mohammedans sub-divided these groups into those born in Burma and those not. A few districts, such as Mandalay, had population groups described as "Others", some large enough to be defined by age, but usually shown as totals of the sexes only.

[51] J. P. Ferguson, "The Society and its Environments", in *Burma: A Country Study*, ed. Frederica M. Bunge, Area Handbook Series, 3rd edition (Washington, DC: US Government, 1983), pp. 94, 95.

[52] UN Manual 4, p. 58. The analysis was repeated using data which included these Hindu and Muslim groups and, due to the smallness of these groups, the results were the same.

[53] It is explained later in the chapter that the result of the calculations should be an even pattern, an approximation to/or between one or two levels of Model Life Tables. A wide spread of levels indicates problems with the data. In the analysis of the 1921–1931 data, seven out of the ten results lay between levels 3 and 5, suggesting that the smoothed data was acceptably accurate.

[54] Roland Pressat, *The Dictionary of Demography*, ed. Christopher Wilson (Oxford: Basil Blackwell, 1985), pp. 4–6.

[55] UN Manual 4, p. 10. See also footnote p. 11.

[56] The problem in the northeast was caused by the exclusion of the Wuntho State from the 1891 Census and its inclusion in later census. From 1901, the area which was formerly the Wuntho State was enumerated as part of Katha District. A small tract was also added to the Shwebo District. The addition of areas of land containing population has the same effect on census survival calculations as immigration; therefore, some form of adjustment was necessary to make the 1891 and 1901 populations of Katha District relatively stable. This balance was achieved by adding to the Katha District population of 1891 an estimate for the population of the Wuntho State, thereby making the district area of the 1891 and 1901 Census the same.

The problem in the southwest margin of the study area was caused by the formation of the Thaton District in 1895. This has already been discussed in Chapter One, and it was calculated that 40 per cent of the area of Thaton had been taken from the Pegu and Shwegyin Districts and 60 per cent from Amherst District. What was required for this analysis was the recreation of the 1891 boundaries in the same place as the 1901 boundaries.

In the 1901 Census there were 156,761 Buddhist females in the Thaton District and the population growth rate was 2.53 per cent per annum. Therefore the Buddhist female population in Thaton in 1891 would be 156,761 less the accumulated population increase of 2.53 per cent per annum or 121,720. But of this 121,720, only 605 had to be added to the total female Buddhist population of the study area as the other 40 per cent was already included in the populations of Pegu and Shwegyin Districts. This 60 per cent, or population of 73,032, was of all ages, and therefore needed assigning to the five year age groups. This was done by multiplying each age group by the new total female Buddhist population (including the 73,032) over the previous total, i.e. 3,038,156 divided by 2,965,124 equals 1.025.

[57] Ansley Johnson Coale and Paul Demeny, *Regional Model Life Tables and Stable Populations* (New York: Academic Press, 1983), pp. 42–5.

[58] UN Manual 4, p. 94.

[59] Ibid., p. 60.

[60] For discussion of bias, see UN Manual 4, p. 61; and for the method of calculating the levels of mortality under ten years, see p. 60.

[61] *RPHAB*, 1930, p. 8.

[62] *RPHAB*, 1930, p. 5; *RPHAB*, 1935, p. 10; *RPHAB*, 1936, p. 13.

[63] *RPHAB*, 1939, p. 9.

CHAPTER 3

[1] *Burma Gazetteer, Vol. A, Bassein District* (Rangoon: 1916), p. 119.

[2] Louis Henry, *Population Analysis and Models*, translated by Etienne van de Walle and Elise F. Jones (London: Edward Arnold, 1976), p. 148.

[3] Roland Pressat, *The Dictionary of Demography*, ed. Christopher Wilson (Oxford: Basil Blackwell, 1985), p. 108.

[4] *Burma Gazetteer, Vol. A, Insein District* (Rangoon: 1914), p. 166. See also *Burma Gazetteer, Vol. A, Syriam District* (Rangoon: 1914), p. 187.

[5] W. T. Gairdner, 'On Infantile Death Rates, in their bearing on Sanitary and Social Science', (1861), p. 15, in *Pamphlets PT.2348-57*, Secretary of State for India Library. It is perhaps worth noting that these opinions come only 15 years after F. Engels published his *The Condition of the Working Class in England*.

[6] Henry S. Shryock and Jacob S. Siegal, *The Methods and Materials of Demography*, condensed ed. Edward G. Stockwell (New York: Academic Press, 1976), p. 235.

[7] *Report on the Sanitary Administration of Burma*, 1909, p. 6.

These reports are generally referred to in the text as annual health reports, and they were issued yearly by the Government Press of Rangoon. From 1870 to 1889, their title was *Report on the Sanitary Administration of British Burma*, and they will be referred to as *RSABB* and the designating year. From 1890 to 1920, their title was as above, and they will be referred to as *RSAB* and the designating year. From 1921 to 1936, the report was titled *Report on the Public Health Administration of Burma*, and will be referred to as *RPHAB* and the designating year. Finally in 1937, the title was changed to *Report on the State of Public Health in Burma*, and will be referred to as *RSPHB* and the designating year.

8 *RSPHB*, 1939, p. 42.
9 Lenore Manderson, "Blame, Responsibility and Remedial Action: Death, Disease and the Infant in Early Twentieth Century Malaya", in *Death and Disease in Southeast Asia*, ed. Norman G. Owen (Singapore: Oxford University Press, 1987), p. 276.
10 League of Nations *Epidemiological Reports*, 1935/36, Vol. 14/15, p. 32.
11 Lado Theodor Ruzicka, "Mortality in India: Past Trends and Future Prospects", in *India's Demography*, ed. Tim Dyson and Nigel Crook (New Delhi: South Asia Publishers Pvt. Ltd., 1984), p. 18.
12 "Public Health and Births and Deaths 1867. British Burma". Extract from the *Proceedings of the Chief Commissioner in the Home Department*. No. 241 (Rangoon: Rangoon Times Press, 1868), p. 51. This was the first annual health report for Burma and will be described hereafter as PHBD.
13 *RSAB*, 1899, p. 9.
14 *RSAB*, 1901, p. 6.
15 *Burma Gazetteer, Vol. A, Bassein District* (Rangoon: 1916), p. 119.
16 *RSAB*, 1904, p. 4.
17 *RSAB*, 1905, p. 4.
18 *RSAB* 1908, Resolution, p. 2.
19 *Burma Gazetteer, Vol. A, Henzada District* (Rangoon: 1915), p. 206.
20 *RSAB*, 1913, p. 8.
21 *RSAB*, 1915, p. 6.
22 *RSAB*, 1916, p. 6.
23 *RSAB*, 1920, p. 9.
24 For further discussion of infant diets, see *RPHAB*, 1928, p. 14; *RPHAB*, 1930, p. 13; RPHAB, 1931, p. 14; RPHAB, 1932, p. 14; RPHAB, 1933, p. 9; and RPHAB, 1934, pp. 9, 10.
25 *RSAB*, 1915, p. 7.
26 *RPHAB*, 1931, p. 15.
27 C. V. Foll, "An Account of some of the Beliefs and Superstitions about Pregnancy, Parturition and Infant Health in Burma", *Journal of Tropical Paediatrics* 5, no. 1 (June 1959): 52.
28 Ibid., p. 53.
29 Ma Ma Tin, "Feeding Patterns of Infants and Young Children in Mandalay Region" (undated paper, probably 1970s). Burma Box, Nutrition Library, London School of Hygiene and Tropical Medicine, p. 4.
30 Cho Nwe Oo, "Nutrition in Pregnant and Lactating Mothers". Paper presented at 2nd Orientation Course in Nutrition for Paediatricians (June 1974), p. 3.
31 Ibid., p. 5. For further discussion, see C. V. Foll, "The Perils of Childhood in Upper Burma", *Journal of Tropical Paediatrics* 4, no. 3 (Dec. 1958): 124, suggesting that the main causes of neonatal deaths were probably local obstetrical practice and the smallness of babies; Jacques M. May, with the collaboration of Irma S. Jarcho, *The Ecology of Malnutrition in the Far and Near East: Food Resources, Habits and Deficiencies* (New York: Hafner Publishing Co., 1961), p. 193, regarding cultural influences on the diet of pregnant women in Burma and Southeast Asia; and FAO, *Report of the Nutrition*

Committee for South and East Asia, Third Meeting, 1953 (Rome: UN FAO, Apr. 1954), p. 9.

32   S. Postmus, "Beri beri of Mother and Child in Burma", *Tropical and Geographical Medicine* 10 (1958): 365.

33   F. Faulkner, "Key Issues in Infant Mortality", *Journal of Tropical Paediatrics and Environmental Child Health* 17, no. 1 (Mar. 1971): 3.

34   S. Postmus, "Diet and Nutritional Condition in Burma", *Burma Medical Journal* 5, no. 4 (Oct. 1957): 27.

35   C. V. Foll and Onmar Khin, "Perinatal Problems in Upper Burma", *Journal of Tropical Medicine and Hygiene* 61 (Sept. 1958): 309.

36   Tin U and Kyaw Myint, eds., "Report of the Peri-natal Mortality and Low Birth Weight Study Project — Burma", SEARO Inter-country Collaborative Project, WHO (Rangoon: Department of Medical Education, 1981), p. 93.

37   J. R. Barva, "Birth Weight, Length and Circumference of the Skull of Infants Born in the Largest Maternity Hospital of Burma", *Burma Medical Journal* 9, no. 1 (Jan 1961): 16.

38   Jane Pryer and Nigel Crook, *Cities of Hunger* (Oxford: Oxfam, 1988), p. 11.

39   Louis Henry, *Population Analysis and Models*, p. 148. See also Tin U and Kyaw Myint, eds., "Report of the Peri-natal Mortality ...". This major study in Hlegu township, near Rangoon, revealed that 50 per cent of neonatal deaths occurred in the first 24 hours and 60 per cent in the first 48 hours. Of the remaining 40 per cent of deaths, infections were the chief cause. This is in a health demonstration centre with twice the normal number of health staff plus additional intervention during the period of the study. It reveals that, when vaccination programmes have eliminated mortality from neonatal tetanus, etc., the neonate still remains highly vulnerable in the first hours of life.

40   Arthur P. Phayre, *Memorandum on the Sparseness of Population in British Burma* (Rangoon: Mission Press, 1862), p. 6.

41   K. N. MacDonald, *The Practice of Medicine Among the Burmese* (Edinburgh: MacLachan and Stewart, 1879), p. 11.

42   Phayre, *Memorandum on the Sparseness of Population*, p. 6.

43   *RSAB*, 1894, p. 28.

44   Foll, "... Beliefs and Superstitions about Pregnancy", p. 56; Foll, "The Perils of Childhood in Upper Burma", p. 124.

45   Ohn Kyi (Dr. Daw), "Beliefs and Practices about Foods and Feeding in Mon State (Moulmein)" (undated paper, probably 1970s); Ma Ma Tin, "Feeding Patterns of Infants ...", p. 2. Both papers are in a collection of undated papers in the Burma Box, Nutrition Library, London School of Hygiene and Tropical Medicine.

46   See discussion in Chapter 4.

47   *RPHAB*, 1928, p. 11.

48   Foll, "... Beliefs and Superstitions about Pregnancy", p. 53.

49   Ma Ma Tin, "Feeding Patterns of Infants ...", p. 4.

50   Sao Yan Naing, "Beliefs and Practices in Nutrition in Northern Shan States" (undated paper, probably 1970s). Burma Box, Nutrition Library, London School of Hygiene and Tropical Medicine.

51 Aung Kyin, "Beliefs and Practices in Nutrition in Central Burma (Magwe)" (undated paper, probably 1970s). Burma Box, Nutrition Library, London School of Hygiene and Tropical Medicine.

52 FAO, *Report of the Nutrition Committee for South and East Asia, Fourth Session*, Tokyo, Japan, 1956 (Rome: UN FAO, 1957), p. 11.

53 Foll, "… Beliefs and Superstitions about Pregnancy", p. 56.

54 Ma Ma Tin, "Feeding Patterns of Infants …", p. 4.

55 Cho Nwe Oo, "Yankin Village Nutrition Promotion Programme", *Burma Medical Journal* 23, nos. 1–4 (Jan.–Dec 1977): 60.

56 Khin-Maung-Naing, Tin-Tin-Oo, Kywe-Thein MS and New-New-Hlaing, "Study on Lactation Performance of Burmese Mothers", *American Journal of Clinical Nutrition* no. 33 (Dec. 1980): 2668.

57 Ibid., p. 2667.

58 Ibid., p. 2668.

59 Tin Tin Oo and Khin Maung Naing, 'A Comparison of Milk Output of Burmese Mothers by Three Different Methods', *Food and Nutrition Bulletin* 4, no. 4 (Dec 1982): 67.

60 Foll, "The Perils of Childhood in Upper Burma", p. 125.

61 Postmus, "Beri beri of Mother and Child in Burma", p. 366.

62 Ibid., p. 367.

63 Pryer and Crook, *Cities of Hunger*, p. 10.

64 Ibid., p. 11.

65 Postmus, "Beri beri of Mother and Child in Burma", p. 367.

66 Pryer and Crook, *Cities of Hunger*, pp. 13, 14.

67 Cho Nwe Oo, "Nutrition in Pregnant and Lactating Mothers", pp. 4, 5.

68 Postmus, "Beri beri of Mother and Child in Burma", p. 366.

69 Sein May Chit, "Nutritional Problems in Burma", p. 6 (undated paper, probably 1970s). Burma Box, Nutrition Library, London School of Hygiene and Tropical Medicine.

70 John Taylor, C. de C. Martin and Thant U, "Preliminary Enquiry into Beri-beri in Burma", *Indian Medical Research Memoirs*, Memoir No. 8 (Mar. 1928), p. 41.

71 FAO, *Rice and Rice Diets: A Nutritional Survey* (Washington: UN FAO, 1948), p. 15.

72 A. Mobsby, "The Nutrition Project, Burma. (WHO)", *Burma Weekly Bulletin* 5, no. 30 (Nov. 1956): 241.

73 FAO, *Report of the Nutrition Committee … Fourth Session*, p. 20.

74 J. W. D. Megau, S. P. Bhattacharji and B. K. Paul, "Further Observations on the Epidemic Dropsy Form of Beri Beri", *Indian Medical Gazette* 63 (Aug. 1928): 419.

75 Kywe Thein, Thane Toe, Tin Tin Oo and Khin Khin Tway, "A Study of Infantile Beri-beri in Rangoon", *Union of Burma Journal of Life Sciences* 1 (1968): 62.

76 Ibid., p. 64. See also Cho Nwe Oo, "Nutrition in Pregnant and Lactating Mothers", for discussion of sub-clinical level of thiamine deficiency in lactating women in Hlegu township.

77 Kywe Thein, et al., "A Study of Infantile Beri-beri in Rangoon", p. 63.

[78] Vinijchaikul K., "Pathological Studies of Acute Infantile Cardiac Beri-beri", *Journal of the Medical Association of Thailand* 47, no. 2 (Feb. 1964): 58.

[79] Kywe Thein, et al., "A Study of Infantile Beri-beri in Rangoon", p. 64.

[80] Postmus, "Diet and Nutritional Condition in Burma", p. 27.

[81] Postmus, "Beri beri of Mother and Child in Burma", p. 368.

[82] PHBD, 1867, p. 51.

[83] *Report on Public Health and Vital Statistics for 1868* (Rangoon: 1870), p. 209. (Hereafter referred to as *RPHVS*.)

[84] *RSABB*, 1870, p. 115.

[85] *RSAB*, 1901, p. 6.

[86] Phayre, *Memorandum on the Sparseness of Population*, p. 6.

[87] William F. B. Laurie, *Our Burmese Wars and Relations with Burma* (London: W. H. Allen & Co., 1880), p. 330.

[88] Ibid., p. 329.

[89] N. K. Kunhikannan, "Infant Feeding in Burma", Current Topics, *Indian Medical Gazette* 55 (July 1920): 265.

[90] FAO, *Report of the Nutrition Committee … Third Meeting*, p. 8.

[91] Ohn Kyi, "Beliefs and Practices about Foods and Feeding …".

[92] Ma Ma Tin, "Feeding Patterns of Infants …", p. 2.

[93] Sao Yan Naing, "Beliefs and Practices in Nutrition in Northern Shan States"; Tin E, "Beliefs and Practices about Foods and Feedings in Kachin State (Myitkyina)" (undated paper, probably 1970s). Burma Box, Nutrition Library, London School of Hygiene and Tropical Medicine.

[94] Po Po, "Nutritional Problems in Childhood", *Burma Medical Journal* 13 (April/July 1965): 100.

[95] Tin Tin Oo and Khin Maung Naing, "Breast Feeding and Weaning Practices for Infants and Young Children in Rangoon", Summary in *DMR Bulletin* 1, no. 3 (Oct. 1986): 33.

[96] Tin Tin Oo and Khin Maung Naing, "Breast Feeding and Weaning Practices for Infants and Young Children in Rangoon, Burma", *Food and Nutrition Bulletin* 7, no. 4 (Dec. 1985): 51.

[97] B. P. Sarin, "Observations on 'Kwashiorkor' or Protein Undernutrition in Rangoon", *Burma Medical Journal* 5, no. 2 (Apr. 1957): 2.

[98] Robert O. Whyte, *Rural Nutrition in Monsoon Asia* (Kuala Lumpur: Oxford University Press, 1974), p. 61.

[99] Kunhikannan, "Infant Feeding in Burma", p. 266.

[100] Sein May Chit, "Nutritional Problems in Burma", p. 1.

[101] Ibid., p. 3.

[102] *RPHAB*, 1930, p. 16.

[103] *RSABB*, 1881, p. 1.

[104] *RSAB*, 1909, p. 6.

[105] *RSAB*, 1915, p. 6.

[106] *RSAB*, 1916, p. 6.

[107] *RPHAB*, 1931, p. 15.

[108] Richard W. B. Ellis in "Infantile Convulsions", *Burma Medical Journal* 4, no. 2 (Apr. 1956): 7–8, differentiates between convulsions in the first 48 hours, and post-48 hours. The first period deaths would be due to anoxia or trauma,

and the neonatal deaths particularly to neonatal tetanus, *B. coli* and *staphylococci*. He suggested that post-neonatal convulsions may be due to infection, hypocalcaemia, infantile beri beri and malaria.

109 R. L. Broadhead, "Tetanus Neonatorum. A Review of Epidemiology, Management and Prevention", *Postgraduate Doctor* 8, no. 7 (July 1985): 456. There would appear to be some breadth of opinion on the incubation of neonatal tetanus. See M. S. Islam, Rahaman M. M., Aziz K. M. S., Munshi M. H., Rahman M. and Patwari Y. P., "Birthcare Practice and Neonatal Tetanus in a Rural Area of Bangladesh", *Journal of Tropical Paediatrics* 28, no. 6 (Dec. 1982): 279, where a common symptom of neonatal tetanus is said to be the inability to suckle within four to five days of birth.

Also, F. D. Schofield, V. M. Tucker and G. R. Westbrook, "Neonatal Tetanus in New Guinea", *British Medical Journal* (23 Sept. 1961): 786, where the first symptom of neonatal tetanus in this survey was the failure to suck between the third and tenth days, and the child must have died by the end of the fourteenth day to be included in the study (relying on oral evidence).

Also, for an example of how age-specific neonatal tetanus can be, see Tom Steel, *The Life and Death of St Kilda* (UK: Fontana, 1975): on the island of Hirta in the outer Hebrides, of 32 male infants born between 1855 and 1876, 25 died of neonatal tetanus, or what the islanders called the "sickness of eight days".

110 Ko Ko U and Khin May Khi, "Epidemiology of Tetanus Neonatorum in Rangoon", *Union of Burma Journal of Life Sciences* 3 (1970): 54.

111 Shwe Oh, "Epidemiology of Neonatal Tetanus in Mandalay Division", Dissertation, Dept. of Preventive and Tropical Medicine, Institute of Medicine 1 (1973–4), p. 36.

112 Gerald L. Mandell, Robert G. Douglas and John E Bennett, eds., *Principles and Practice of Infectious Disease* (New York: J. Wiley and Sons, 1979), p. 1355.

113 Ko Ko U and Khin May Khi, "Epidemiology of Tetanus Neonatorum in Rangoon", p. 55.

114 Mandell, et al., eds., *Principles and Practice of Infectious Disease*, p. 1355.

115 John B. Wyon and John E. Gordon, *The Khanna Study* (Harvard: Harvard University Press, 1971), p. 184.

116 M. S. Islam, et al., "Birthcare Practice ...", p. 300.

117 *RPHVS*, 1868, p. 60.

118 *RSAB*, 1913, p. 8.

119 *RSAB*, 1914, p. 9.

120 *RSAB*, 1915, p. 6.

121 *RSAB*, 1916, p. 6.

122 *RSAB*, 1915, p. 6.

123 PHBD, 1867, p. 61. See also Shwe Oh, "Epidemiology of Neonatal Tetanus in Mandalay Division", and Ko Ko U and Khin May Khi, "Epidemiology of Tetanus Neonatorum in Rangoon", for discussions of seasonality of neonatal tetanus. The peak in Rangoon occurred in June, during the rains, and this was also true for Mandalay. But births also peak in that season, probably due to the Buddhist Lent (when no marriages take place) leading to a marriage peak in November. Both the Rangoon and Mandalay studies

also found a higher incidence of males than females; but all these cases were hospital admissions, so this may reflect more care being given to male babies than female, and not the disease incidence.

124 *RSAB*, 1913, p. 7.
125 *RSAB*, 1920, p. 9.
126 *RSAB*, 1920, Resolution, Rangoon, p. 5.
127 *RSAB*, 1894, p. 28.
128 *RPHAB*, 1931, p. 16.
129 *RSAB*, 1920, p. 9.
130 Foll, "... Beliefs and Superstitions about Pregnancy", p. 55.
131 Shwe Oh, "Epidemiology of Neonatal Tetanus in Mandalay Division", p. 45.
132 Ibid., p. 46; Ko Ko U and Khin May Khi, "Epidemiology of Tetanus Neonatorum in Rangoon", p. 186.
133 PHBD, 1867, p. 74.
134 Ibid., p. 90.
135 *RPHVS*, 1868, p. 208.
136 *RSAB*, 1910, p. 5.
137 *RSAB*, 1910, p. 6.
138 *RSAB*, 1913, p. 8.
139 *RPHAB*, 1924, p. 12.
140 P. C. Banerjee, "Report of a Measles Survey in Sagaing", *Burma Medical Journal* 16, no. 4 (Oct. 1968): 219. In this survey, Dr Banerjee found a history of 82 attacks among 633 infants, or 13 per cent, of which five were fatal.
141 *RPHAB*, 1921, p. 13.
142 A. Tomkins, G. Mann and S. Khanum, "New Approaches Toward the Prevention of Measles", *Postgraduate Doctor* 2, no. 1 (1986): 5.
143 B. P. Sarin, "The Treatment of Acute Diarrhoea in Infants", *Burma Medical Journal* 4, no. 4 (Oct. 1956). Dr Sarin noted in his paper that "undernutrition and prematurity predispose to diarrhoeas, as these infants have a lowered functional capacity and poor resistance to infection".
144 B. E. R. Symonds, "Clinical Studies on South Trinidadian Children. 11. The Treatment of Neonatal Tetanus", *Journal of Tropical Paediatrics* 6, no. 1 (June 1960): 13.
145 G. T. Strickland, *Hunter's Tropical Medicine* (London: W.B. Saunders and Co., 1984), p. 17.
146 Ibid., p. 315. See also p. 973 for confirmation that *E. coli* is found in Southeast Asia.
147 *RSAB*, 1909, p. 6.
148 *RSAB*, 1910, p. 6.
149 *RPHVS*, 1868, p. 60; *RPHAB*, 1927, p. 29; *RPHAB*, 1928, p. 27.
150 *RPHAB*, 1924, p. 13.
151 *RPHAB*, 1931, p. 16.
152 *RSPHB*, 1937, p. 44; 1938, p. 44.
153 *Burma Gazetteer, Vol. A. Yamethin District* (Rangoon: 1934), p. 159.
154 Paul D. Hoeprich, ed., *Infectious Diseases: A Guide to the Understanding and Management of Infectious Processes* (Hagerstown, MD: Harper and Row, 1983), p. 618.

155 Ibid., p. 619.
156 Mandell, et al., eds., *Principles and Practice of Infectious Disease*, p. 1328.
157 *RSAB*, 1916, p. 6.
158 *RSAB*, 1893, p. 27. *RSAB*, 1894, p. 30. So great was the panic in Mandalay that a petition was sent to the Sanitary Commissioner asking him to take steps to remedy the "growing evil".
159 *RSAB*, 1892, p. 29.
160 *RSAB*, 1919, p. 8.
161 Samuel R. Christophers, John A. Sinton and Gordon Covell, *How To Do a Malaria Survey*, Health Bulletin No. 14 (Government of India Central Publications Branch, 1928), p. 119.
162 John A. Sinton, *What Malaria Costs India*, Health Bulletin No. 26, Malaria Bureau No. 13 (Simla: Government of India Press, 1939), p. 2.
163 Ibid., pp. 8, 9.
164 John A. Sinton, *What Malaria Costs India* (1939), p. 10.
165 C. A. Bentley, *Malaria and Agriculture in Bengal*, Government of Bengal Public Health Department (Calcutta: Bengal Secretariat Book Depot, 1925).
166 G. J. Ebrahim, "Editorial: Malaria in Childhood", *Journal of Tropical Paediatrics* 30, no. 4 (Aug. 1984): 194.
167 Ibid.
168 *RSABB*, 1883, p. 12.
169 E. Meyer, "Depression et Malaria à Sri-Lanka 1925–1939", Vol. 1, Thesis, Écoles des Hautes Études en Science Sociales, (1980), p. 214.
170 Ibid., p. 220.
171 *RSAB*, 1909, p. 6.
172 *RSAB*, 1910, p. 6.
173 *RSAB*, 1909, p. 4.
174 *RSAB*, 1910, p. 5.
175 *RSAB*, 1917, pp. 10, 11.
176 *RSAB*, 1916, p. 11. The figure for Kyaukse district has been taken from 1917, p. 11, as the figure given for Kyaukse in 1916 is 83 only, and this would appear to be a printing error.
177 Ibid., p. 10.
178 *RSAB*, 1917, p. 11.
179 Ibid., p. 12.
180 J. G. Scott and J. P. Hardiman, *Gazetteer of Upper Burma and the Shan States*, Part 2, Vol. 1 (Rangoon: 1901), p. 507.
181 *RPHAB*, 1926, p. 9.
182 *RPHAB*, 1930, p. 13.
183 *RPHAB*, 1929, p. 9; *RPHAB*, 1931, p. 16; *RPHAB*, 1933, p. 8; *RSPHB*, 1938, p. 44; *RSPHB*, 1939, p. 42; Maung Tin, *Report on the Malaria Survey of Kya-In Township, Amherst District* (Rangoon: 1941), p. 29.
184 N. P. O'Gorman Lalor, *Investigation of Malaria at Kyaukpyu* (Rangoon: 1912), p. 4.
185 N. P. O'Gorman Lalor, *Investigation of Malaria in the District of Katha* (Rangoon: 1913), p. 2.
186 Ma Htay Nwe, "Malaria in Children in Lashio Township", *Burma Medical Journal* 26, no. 3 (Sept. 1980): 164, 165.

187 Ibid., p. 163.
188 *RSPHB*, 1938, p. 42.
189 League of Nations Health Organisation, *Intergovernmental Conference of Far-Eastern Countries on Rural Hygiene, Preparatory Papers, 2. Note on Medical Organisation in Burma* (Geneva: 15 Mar. 1937), p. 45.
190 Ibid., p. 43.
191 *RSAB*, 1917, p. 6.
192 *RPHAB*, 1934, p. 35.
193 *RSAB*, 1906, p. 4.
194 *RPHAB*, 1929, p. 10.
195 *RPHAB*, 1928, p. 14.
196 *RSAB*, 1920, p. 11.
197 *RPHAB*, 1935, p. 44.
198 *RPHAB*, 1922, p. 15.
199 *RSPHB*, 1939, p. 43.
200 *RPHAB*, 1931, p. 16.
201 *RPHAB*, 1929, p. 11.
202 *RPHAB*, 1931, pp. 17, 19.
203 *RSPHB*, 1939, p. 43.
204 *RPHAB*, 1929, p. 10; *RPHAB*, 1930, p. 15.
205 *RPHAB*, 1932, p. 50.
206 "Notes and News: Infant Death Rate in Burma", *Journal of Tropical Medicine and Hygiene* 17 (1914): 350.
207 Evans Col., "Burma Hospitals. Extract from Annual Report", *Indian Medical Gazette* 50 (Oct. 1915): 392.
208 *RPHAB*, 1927, p. 17; *RSAB*, 1916, p. 4.
209 *RPHAB*, 1929, pp. 59–61.
210 *RSAB*, 1915, p. 7.
211 *RSAB*, 1920, p. 11.

CHAPTER 4

1 Roland Pressat, *The Dictionary of Demography*, ed. Christopher Wilson (Oxford: Basil Blackwell, 1985), p. 76.
2 Melford E. Spiro, *Kinship and Marriage in Burma* (Berkeley: University of California Press, 1977), p. 107.
3 Mi Mi Khaing, *The World of Burmese Women* (London: Zed Books Ltd., 1984), p. 16; Spiro, *Kinship and Marriage in Burma*, p. 259.
4 Spiro, *Kinship and Marriage in Burma*, p. 84.
5 Ibid., p. 84; Mi Mi Khaing, *The World of Burmese Women*, p. 15.
6 Mi Mi Khaing, *The World of Burmese Women*, p. 26.
7 Father Sangermano, *A Description of the Burmese Empire*, transl. William Tandy. Originally published in Rome by Oriental Translation Fund of Great Britain and Ireland in 1833. (New York: Augustus M. Kelley, 1969), p. 165.
8 Mi Mi Khaing *The World of Burmese Women*, p. 34. C. Mougne, in a paper given to the British Society for Population Studies at City University, London on 12 July 1985, described a very similar matrilocal agreement in northern Thai villages. The son-in-law, while staying with the bride's parents, is known as the "work buffalo".

9   White, Herbert Thirkell, *A Civil Servant in Burma* (London: Edward Arnold, 1913), p. 70. It is difficult to assess the credibility of White's statements because, on the same page, he stated that jealousy was a prevalent vice and "many die for love" in Burma.

10   Tin U and Kyaw Myint, eds., "Report of the Peri-natal Mortality and Low Birth Weight Study Project — Burma", SEARO Inter-country Collaborative Project, WHO (Rangoon: Department of Medical Education, 1981), p. 37.

11   C. J. R. Francis and U. E. K. Mamsa, "Age of Puberty in the Burmese Male and Female", *Union of Burma Journal of Life Sciences* 3 (1970): 178.

12   Ansley Johnson Coale and Paul Demeny, "Methods of Estimating Basic Demographic Measures from Incomplete Data", *Population Studies* no. 42 (New York: UN Department of Economic and Social Affairs, 1967), pp. 96, 97.

13   Arthur P. Phayre, *Memorandum on the Sparseness of Population in British Burma* (Rangoon: Mission Press, 1862), p. 5.

14   Susan C. M. Scrimshaw, "Infant Mortality and Behaviour in the Regulation of Family Size", *Population and Development Review* 4, no. 3 (Sept. 1978), p. 389.

15   Tin Tin Nyunt, "Estimation of Vital Rates for Burma and Their Effects on the Future Size of the Population". MA thesis, Australian National University, Dept. of Demography, Research School of Social Sciences (Canberra: ANU, Sept. 1978), p. 71.

16   Ibid., p. 71.

17   John Charles Caldwell, "The Mechanisms of Demographic Change in Historical Perspective", *Population Studies* 35, no. 1 (Mar. 1981): 14.

18   Ibid., p. 15.

19   June Nash and Manning Nash, "Marriage, Family, and Population Growth in Upper Burma", *Southwestern Journal of Anthropology* 19, no. 3 (1963): 257.

20   Anthony Reid, "Low Population Growth and its Causes in Pre-Colonial Southeast Asia"; Norman G. Owen, "Toward a History of Health in Southeast Asia", both in *Death and Disease in Southeast Asia*, ed. Norman G. Owen (Singapore: Oxford University Press, 1987), pp. 39 and 40, and p. 11, respectively.

21   Sarah B. Hanley and Kozo Yamamura, *Economic and Demographic Change in Pre-Industrial Japan 1600–1868* (Princeton: Princeton University Press, 1977), p. 324. See this work for a discussion of the regulation of family size in Tokugawa, Japan, through delayed marriage, high percentage of non-married, abortion and infanticide.

22   For a discussion of population and adjustment in Europe and Asia, see Edward A. Wrigley, *Population and History* (London: Weidenfeld and Nicolson, 1969); and Hanley and Yamamura, *Change in Pre-Industrial Japan*.

23   Pressat, *The Dictionary of Demography*, p. 21.

24   *Journal of Tropical Paediatrics*, "Contraceptive Effect of Breast Feeding", 28, no. 1 (Feb. 1982) Editorial, p. iii.

25   John B. Wyon and John E. Gordon, *The Khanna Study* (Harvard: Harvard University Press, 1971), pp. 168, 169.

26   Ibid., p. 169.

27 Michel Carael, "Relations between Birth Intervals and Nutrition in Three Central African Populations (Zaire)", in *Nutrition and Human Reproduction*, ed. W. Henry Mosely (New York: Plenum Press, 1978), p. 379.

28 Robert O. Whyte, *Rural Nutrition in Monsoon Asia* (Kuala Lumpur: Oxford University Press, 1974), p. 13.

29 Scrimshaw, "Infant Mortality and Behaviour in the Regulation of Family Size", p. 395.

30 Phayre, *Memorandum on the Sparseness of Population*, p. 5.

31 Nash and Nash, "Marriage, Family, and Population Growth ...", p. 265.

32 Pressat, *The Dictionary of Demography*, p. 140.

33 Ibid., p. 140.

34 *Report on Public Health and Vital Statistics for 1868* (Rangoon: 1870), pp. 47, 48. Hereafter referred to as *RPHVS*.

35 C. V. Foll, "An Account of some of the Beliefs and Superstitions about Pregnancy, Parturition and Infant Health in Burma", *Journal of Tropical Paediatrics* 5, no. 1 (June 1959): 54.

36 Ibid., p. 123.

37 Sangermano, *A Description of the Burmese Empire*, p. 165.

38 Whyte, *Rural Nutrition in Monsoon Asia*, p. 64.

39 Spiro, *Kinship and Marriage in Burma*, p. 219.

40 Keith Norman MacDonald, *The Practice of Medicine Among the Burmese* (Edinburgh: MacLachan and Stewart, 1879), p. 54.

41 C. Mougne, "An Ethnography of Reproduction: Changing Patterns of Fertility in a Northern Thai Village" in *Nature and Man in South East Asia*, ed. P. A. Stott (London: School of Oriental and African Studies, 1978), p. 80.

42 Ibid., p. 81.

43 Foll, "... Beliefs and Superstitions about Pregnancy", p. 54.

44 Ibid., p. 55.

45 *Report on the Sanitary Administration of Burma*, 1914, p. 9. These reports are generally referred to in the text as annual health reports, and they were issued yearly by the Government Press of Rangoon. From 1870 to 1889, their title was *Report on the Sanitary Administration of British Burma*, and they will be referred to as *RSABB* and the designating year. From 1890 to 1920, their title was as above, and they will be referred to as *RSAB* and the designating year. From 1921 to 1936, the report was titled *Report on the Public Health Administration of Burma* and will be referred to as *RPHAB* and the designating year. Finally in 1937, the title was changed to *Report on the State of Public Health in Burma* and will be referred to as *RSPHB* and the designating year.

46 *RSAB*, 1914, p. 9.

47 *RSAB*, 1918, p. 3.

48 *RPHVS*, 1868, p. 209.

49 B. P. Sarin, "Observations on 'Kwashiorkor' or Protein Undernutrition in Rangoon", *Burma Medical Journal* 5, no. 2 (Apr. 1957): 1.

50 G. Thomas Strickland, *Hunter's Tropical Medicine* (London: W. B. Saunders and Co., 1984), p. 837.

51 *RSABB*, 1873, p. 26.

52 Dr Daw Ohn Kyi, "Beliefs and Practices about Foods and Feeding in Mon State (Moulmein)" (undated paper, probably 1970s). Burma Box, Nutrition Library, London School of Hygiene and Tropical Medicine.
53 Ma Ma Tin, "Feeding Patterns of Infants and Young Children in Mandalay Region" (undated paper, probably 1970s). Burma Box, Nutrition Library, London School of Hygiene and Tropical Medicine, p. 3.
54 Ibid., p. 3.
55 Po Po, "Nutritional Problems in Childhood", *Burma Medical Journal* 13 (April/ July 1965): 100.
56 Kywe-Thein, Tin-U, Tin-Tin-Oo and Khin-Kyi-Nyunt, "An Epidemiological Study of Protein Calorie Malnutrition in Rangoon", *Union of Burma Journal of Life Sciences* 4 (1971): 569, 572.
57 Cho Nwe Oo, "Prevalence of Protein Calorie Malnutrition in Burma", *Burma Medical Journal* 21, no. 4 (Oct. 1975): 4.
58 Dr Daw Sein May Chit "Nutritional Problems in Burma" (undated paper, probably 1970s). Burma Box, Nutrition Library, London School of Hygiene and Tropical Medicine, pp. 7, 8.
59 S. Postmus, "Diet and Nutritional Condition in Burma", *Burma Medical Journal* 5, no. 4 (Oct. 1957): 27.
60 Cho Nwe Oo, "Yantein Village Nutrition Promotion Programme", *Burma Medical Journal* 23, nos. 1–4 (Jan.–Oct. 1977): 53.
61 B. O. Binns, "Analysis of Pre-war Diet in Burma", undated paper (probably 1946/1947), stamped "UT.29/X". Nutrition Dept., London School of Hygiene and Tropical Medicine.
62 Cho Nwe Oo, "Yantein Village Nutrition Promotion Programme", p. 55.
63 Binns, "Analysis of Pre-war Diet in Burma".
64 Cho Nwe Oo, "Yantein Village Nutrition Promotion Programme", p. 55.
65 Ma Ma Tin, "Feeding Patterns of Infants …", p. 3.
66 For a full discussion, see Amartya Kumar Sen, *Poverty and Famines: An Essay on Entitlement and Deprivation* (Oxford: Clarendon Press, 1981).
67 U Maung Gale, *Reports on the Dietary and Nutritional Surveys Conducted in Certain Areas of Burma* (Rangoon: Superintendent of Government Printing and Stationery, 1948), pp. 6, 7.
68 Ibid., p. 34.
69 Ibid., p. 132.
70 Ibid., p. 156.
71 Ibid., p. 141.
72 *RSAB*, 1913, p. 16.
73 *RPHAB*, 1931, p. 52.
74 Ibid., p. 52.
75 *RPHAB*, 1936, p. 50.
76 League of Nations Health Organisation, *Intergovernmental Conference of Far-Eastern Countries on Rural Hygiene. Preparatory Papers, 2.* (Geneva: League of Nations, 1937), p. 38.
77 *RPHAB*, 1925, p. 27.
78 *RSPHB*, 1939, p. 47.
79 *RPHAB*, 1927, p. 37.

80 *RSPHB*, 1937, p. 49.
81 John Taylor, C. de C. Martin and Thant U, "Preliminary Enquiry into Beri-beri in Burma", *Indian Medical Research Memoirs*, Memoir no. 8 (Mar. 1928): 18.
82 Ibid., p. 28.
83 Ibid., p. 29.
84 T. E. Tupasi, "Nutrition and Acute Respiratory Infection", in *Acute Respiratory Infections in Childhood*, ed. R. M. Douglas and E. Kerby-Easton. (Adelaide: University of Adelaide, 1985), p. 68.
85 Ibid.
86 FAO, *Rice and Rice Diets. A Survey* (Washington: UN FAO, 1948), p. 15.
87 Tupasi, "Nutrition and Acute Respiratory Infection", p. 68.
88 *RSAB*, 1919, p. 16.
89 *RPHAB*, 1921, p. 18.
90 *RPHAB*, 1926, p. 23.
91 Asa Crawford Chandler, "The Prevalence and Epidemiology of Hookworm and other Helminthic Infections in India. Part VI. BURMA", *Indian Journal of Medical Research* 14 (1926–7): 733–44.
92 Ibid., p. 736.
93 Ibid., p. 741.
94 Ibid., pp. 741, 742.
95 *Annual Report on Hospitals and Dispensaries in Burma, 1934,* and *Triennial Review for the Years 1932–34* (Rangoon: Superintendent of Government Printing and Stationery, 1935), p. 9.
96 Kyaw Win, "A Report on Intestinal Helminthic Infections in Mon State", *Burma Medical Journal* 22, no. 3 and 4 (July/Oct. 1976): 31.
97 Ba Tun U and Ko Ko U, "Some Observations on the Helminthic Infestations of the Burmese Village Community", *Burma Medical Journal* 16, no. 2 (Apr. 1968): 122.
98 C. V. Foll, "The Perils of Childhood in Upper Burma", *Journal of Tropical Paediatrics* 4, no. 3 (Dec. 1958): 126.
99 Kenneth H. Brown, R. H. Gilman, M. Khatun and Ahmed M. G., "Absorption of macro-nutrients from a rice-vegetable diet before and after treatment of ascariasis in children", *American Journal of Clinical Nutrition* no. 33 (1980): 1978.
100 L. S. Stephenson, D. W. T. Crompton, M. C. Latham, S. E. Arnold, and A. A. S. Jansen, "Evaluation of a Four Year Project to Control Ascaris Infection in Children in Two Kenyan Villages", *Journal of Tropical Paediatrics* 29, no. 3 (June 1983): 175.
101 Gerald L. Mandell, Robert G. Douglas and John E. Bennett, eds., *Principles and Practice of Infectious Disease* (New York: J. Wiley and Sons, 1979), p. 2144.
102 Strickland, *Hunter's Tropical Medicine*, p. 17.
103 *RPHVS*, 1868, p. 209.
104 *RSABB*, 1880, Resolution accompanying the Report, p. 3.
105 *RSAB*, 1894, p. 28.
106 Soe Soe Aye, "Morbidity Pattern of Children at Rangoon Children Hospital", *Burma Medical Journal* 25, no. 1 (Jan. 1979): 13.

107 Ma Ma Tin, "Morbidity Pattern Seen in the Department of Child Health, General Hospital, Mandalay", *Burma Medical Journal* 20, no. 1 (Jan. 1972): 14.
108 WHO, Interim Programme Report, 1986, 'Control of Diarrhoeal Diseases', WHO/CDD/87.26, p. 10.
109 Ibid., p. 39.
110 Soe Soe Aye, "Morbidity Pattern of Children ...", p. 21.
111 "Public Health and Births and Deaths 1867. British Burma", Extract from the *Proceedings of the Chief Commissioner in the Home Department* No. 241 (Rangoon: Rangoon Times Press, 1868), p. 74. This was the first annual health report for Burma and will be described hereafter as PHBD.
112 Ibid., p. 90.
113 *RPHVS*, 1868, p. 209.
114 *RPHAB*, 1932, p. 28.
115 Ma Ma Tin, "Morbidity Pattern Seen ...", p. 17.
116 *RSAB*, 1915, p. 15.
117 S. Lyle Cummins, "The Tuberculosis of Tropical Countries", *Indian Medical Gazette* 74 (Sept. 1939): 515.
118 Ibid., p. 515.
119 *RPHVS*, 1868, p. 209.
120 Ibid., p. 156.
121 PHBD, 1867, p. 12.
122 Ibid., p. 48.
123 *RPHVS*, 1868, p. 45.
124 *RSAB*, 1910, p. 5.
125 P. C. Banerjee, "Report of a Measles Survey in Sagaing", *Burma Medical Journal* 16, no. 4 (Oct. 1968): 219.
126 Ibid., p. 220.
127 *RSAB*, 1910, p. 17.
128 *RSAB*, 1912, p. 15.
129 Mandell, et al., eds., *Principles and Practice of Infectious Disease*, p. 1334.
130 Cheng Siok-Hwa, *The Rice Industry of Burma, 1852–1940* (Kuala Lumpur: University of Malaya Press, 1968), pp. 77–94.
131 *RSAB*, 1918, p. 12.
132 Ibid., p. 14.
133 Ibid., p. 13.
134 *RSAB*, 1912, p. 11.
135 Ibid., p. 11.
136 Ibid., p. 11.
137 *RSAB*, 1915, p. 13.
138 *RSAB*, 1917, p. 13
139 Ibid., p. 13.
140 Ibid., p. 12.
141 *RSPHB*, 1939, p. 39.
142 *RPHAB*, 1936, p. 40.
143 John A. Sinton, *What Malaria Costs India*, Health Bulletin no. 26, Malaria Bureau no. 13 (Simla: Government of India Press, 1939), p. 8.

[144] M. Kandiah, M. Lee, T. K. Ng, and Y. H. Chong, "Malnutrition in Malaria Endemic Villages of Bengkoka Peninsula, Sabah", *Journal of Tropical Paediatrics* 30, no. 1 (Feb. 1984): 26.

[145] Ibid., p. 24.

CHAPTER 5

[1] Norman G. Owen, "Measuring Mortality in the Nineteenth Century Philippines", in *Death and Disease in Southeast Asia*, ed. Norman G. Owen (Singapore: Oxford University Press, 1987), p. 91.

[2] *Shorter Oxford English Dictionary on Historical Principles*, Vol. II (Oxford: 1983), p. 2396.

[3] See John Snow's monograph on cholera, mentioned in *Epidemiology, Man and Disease* by John P. Fox, Carrie E. Hall and Lila R. Elveback (New York: Macmillan, 1970); William H. McNeill, *Plagues and Peoples* (Harmondsworth: Penguin, 1979), p. 252, for a description of cholera in Hamburg.

[4] *Report on the Sanitary Administration of British Burma*, 1888, p. 4.
These reports are generally referred to in the text as annual health reports, and they were issued yearly by the Government Press of Rangoon. From 1870 to 1889, their title was *Report on the Sanitary Administration of British Burma*, and they will be referred to as *RSABB* and the designating year. From 1890 to 1920, their title was as above, and they will be referred to as *RSAB* and the designating year. From 1921 to 1936, the report was titled *Report on the Public Health Administration of Burma* and will be referred to as *RPHAB* and the designating year. Finally in 1937, the title was changed to *Report on the State of Public Health in Burma* and will be referred to as *RSPHB* and the designating year.

[5] Gerald L. Mandell, Robert G. Douglas and John E. Bennett, eds., *Principles and Practice of Infectious Disease* (New York: J. Wiley and Sons, 1979), p. 209.

[6] Ibid., p. 211.

[7] William H. McNeill, *Plagues and Peoples* (Harmondsworth: Penguin, 1979), p. 240.

[8] Father Sangermano, *A Description of the Burmese Empire*, translated by William Tandy. Originally published in Rome by Oriental Translation Fund of Great Britain and Ireland in 1833. (New York: Augustus M. Kelley, 1969), p. 168.

[9] R. Glass, S. Becker, M. Huq, B. Stoll, M. Khan, M. Merson, J. Lee and R. Black, "Endemic Cholera in Rural Bangladesh 1966–1980", *American Journal of Epidemiology* 116, no. 6 (1982): 967; J. Miller, Richard G. Feachem and B. S. Drasar, "Cholera Epidemiology in Developed and Developing Countries", *Lancet* (2 Feb. 1985): 261–3. The epidemiology of cholera could be said to have started with John Snow's famous monograph on cholera published in 1855. This identified a living cell as the cause of cholera and argued that its transmission was by direct contact, or by contaminated food or water. This theory was resisted by the "miasmic" medical opinion at the time. See John P. Fox, Carrie E. Hall and Lila R. Elveback, *Epidemiology, Man and Disease* (New York: Macmillan, 1970).

[10] Glass, et al., "Endemic Cholera in Rural Bangladesh", p. 967; Miller, et al., "Cholera Epidemiology ...", pp. 261, 263.

11 Victor B. Lieberman, *Burmese Administrative Cycles: Anarchy and Conquest c 1580–1760* (Princeton: Princeton University Press, 1984), p. 20. In his discussion of the factors affecting population growth in sixteenth-century Upper Burma, Lieberman mentions cholera, plague, malaria and smallpox.

12 HMSO, *Statistical Report on the Sickness, Mortality and Invaliding Among Her Majesty's Troops Serving in Ceylon, the Tenasserim Provinces and the Burmese Empire* (London: HMSO, 1841), p. 13.

13 David Nokes, *Jane Austen: A Life* (London: Fourth Estate, 1997), p. 525. There were British deaths from cholera during the second Britain–Burma War also. One of these was Jane Austen's brother, Admiral Charles Austen, who died while on active service up the Irrawaddy River in 1852.

14 See *RSABB*, 1877, 1878, 1881, 1882; *RSAB*, 1917; *RPHAB*, 1934.

15 *RSABB*, 1882, p. 27.

16 *RSAB*, 1918, p. 7.

17 *RSABB*, 1883, p. 8.

18 *RSABB*, 1875, p. 41.

19 *RSABB*, 1870, pp. 4, 6.

20 *RSABB*, 1878, p. 4.

21 Ibid., p. 6.

22 *RSAB*, 1908, p. 8.

23 *RPHAB*, 1929, p. 13.

24 See David Arnold, "Cholera Mortality in British India 1817–1914", in *India's Historical Demography: Studies in Famine, Disease and Society*, ed. Tim Dyson (London: Curzon Press, 1989), for discussion of the role of migrants in cholera epidemics.

25 *RSAB*, 1907, p. 7.

26 HMSO, *Report of the Royal Commission on Labour in India* (London: HMSO, June 1931), p. 429.

27 Ibid., p. 427.

28 Ibid., pp. 434, 435.

29 Ibid., p. 433.

30 Ibid., p. 442.

31 Ibid., p. 431.

32 *RSABB*, 1878, p. 6.

33 *RSABB*, 1877, p. 30.

34 *RSAB*, 1919, p. 7.

35 *RPHAB*, 1932, p. 86.

36 *RSAB*, 1908, p. 10.

37 Ibid., p. 10.

38 Ibid., pp. 10, 8.

39 *RSAB*, 1918, p. 7.

40 *RPHAB*, 1930, p. 19.

41 *RSABB*, 1876, pp. 47, 54.

42 *RSABB*, 1872, p. 38.

43 Mandell, et al., eds., *Principles and Practice of Infectious Disease*, p. 1216.

44 *RPHAB*, 1924, p. 30.

45 *RSAB*, 1902, p. 11.

⁴⁶ *RSAB*, 1903, p. 16.
⁴⁷ *RSAB*, 1898, Appendices, p. xxx.
⁴⁸ *RSABB*, 1895, p. 38.
⁴⁹ *RSPHB*, 1938, p. 31.
⁵⁰ Ibid., p. 36.
⁵¹ Ibid., p. 37.
⁵² Arnold, "Cholera Mortality in British India …", p. 33.
⁵³ McNeill, *Plagues and Peoples*, p. 144.
⁵⁴ Ibid., p. 144.
⁵⁵ Terence H. Hull, "Plague in Java", in *Death and Disease in Southeast Asia*, ed. Norman G. Owen, p. 212.
⁵⁶ Ibid., p. 214. Hull reports that in Java, researchers found that rural housing, with rafters and thatched roofs, made it easier for the rat flea to transfer to humans than in brick-walled town houses with rat burrows underneath. Also see *Burma Gazetteer, Vol. A, Mandalay District* (Rangoon: 1928), p. 75.
⁵⁷ *RSAB*, 1907, p. 11.
⁵⁸ *RSAB*, 1908, p. 5.
⁵⁹ *RSAB*, 1914, p. 11; *RSAB*, 1910, p. 7.
⁶⁰ *RPHAB*, 1923, p. 20.
⁶¹ *RSPHB*, 1939, p. 16.
⁶² *RPHAB*, 1930, p. 25.
⁶³ *RSAB*, 1917, p. 14.
⁶⁴ Ibid., p. 8.
⁶⁵ Ibid.
⁶⁶ *RSAB*, 1898, p. 31.
⁶⁷ *RSAB*, 1900, pp. 15–21.
⁶⁸ *RSAB*, 1906, p. 10.
⁶⁹ Ibid., p. 9.
⁷⁰ *RSAB*, 1905, Resolution, p. 2.
⁷¹ *RSAB*, 1906, p. 19.
⁷² *RSAB*, 1907, p. 17.
⁷³ *RSAB*, 1909, p. 19.
⁷⁴ *RSAB*, 1913, Resolution, p. 2; HMSO, *Correspondence Regarding Measures for the Prevention of Plague. East India (Plague)* (London: HMSO, 1907), p. 37.
⁷⁵ *RSAB*, 1916, p. 16.
⁷⁶ *RSABB*, 1870, p. 80.
⁷⁷ *RSAB*, 1905, pp. 8, 9; *RSAB*, 1907, pp. 11–3; *RSAB*, 1918, p. 8.
⁷⁸ *RSAB*, 1906, p. 11.
⁷⁹ *RSAB*, 1909, p. 12.
⁸⁰ Ibid., p. 13.
⁸¹ *RSAB*, 1910, p. 9.
⁸² *RSAB*, 1911, p. 17.
⁸³ Ibid., p. 10.
⁸⁴ Ibid., p. 11.
⁸⁵ Ibid., p. 12.
⁸⁶ Ibid., p. 16.
⁸⁷ Ibid., p. 17.

88 *RSAB*, 1913, p. 9.
89 *RSAB*, 1917, p. 9.
90 *RSAB*, 1926, p. 20.
91 Daniel George Edward Hall, *A History of South-East Asia*, 4th edition (Basingstoke: Macmillan, 1981), p. 782.
92 *RSAB*, 1928, p. 20.
93 *RSAB*, 1922, p. 19.
94 *Notes on Sanitary Organisation and Development in Burma* (Rangoon: Superintendent of Government Printing, 1915), p. 13.
95 Ibid., pp. 4, 5; *RSAB*, 1912, p. 14.
96 *RPHAB*, 1928, p. 34; *RPHAB*, 1929, p. 30.
97 *RPHAB*, 1928, p. 35.
98 *RPHAB*, 1931, pp. 50, 51.
99 *RSPHB*, 1939, p. 30.
100 *RPHAB*, 1924, p. 30.
101 *RPHAB*, 1936, p. 65.
102 *RPHAB*, 1932, p. 54.
103 *RSPHB*, 1938, pp. 29, 30.
104 McNeill, *Plagues and Peoples*, p. 138.
105 Ibid., p. 128.
106 Barend Jan Terwiel, "Asiatic Cholera in Siam: Its First Occurrence and the 1820 Epidemic", in *Death and Disease in Southeast Asia*, ed. Norman G. Owen, p. 147.
107 Peter Gardiner and Mayling Oey, "Morbidity and Mortality in Java, 1880–1940: The Evidence of the Colonial Reports", in *Death and Disease in Southeast Asia*, ed. Norman G. Owen, p. 61.
108 Barbara Lovric, "Bali: Myth, Magic and Morbidity", in *Death and Disease in Southeast Asia*, ed. Norman G. Owen, p. 125.
109 Ann B. Jannetta, *Epidemics and Mortality in Early Modern Japan* (Princeton: Princeton University Press, 1987).
110 Lieberman, *Burmese Administrative Cycles*, p. 20. See footnote re smallpox.
111 *RSABB*, 1879, p. 27; also *Burma Gazetteer, Vol. A, Insein District* (1914), p. 169, and *Burma Gazetteer, Vol. A, Syriam District*, p. 189.
112 Jannetta, *Epidemics and Mortality in Early Modern Japan*, p. 64.
113 *RSABB*, 1879, p. 18.
114 Ibid., p. 26.
115 *RSAB*, 1897, p. 18.
116 *RSAB*, 1915, p. 9; *RSAB*, 1916, p. 7.
117 *RSAB*, 1915, p. 9.
118 *RSAB*, 1907, p. 9.
119 *Notes on Sanitary Organisation and Development in Burma*, (1915), p. 9.
120 *RPHAB*, 1925, p. 15.
121 *RPHAB*, 1926, p. 17.
122 *RSAB*, 1899, p. 20.
123 *RSAB*, 1905, p. 7.
124 Ibid., p. 7.
125 *RSAB*, 1910, p. 20.

126 *RPHAB*, 1922, p. 17.
127 John R. Paul, *Clinical Epidemiology* (Chicago: University of Chicago Press, 1958), p. 28.
128 "Public Health and Births and Deaths 1867. British Burma". Extract from the *Proceedings of the Chief Commissioner in the Home Department*. No. 241 (Rangoon: Rangoon Times Press, 1868), p. 61.
129 Ibid., p. 78.
130 *Report on Public Health and Vital Statistics for 1868* (Rangoon: Chief Commissioner's Office Press, 1870), p. 15. Hereafter referred to as *RPHVS*.
131 Ibid., pp. 16, 17.
132 *RSABB*, 1882, p. 13.
133 *RSABB*, 1883, p. 16.
134 *RSAB*, 1904, p. 10.
135 *RSAB*, 1916, p. 13.
136 *RPHAB*, 1931, p. 32.
137 *RSAB*, 1908, p. 12.
138 *RSAB*, 1919, p. 15.
139 *RSAB*, 1920, p. 15.
140 *RPHAB*, 1923, p. 28.
141 *RPHAB*, 1926, p. 22.
142 *RPHAB*, 1928, p. 5.
143 W. G. King, "Prevention of the Spread of Tuberculosis in Burma", *Indian Medical Gazette* 45, Supplement (1910): 5.
144 Ibid., p. 7.
145 *RPHAB*, 1932, p. 29.
146 *RPHAB*, 1934, p. 20.
147 S. Lyle Cummins, "The Tuberculosis of Tropical Countries", *Indian Medical Gazette* 74 (Sept. 1939): 515.
148 *RPHVS*, 1868, p. 186.
149 King, "Prevention of the Spread of Tuberculosis", p. 5.
150 *RPHAB*, 1928, p. 25.
151 Ibid., p. 25.
152 *RPHAB*, 1931, p. 32.
153 *RSAB*, 1915, p. 14.
154 *RSPHB*, 1938, pp. 25, 28.
155 *RPHAB*, 1936, p. 24; *RSPHB*, 1937, p. 28; *RSPHB*, 1939, p. 27.
156 Thein Aung, "ARI in Childhood in Burma — What Happens Now?", in *Acute Respiratory Infections in Childhood*, ed. R. M. Douglas and E. Kerby-Easton (Adelaide: University of Adelaide, 1985), p. 1.
157 *RPHAB*, 1932, p. 28.
158 Colin Brown, "The Influenza Pandemic of 1918 in Indonesia", in *Death and Disease in Southeast Asia*, ed. Norman G. Owen, p. 236.
159 *RSAB*, 1918, p. 10.
160 Ibid., p. 10.
161 Ibid., p. 1.
162 Ibid., p. 12.
163 Amartya Kumar Sen, *Poverty and Famines: An Essay on Entitlement and Deprivation* (Oxford: Clarendon Press, 1981), p. 215.

164 Brown, "The Influenza Pandemic of 1918", p. 235.
165 Ibid., p. 242. Also see Mandell, et al., eds., *Principles and Practice of Infectious Disease*, p. 856: The pulmonary complications of viral pneumonia are thought to have been more common in the adult age group (including the young and healthy) than in children, which might help to explain this high adult mortality in Burma. Also see *RSAB*, 1918, p. 17: The medical authorities found that in the majority of fatalities, death was due to "lung complications" such as bronchitis, pleurisy and pneumonia.
166 *RSAB*, 1918, p. 10.
167 Ibid., pp. 10–2.
168 *RPHAB*, 1921, Resolution, p. 4.
169 *RSAB*, 1918, p. 13.
170 Ibid., p. 18.
171 Ibid., p. 14.
172 Ibid., p. 18
173 Ibid., p. 15.
174 Ibid., p. 14.
175 Ibid., p. 22.
176 Ibid.
177 Ibid., p. 15.
178 Ibid.
179 Ibid., p. 11.
180 Ibid., p. 16.
181 Ibid., p. 12.
182 Ibid., Resolution, p. 1.
183 *RSAB*, 1910, p. 17.
184 Ibid.
185 *RSPHB*, 1937, p. 28.
186 *RPHAB*, 1930, p. 34.
187 *RPHAB*, 1926, p. 24.
188 *RSAB*, 1912, p. 11.
189 *RPHAB*, 1928, p. 26.
190 *RSPHB*, 1939, p. 28.
191 *RSPHB*, 1938, p. 29; *RPHAB*, 1935, p. 25; *RPHAB*, 1934, p. 21.
192 *RPHAB*, 1936, p. 26.
193 *RSAB*, 1913, p. 13.
194 *RPHAB*, 1924, p. 27.
195 *RPHAB*, 1930, p. 34; *RPHAB*, 1927, p. 27.
196 *RSPHB*, 1937, p. 29.
197 *RSPHB*, 1939, p. 29.
198 J. G. Scott and J. P. Hardiman, *Gazetteer of Upper Burma and the Shan States. Part 2*, Vol. 2 (Rangoon: Superintendent of Government Printing, 1900), p. 116.
199 *Imperial Gazetteer of India, Burma*, Vol. 2 (Calcutta: 1908), p. 63.
200 *Burma Gazetteer, Vol. A, Syriam District*, p. 107; *Burma Gazetteer, Vol. A, Insein District*, p. 76.
201 Hall, *A History of South-East Asia*, p. 640.

202 *Imperial Gazetteer of India, Burma,* Vol. 2, (1908), p. 63.
203 *Burma Gazetteer, Vol. A, Tharrawaddy District,* pp. 28, 29.
204 Ibid., p. 39.
205 *Burma Gazetteer, Vol. A, Shwebo District,* p. 142.
206 Ibid.
207 Scott and Hardiman, *Gazetteer of Upper Burma,* Vol. 2, p. 265.
208 *Burma Gazetteer, Vol. A, Shwebo District,* p. 142.
209 *Burma Gazetteer, Vol. A, Lower Chindwin District,* pp. 149, 150.
210 *Imperial Gazetteer of India, Burma,* Vol. 2, p. 266.
211 *Census of India 1901,* Vol. 1, Pt. 1, Report (Calcutta: Superintendent of Government Printing, 1903), p. 59.
212 Charles L. Keeton, *King Thebaw and the Ecological Rape of Burma* (New Delhi: Manohar Book Service, 1974), pp. 156, 157.
213 Ibid., p. 345.
214 *Imperial Gazetteer of India, Burma,* Vol. 2, p. 298.
215 *Burma Gazetteer, Vol. A, Kyaukse District,* p. 35.
216 *Burma Gazetteer, Vol. A, Mandalay District,* p. 79.
217 *RPHAB,* 1934, p. 1.
218 *RPHAB,* 1932, p. 2.
219 *RSPHB,* 1937, p. 1.
220 *RPHAB,* 1926, p. 2.
221 *Burma Gazetteer, Vol. A, Thayetmyo District,* p. 46.
222 Sen, *Poverty and Famines,* p. 216.

CHAPTER 6

1   Jacques M. May, with the collaboration of Irma S. Jarcho, *The Ecology of Malnutrition in the Far and Near East: Food Resources, Habits and Deficiencies* (New York: Hafner Publishing Co., 1961), p. 6.
2   Anthony Reid, *Southeast Asia in the Age of Commerce 1450–1680,* Vol. 1, "The Lands Below the Winds" (New Haven: Yale University Press, 1988–93), p. 5.
3   George Coedès, *The Indianized States of Southeast Asia.* Transl. Susan Brown Cowing, ed. Walter F. Vella (Honolulu: University Press of Hawaii, 1968), p. 63.
4   Victor B. Lieberman, *Burmese Administrative Cycles: Anarchy and Conquest c 1580–1760* (Princeton: Princeton University Press, 1984), p. 18.
5   Lieberman, *Burmese Administrative Cycles,* pp. 17, 19.
6   Cheng Siok-Hwa, *The Rice Industry of Burma, 1852–1940* (Kuala Lumpur: University of Malaya Press, 1968), pp. 241, 243.
7   See Cheng, *The Rice Industry of Burma,* and M. S. I. Diokno, "British Firms and the Economy of Burma, with Special Reference to the Rice and Teak Industries, 1917–1937", PhD Thesis, University of London (May 1983) for full discussion.
8   Cheng, *The Rice Industry of Burma,* p. 81.
9   Ibid., p. 83.
10 Ibid., p. 94.
11 Ibid., pp. 253, 256.
12 Ibid., p. 83.

13 Ibid., p. 93.
14 Ibid., p. 88.
15 Ibid., p. 84.
16 Ibid., p. 200.
17 Ibid., p. 106.
18 Ibid., p. 108.
19 FAO, *Rice and Rice Diets. A Nutritional Survey* (Washington: UN FAO, 1948), p. 2.
20 Ibid., p. 14.
21 Ibid.
22 Ibid., p. 15.
23 Pe Kyin, *The Nutritive Value of Burmese Foods* (Rangoon: Directorate of Health Services, 1967), pp. 40–3.
24 Cheng, *The Rice Industry of Burma*, p. 200.
25 *Report on the Public Health Administration of Burma* 1923, p. 40.
   These reports are generally referred to in the text as annual health reports, and they were issued yearly by the Govt. Press of Rangoon. From 1870 to 1889, their title was *Report on the Sanitary Administration of British Burma*. From 1890 to 1920, their title was *Report on the Sanitary Administration of Burma*, and they will be referred to as *RSAB* and the designating year. From 1921 to 1936, the report was titled as above, and will be referred to as *RPHAB* and the designating year. Finally in 1937, the title was changed to *Report on the State of Public Health in Burma*, and will be referred to as *RSPHB* and the designating year.
26 FAO, *Rice and Rice Diets*, p. 18.
27 Ibid., p. 64.
28 Ibid., p. 60.
29 Ibid., p. 14.
30 "Public Health and Births and Deaths 1867. British Burma". Extract from the *Proceedings of the Chief Commissioner in the Home Department*. No. 241 (Rangoon: Rangoon Times Press, 1868), p. 18. This was the first annual health report for Burma.
31 *RSAB*, 1919, p. 15; *RPHAB*, 1921, p. 13; *RPHAB*, 1922, p. 22; *RPHAB*, 1932, p. 30.
32 *RSAB*, 1919, p. 15.
33 Ibid.
34 *RSAB*, 1908, p. 17.
35 William L. Braddon, "Beri Beri, Its Cause, Symptoms, Diagnosis, Treatment, Pathology, and Prevention", in *Transactions of the Bombay Medical Congress 1909*, ed. W. E. Jennings (Bombay: Bennet, Coleman and Co., undated). The experiments described by Braddon were disgraceful, when judged by even the most lax of medical ethics. From December 1905 to June 1908, the patients at a lunatic asylum in Kuala Lumpur were divided into two groups. One group was fed on "cured" (i.e. parboiled) rice; the other ate "uncured" (highly milled) rice. It was found that beri beri attacked only those patients who ate "uncured" rice as their staple diet.
36 *RSAB*, 1911, p. 19.

[37] William L. Braddon, "Beri Beri, Its Cause, Symptoms, Diagnosis, Treatment, Pathology, and Prevention", in *Transactions of the Bombay Medical Congress 1909*, ed. W. E. Jennings (Bombay: Bennet, Coleman and Co., undated), p. 273.

[38] *RSAB*, 1913, p. 10; *RSAB*, 1918, p. 19.

[39] John Taylor, C. de C. Martin and Thant U, "Preliminary Enquiry into Beri-beri in Burma", *Indian Medical Research Memoirs*, Memoir No. 8 (Mar. 1928): 13.

[40] J. H. Williams, *Elephant Bill* (London: Penguin, 1964), p. 48.

[41] Taylor, et al., "Preliminary Enquiry into Beri-beri ...", p. 22.

[42] G. G. Jolly, "Beri Beri in Cheduba Island, Arakan, Burma", *Indian Medical Gazette* 65 (July 1930): 385.

[43] Taylor, et al., "Preliminary Enquiry into Beri-beri ...", p. 26.

[44] Ibid., p. 25.

[45] Ibid., p. 22.

[46] Ibid., p. 24.

[47] Ibid., p. 20.

[48] *Atta* flour is a semi-refined Indian flour made from durum wheat with some of the bran removed. Some brands of *atta* flour are considered wholemeal with only the husk removed while other brands are mixed with very finely-milled *maida* flour.

[49] *RSAB*, 1909, p. 18.

[50] *RSAB*, 1913, p. 13.

[51] Ibid.

[52] *RPHAB*, 1922, p. 22.

[53] *RPHAB*, 1923, p. 29.

[54] *RPHAB*, 1929, p. 20.

[55] *RPHAB*, 1930, p. 32.

[56] *RPHAB*, 1931, p. 33.

[57] *RPHAB*, 1922, p. 23.

[58] HMSO, *Report of the Royal Commission on Labour in India* (London: HMSO, June 1931), pp. 429, 431.

[59] *RPHAB*, 1931, p. 33.

[60] *RPHAB*, 1932, p. 30.

[61] *RPHAB*, 1935, p. 27.

[62] Ibid.

[63] Taylor, et al., "Preliminary Enquiry into Beri-beri ...", pp. 31–37. The figures for average urban Burmese, Muslim or better off Hindus were the approximate average weight of rice consumed by these groups from eight towns, namely Bassein, Pegu, Prome, Toungoo, Meiktila, Myingyan, Thayetmyo, and Mandalay.

[64] Ibid., p. 39.

[65] Ibid., p. 31.

[66] *RSAB*, 1910, p. 17.

[67] *RSAB*, 1919, p. 15.

[68] *Union of Burma Report by the Inter-Departmental Committee on Nutrition for National Defence* (May 1963), p. 150.

69 Ibid., p. 150.
70 *RPHAB*, 1931, p. 33.
71 *RPHAB*, 1935, p. 27.
72 *RSPHB*, 1937, p. 17.
73 *RSPHB*, 1938, p. 18.
74 Taylor, et al., "Preliminary Enquiry into Beri-beri ...", p. 44.
75 Ibid., p. 43.
76 Ibid., p. 14.
77 Ibid., p. 37.
78 Ibid.
79 Ibid., p. 39.
80 Cheng, *The Rice Industry of Burma*, p. 108.
81 *RSPHB*, 1939, p. 52.
82 Michael Warboys, "Science and British Colonial Imperialism 1895–1940",
    D. Phil. thesis, University of Sussex (1979), p. 382.
83 *RSPHB*, 1938, p. 56.
84 U Maung Gale, *Reports on the Dietary and Nutritional Surveys Conducted in
    Certain Areas of Burma* (Rangoon: Superintendent of Government Printing
    and Stationery, 1948), p. 2. The report notes that food values were taken
    largely from Health Bulletin No. 23 (1937) and Shanghai Foods (1937).
85 The occupational descriptions are those used in U Maung Gale, *Reports on
    the Dietary and Nutritional Surveys*, p. 1.
86 Ibid., p. 3.
87 Ibid., p. 5.
88 Robert O. Whyte, *Rural Nutrition in Monsoon Asia* (Kuala Lumpur: Oxford
    University Press, 1974), p. 94.
89 S. Postmus, "Diet and Nutritional Condition in Burma", *Burma Medical
    Journal* 5, no. 4 (Oct. 1957): 25.
90 S. Postmus, "Beri beri of Mother and Child in Burma", *Tropical and
    Geographical Medicine* 10 (1958): 366.
91 U Maung Gale, *Reports on the Dietary and Nutritional Surveys*, p. 61.
92 Taylor, et al., "Preliminary Enquiry into Beri-beri ...", pp. 68–73.
93 U Maung Gale, *Reports on the Dietary and Nutritional Surveys*, p. 76.
94 Ibid., p. 76.
95 Ibid., p. 80.
96 Taylor, et al., "Preliminary Enquiry into Beri-beri ...", pp. 68–73. Taylor,
    et al., used data from six towns: Bassein, Pegu, Prome, Toungoo, Meiktila,
    and Myingyan. The figures quoted here are the upper and lower levels of
    those averages.
97 B. O. Binns, "Analysis of Pre-war Diet in Burma", undated paper (probably
    1946/1947), stamped "UT.29/X". Nutrition Dept., London School of Hygiene
    and Tropical Medicine.
98 Postmus, "Diet and Nutritional Condition in Burma, p. 23.
99 FAO, *Rice and Rice Diets*, p. 15. It must be understood that all these estimates
    are based on averaged figures from experimental work. Also that the levels
    of thiamine depend on the condition of the rice grain and that degrees of
    milling, whether hand pounding or machine, also cause variations. But
    these fluctuations do not weaken the basic argument.

100 R. G. Chitre and Tin Tin Oo, "Role of Nutrition in Disease", *Burma Medical Journal* 5, no. 2 (Apr. 1957): 27.

101 Binns, "Analysis of Pre-war Diet in Burma".

102 Taylor, et al., "Preliminary Enquiry into Beri-beri ...", pp. 68–73.

103 G. G. Jolly, "The Use of Germinated Pulse and Beans in the Natural Dietary of the Burmese", *Indian Medical Gazette* 58 (June 1923): 255–6.

104 For full discussion of the interactions and predisposition of deficiency states to infections, see T. E. Tupasi, "Nutrition and Acute Respiratory Infection", in *Acute Respiratory Infections in Childhood*, ed. R. M. Douglas and E. Kerby-Eaton (Adelaide, SA: Department of Community Medicine University of Adelaide, 1985), p. 68.

105 See Chitre and Tin Tin Oo, "Role of Nutrition in Disease"; *Union of Burma Report by the Inter-Departmental Committee on Nutrition for National Defence*; Sein May Chit, "Nutritional Problems in Burma" (undated paper, probably 1970s), Burma Box, Nutrition Library, London School of Hygiene and Tropical Medicine; Pe Kyin, *The Nutritive Value of Burmese Foods*; Ba Tin, "Nutritional Status of Rural and Urban Community in Burma". Dissertation, D.P. and T.M., Institute of Medicine 1, Rangoon (1969).

106 Chitre and Tin Tin Oo, "Role of Nutrition in Disease", p. 29.

107 *Union of Burma Report by the Inter-Departmental Committee on Nutrition for National Defence*, pp. 49, 54, 91, 118.

108 Ibid., p. 28.

109 Ba Tin, "Nutritional Status of Rural and Urban Community in Burma", pp. 28, 30, 33.

110 Sein May Chit, "Nutritional Problems in Burma", p. 5.

111 Ibid., p. 3.

112 FAO, *Report of the Nutrition Committee for South and East Asia, Fourth Session*, Tokyo, Japan, 1956 (UN FAO, 1957), p. 9.

113 FAO, *Rice and Rice Diets*, p. 21.

114 League of Nations Health Organisation, *Intergovernmental Conference of Far-Eastern Countries on Rural Hygiene. Preparatory Papers. Report of the Malayan Delegation* (Geneva: 1937).

115 C. E. Cobb, "Beri Beri and Rice Control in Malaya", *Indian Medical Gazette* 59 (Aug. 1924): 401, 402.

116 Ibid., p. 401.

117 Ibid., p. 402.

118 D. J. Steinberg, ed., *In Search of Southeast Asia* (Honolulu: University of Hawaii Press, 1985), p. 242.

119 Charles Robequain, *The Economic Development of Indo-China*, transl. Isabel A. Ward (Oxford: Oxford University Press, 1944), p. 277.

120 League of Nations Health Organisation, *Report of the Intergovernmental Conference of Far-Eastern Countries on Rural Hygiene, held at Bandoeng (Java), 3rd–13th August, 1937*, p. 89.

121 David J. Wyler and Louis H. Miller, "Plasmodium Species (Malaria)", in *Principles and Practice of Infectious Disease*, ed. Gerald L. Mandell, R. Gordon Douglas and John E. Bennett (New York: J. Wiley and Sons, 1979), p. 2097.

122 Lieberman, *Burmese Administrative Cycles*, p. 18.
123 Ibid., p. 17, quoting Adas.
124 G. T. Strickland, *Hunter's Tropical Medicine* (London: W.B. Saunders and Co., 1984), pp. 527, 528.
125 Wyler and Miller, "Plasmodium Species (Malaria)", in *Principles and Practice of Infectious Disease*, p. 2097.
126 Ibid., p. 2101.
127 Ibid., p. 2098.
128 Ibid., p. 2100.
129 *RSAB*, 1914–1939.
130 R. C. Robertson, "A Malaria Survey on the China–Burman Highway", *Transactions of the Royal Society of Tropical Medicine and Hygiene* 34, no. 4 (Jan. 1941): 320, 329.
131 Ibid., p. 320.
132 *RPHAB*, 1924, p. 8.
133 *RSAB*, 1912, p. 11.
134 Daniel George Edward Hall, *A History of South-East Asia*, 4th edition (Basingstoke: Macmillan, 1981), p. 157.
135 *Burma Gazetteer, Vol. A, Kyaukse District* (Rangoon: 1925), p. 35.
136 Ibid., p. 74
137 Public Works Department, Burma, *Ye-u Canal Project Revised Estimate 1908* (Rangoon: Government Printing and Stationery, 1909), p. 2.
138 Ibid., p. 5.
139 *Descriptive Account of Irrigation Works — Canal and Tank Systems — in Burma* (Rangoon: Superintendent of Government Printing, 1914), p. 3.
140 R. B. Smart, *Report on the Reclassification of the Soil in the Area Irrigated from the Shwebo Canal in the Shwebo District* (Rangoon: 1917), p. 9.
141 *Burma Gazetteer, Vol. A, Kyaukse District* (Rangoon: 1925), p. 74.
142 Ibid., p. 76.
143 Interview with Dr U Myint Swe, Team Leader (Malaria), Mandalay Division, on 9 July 1987, quoting personal comment by U Thang Maung of an old Burmese saying.
144 Khin-Maung-Kyi, "Malaria Vectors in Burma. 2", *Union of Burma Journal of Life Sciences* 3 (1970): 219, 220, 222.
145 Khin-Maung-Kyi, "The Anopheline Mosquitoes of Burma. 1. Subgenus Anopheles Meigen Series Anopheles and Myzorhyneus Edwards", *Union of Burma Journal of Life Sciences* 4 (1971): 288.
146 Khin-Maung-Kyi, "Malaria Vectors in Burma. 3" *Union of Burma Journal of Life Sciences* 5 (1972): 81, 82, 89.
147 Khin-Maung-Kyi, "The Anopheline Mosquitoes of Burma. 3", *Union of Burma Journal of Life Sciences* 4 (1971): 474.
148 Khin Maung Kyi U, "Rapid and Efficient Methods for Sampling Anopheline Populations in Insecticide Treated Areas", *Burma Medical Journal* 12 (Oct. 1964): 130.
149 Khin-Maung-Kyi, "Malaria Vectors in Burma. 1", *Union of Burma Journal of Life Sciences* 3 (1970): 205.

[150] M. Postiglione and V. Venkat Rao, "Malaria in Burma, A Review", *Indian Journal of Malariology* 10 (4 Dec. 1956): 284, and p. 283, which refers to D. G. R. Fox, "The Anopheline Mosquitoes of Burma", thesis, Cambridge University (1949).

[151] D. G. R. Fox, "The Anopheline Mosquitoes of Burma", p. 284.

[152] Khin-Maung-Kyi, "Malaria Vectors in Burma. 1", p. 211.

[153] Maung Tin, *Report on the Malaria Survey of Kya-in Township, Amherst District* (Rangoon: 1941), p. 26.

[154] Ibid., p. 29.

[155] *Burma Gazetteer, Vol. A, Kyaukse District* (Rangoon: 1925), p. 67.

[156] Maung Tin, *Malaria Survey of Kya-in Township*, p. 26.

[157] R. K. Singh, *Report on a Malaria Survey of Kengtung Town, Southern Shan States, Burma* (Rangoon: Government Press, 1940), p. 9.

[158] *RSPHB*, 1939, p. 40.

[159] League of Nations Health Organisation. *Intergovernmental Conference of Far-Eastern Countries on Rural Hygiene. Report by the Preparatory Committee* (Geneva: 1937), p. 76.

[160] League of Nations Health Organisation. *Intergovernmental Conference of Far-Eastern Countries on Rural Hygiene. Preparatory Papers: Report of the Philippines* (Geneva: Apr. 1937), p. 11.

[161] League of Nations Health Organisation. *Report of the Intergovernmental Conference ...*, p. 93.

[162] Ibid., p. 92.

[163] N. P. O'Gorman Lalor, *Investigation of Malaria in the District of Katha* (Rangoon: Superintendent of Government Printing, 1913), p. 8 (Chart No. 1).

[164] Ibid., p. iii.

[165] Postiglione and Venkat Rao, "Malaria in Burma, A Review", p. 283.

[166] *Proceedings of the Government of Burma in the Home (Medical) Department, Burma, (June 1911–Sept 1912)*, File 5/2, 11, Part B.

[167] *RSAB*, 1912, p. 11.

[168] W. G. King, *Information Supplied for the Simla Anti-Malarial Conference of 1909* (Rangoon: Superintendent of Government Printing, 1909), p. 18.

[169] *Annual Report of the Provincial Malarial Committee, Burma* (Rangoon: Superintendent of Government Printing, 1912) Appendix 1, p. 3.

[170] Strickland, *Hunter's Tropical Medicine*, p. 528.

[171] N. P. O'Gorman Lalor, *Spleen Census of the Province of Burma, with a Malarial Map of the Province and a Preliminary Note on Blackwater Fever* (Rangoon: Government Printing, 1912), pp. 1, 2, 8.

[172] Samuel R. Christophers and C.A. Bentley, "The Human Factor. An Extension of our Knowledge Regarding the Epidemiology of Malarial Disease", in *Transactions of the Bombay Medical Congress 1909*, ed. W. E. Jennings (Bombay: Bennet, Coleman & Co., undated), p. 80.

[173] *RSAB*, 1917, p. 11.

[174] *RSAB*, 1917, pp. 12, 13.

[175] Christophers and Bentley, "The Human Factor ...", p. 80.

[176] Ronald Ross, *The Prevention of Malaria* (London: John Murray, 1910), p. 197.

[177] Patrick Hehir, *Prophylaxis of Malaria in India* (Allahabad: Pioneer Press, 1910), p. 31.

[178] John A. Sinton, *What Malaria Costs India*, Health Bulletin No. 26, Malaria Bureau No. 13 (Simla: Govt. of India Press, 1939), p. 7.

[179] O'Gorman Lalor, *Spleen Census of the Province of Burma*, p. 8.

[180] King, *Information Supplied for the Simla Anti-Malarial Conference*, p. 23.

[181] M. Jafar, "Malaria in Mingaladon Cantonment, Burma", *Indian Medical Gazette* 67 (Sept. 1932): 495.

[182] Mya Than, "Anti-Malaria Programme in Burma", dissertation, D.P. and T.M., School of Preventive and Tropical Medicine, Rangoon (1975), p. 73.

[183] "Report of a Committee Convened for the Co-ordination of Policy Regarding the Prevention of Malarial Conditions Produced During the Construction of Roads and Railways", *Indian Journal of Malariology* 1 (2 June 1947): 253–63.

[184] Ba Maw, (Dr.), Sedawgyi Dam Project Area, Project Medical Hospital, Monthly Report for Malaria, 1981 to 1986 (undated).

CONCLUSION

[1] Peter Boomgaard and A. J. Gooszen, *Changing Economy in Indonesia*, Vol. II (Amsterdam: Royal Tropical Institute, 1991), p. 82.

[2] Ibid., pp. 55, 57, 58, 60.

[3] Ibid., pp. 49, 50.

[4] Ibid., p. 56.

[5] Ibid., p. 57.

[6] Ibid., p. 57.

[7] Ibid., p. 59.

[8] Ibid., p. 59.

[9] Ibid., p. 60.

Glossary

Kwin	Transfer of territory between administrative districts.
Lakh	One hundred thousand of a traditional number system, with separators in a different position, for example 450,681 rupees is approximately four and a half lakhs or written as 4,50,681.
Mahamuni	Festival held in Mandalay, presumed to be named after the town in Arakan.
Mahathayayawgyi	A famine which occurred in 1824–25.
Myook	Township officer appointed under the British.
Noe Myet	Condition suffered by a weanling (due to protein malnutrition) when its mother becomes pregnant.
Sit-tan	Administrative records assembled by the Burmese kings in 1783 and 1826.
Thathameda	Head tax.
Thugyi	Headman of a village or township.
Thungena	A childhood disease.
Wunthanu Athins	Village nationalist organisations widespread in the 1920s and early 1930s.

Bibliography

Adas, Michael, "Agrarian Development in the Plural Society. 1852–1941". University of Wisconsin, University Microfilms, 1971.

——, *The Burma Delta: Economic Development and Social Change on an Asian Rice Frontier 1852–1941*. Madison: University of Wisconsin Press, 1974.

Andrus, James Russell, *Burmese Economic Life*. Stanford: Stanford University Press, 1948.

Annual Report of the Provincial Malarial Committee, Burma. Rangoon: Superintendent of Government Printing, 1912.

Annual Report on Hospitals and Dispensaries in Burma, 1934, and *Triennial Review for the Years 1932–34*. Rangoon: Superintendent of Government Printing and Stationery, 1935.

Arnold, David, "Cholera Mortality in British India 1817–1914", in *India's Historical Demography: Studies in Famine, Disease and Society*, edited by Tim Dyson. London: Curzon Press, 1989.

Aung Kyin, "Beliefs and Practices in Nutrition in Central Burma (Magwe)". Undated paper, probably 1970s. Burma Box, Nutrition Library, London School of Hygiene and Tropical Medicine.

Aung Myint Thein, "Estimation of Infant and Childhood Mortality from Burma's First Stage Census: 1953". MSc Demography project paper, London School of Economics and Political Science, July 1975.

Ba Maw, (Dr), Sedawgyi Dam Project Area, Project Medical Hospital, Monthly Report for Malaria, 1981 to 1986 (undated).

Banerjee, P. C., "Report of a Measles Survey in Sagaing", *Burma Medical Journal* 16, no. 4 (Oct. 1968).

Ba Tin, "Nutritional Status of Rural and Urban Community in Burma". Dissertation, D.P. and T.M., Institute of Medicine 1, Rangoon, 1969.

Ba Tun U and Ko Ko U, "Some Observations on the Helminthic Infestations of the Burmese Village Community". *Burma Medical Journal* 16, no. 2 (Apr. 1968).

Barva, J. R., "Birth Weight, Length and Circumference of the Skull of Infants Born in the Largest Maternity Hospital of Burma", *Burma Medical Journal* 9, no. 1 (Jan. 1961).

Baxter, J., *Report on Indian Immigration*. Rangoon: Superintendent of Government Printing and Stationery, 1941.

Benjamin, Bernard, *The Population Census*. London: Heinemann, 1970.

Bentley, C. A., *Malaria and Agriculture in Bengal*. Calcutta: Government of Bengal Public Health Department, Bengal Secretariat Book Depot, 1925.

Binns, B. O., "Analysis of Pre-war Diet in Burma". Undated paper, probably 1946/1947, stamped "UT.29/X". Nutrition Department, London School of Hygiene and Tropical Medicine.

Boomgaard, Peter and A. J. Gooszen, *Changing Economy in Indonesia*, Vol. II. Amsterdam: Royal Tropical Institute, 1991.

Braddon, William Leonard, "Beri Beri, Its Cause, Symptoms, Diagnosis, Treatment, Pathology, and Prevention", in *Transactions of the Bombay Medical Congress 1909*, edited by W. E. Jennings. Bombay: Bennet, Coleman and Co., undated.

Breman, Jan C., "Java: Population Growth and Demographic Structure". *Tijdschrift van het Koninklijk Nederlandsch Aardrijkskundig Genootschap* 80, no. 3 (1963): 252–303.

Broadhead, R. L., "Tetanus Neonatorum: A Review of Epidemiology, Management and Prevention", *Postgraduate Doctor* 8, no. 7 (July 1985).

Brown, Colin, "The Influenza Pandemic of 1918 in Indonesia", in *Death and Disease in Southeast Asia*, edited by Norman G. Owen. Singapore: Oxford University Press, 1987.

Brown, Kenneth H., R. H. Gilman, M. Khatun and Ahmed M. G., "Absorption of macro-nutrients from a rice-vegetable diet before and after treatment of ascariasis in children", *American Journal of Clinical Nutrition* 33, no. 9 (September 1980): 1975–82.

Burma Gazetteer, Vol. A, Bassein District. Rangoon: 1916.

———, *Henzada District*. Rangoon: 1915.

———, *Insein District*. Rangoon: 1911.

———, *Insein District*. Rangoon: 1914.

———, *Kyaukse District*. Rangoon: 1925.

———, *Lower Chindwin District*. Rangoon: 1912.

———, *Mandalay District*. Rangoon: 1928.

———, *Pegu District*. Rangoon: 1911.

———, *Shwebo District*. Rangoon: 1929.

———, *Syriam District*. Rangoon: 1911.

———, *Syriam District*. Rangoon: 1914.

———, *Tharrawaddy District*. Rangoon: 1959.

———, *Thayetmyo District*. Rangoon: 1911.

———, *Toungoo District*. Rangoon: 1914.

———. *Yamethin District*, Rangoon: 1934.

Burma Gazetteer, Vol. B, Insein District No. 6. Rangoon: 1913.

———, *Katha District*. Rangoon: 1913.

———, *Maubin District No. 14*. Rangoon: 1912.

———, *Myaungmya District No. 13*. Rangoon: 1912.

———, *Myingyan District No. 38*. Rangoon: 1913.

———, *Myingyan District No. 40*. Rangoon: 1924.

———, *Tharrawaddy District No. 8*. Rangoon: 1912.

———, *Yamethin District No. 39*. Rangoon: 1924.

Burney H., Harvey G.E. (ed.), "On the Population of the Burman Empire", *Journal of the Burma Research Society* 31, Part 1 (Apr. 1941).

Bwibo, N., "The Role of Neonatal Infection in Neonatal and Childhood Mortality", *Journal of Tropical Paediatrics and Environmental Child Health* 17, no. 3 (1971).

Caldwell, John Charles, "The Mechanisms of Demographic Change in Historical Perspective", *Population Studies* 35, no. 1 (Mar. 1981). Reprinted in *The Economics of the Family*, edited by Nancy Folbre. Cheltenham: E. Elgar Pub. Ltd, c. 1996.

Carael, Michel, "Relations between Birth Intervals and Nutrition in Three Central African Populations (Zaire)", in *Nutrition and Human Reproduction*, edited by W. Henry Mosely. New York: Plenum Press, 1978.

Census of British Burma 1872, Report. Rangoon: Government Press, 1875.

Census of British Burma 1881, Report, Vol. 1. London: Eyre and Spottiswoode, 1883.

Census of Burma 1891, Report.

Census of India 1891, General Tables for the British Provinces and Feudatory States, Vol. 2, Statistics. London: Eyre and Spottiswoode, 1892.

Census of India 1901, Vol. 1, Part 1, Report. Calcutta: Superintendent of Government Printing, 1903.

———, *Vol. 1-A, India, Part 2, Tables*. Calcutta: Superintendent of Government Printing, 1903.

Census of India 1901, Vol. 12-C, Burma Part 4, Upper Burma Provincial Tables, (Rangoon: Superintendent of Government Printing, 1905).

Census of India 1911, Vol. 9, *Burma, Part 2, Tables*. Calcutta: Superintendent of Government Printing, 1912

Census of India 1931, Vol. 11, Burma, Part 2, Tables. Rangoon: Supt. of Government Printing, 1933.

Chandler, Asa Crawford, "The Prevalence and Epidemiology of Hookworm and other Helminthic Infections in India. Part VI. BURMA", *Indian Journal of Medical Research* 14 (1926–7).

Cheng Siok-Hwa, *The Rice Industry of Burma, 1852–1940*. Kuala Lumpur: University of Malaya Press, 1968.

Chitre, R. G. and Tin Tin Oo, "Role of Nutrition in Disease", *Burma Medical Journal* 5, no. 2 (Apr. 1957).

Cho Nwe Oo, "Nutrition in Pregnant and Lactating Mothers". Paper presented at 2nd Orientation Course in Nutrition for Paediatricians (June 1974).

———, "Prevalence of Protein Calorie Malnutrition in Burma", *Burma Medical Journal* 21, no. 4 (Oct. 1975).

———, "Yantein Village Nutrition Promotion Programme", *Burma Medical Journal* 23 (Jan. to Oct. 1977)

Christophers, Samuel Rickard and C. A. Bentley, "The Human Factor. An Extension of our Knowledge Regarding the Epidemiology of Malarial Disease", in *Transactions of the Bombay Medical Congress 1909*, edited by W. E. Jennings. Bombay: Bennet, Coleman and Co., undated.

Christophers, Samuel R., John A. Sinton and Gordon Covell, *How To Do a Malaria Survey*, Health Bulletin No. 14. Government of India Central Publications Branch, 1928.

Cipolla, Carlo M., *The Economic History of World Population*. London: Penguin, 1974.

Clarke, J. I., *Population Geography and the Developing Countries*. Oxford: Pergamon Press, 1971.

Coale, Ansley Johnson and Paul Demeny, "Methods of Estimating Basic Demographic Measures from Incomplete Data", *Population Studies* no. 42. Usually known as UN Manual 4. New York: UN Department of Economic and Social Affairs, 1967.

_____, *Regional Model Life Tables and Stable Populations*. New York: Academic Press, 1983.

Cobb, C. E., "Beri Beri and Rice Control in Malaya", *Indian Medical Gazette* 59, (Aug. 1924).

Coedès, George, *The Indianized States of Southeast Asia*. Translated by Susan Brown Cowing and edited by Walter F. Vella. Honolulu: University Press of Hawaii, 1968.

Cox, Hiram, *Journal of a Residence in the Burman Empire*. London: G. & W. B. Whittaker, 1821.

Cummins, Stevenson Lyle, "The Tuberculosis of Tropical Countries", *Indian Medical Gazette* 74 (Sept. 1939): 513–6.

Davis, Kingsley, "Population Policy and the Theory of Reproductive Motivation", in *Essays of Economic Development and Cultural Change in Honour of Bert E. Hoselitz*, edited by M. Nash. Chicago: University of Chicago Press, 1977.

_____, *The Population of India and Pakistan*. Princeton: Princeton University Press, 1951.

Descriptive Account of Irrigation Works — Canal and Tank Systems — in Burma. Rangoon: Superintendent of Government Printing, 1914.

Diokno, M. S. I., "British Firms and the Economy of Burma, with Special Reference to the Rice and Teak Industries, 1917–1937". PhD thesis, University of London, May 1983.

Dobby, Ernest Henry George, *Southeast Asia*. London: University of London Press, 1950.

Dodge, N. N., "Population Estimates for the Malay Peninsula in the Nineteenth Century, with Special Reference to the East Coast States", *Population Studies* 34, no. 3 (Nov. 1980).

Dyson, Tim, *India's Historical Demography: Studies in Famine, Disease and Society*. London: Curzon Press, 1989.

_____, "Preliminary Demography of 1981 Census", *Economic and Political Weekly* 16, no. 3 (1981): 1349–56.

Ebrahim, G. J., "Malaria in Childhood", *Journal of Tropical Paediatrics* 30, no. 4 (Aug. 1984) Editorial.

Economic and Social Board, *A Study of the Economic and Social History of Burma*, Part 3, Administration Report. Rangoon: Office of the Prime Minister, 1957.

Ellis, Richard White Bernard, "Infantile Convulsions", *Burma Medical Journal* 4, no. 2 (Apr. 1956).

Evans, Col., "Burma Hospitals. Extract from Annual Report", *Indian Medical Gazette* 50 (Oct. 1915).

FAO, *Rice and Rice Diets: A Survey*. Washington: UN FAO, 1948.

_____, *Report of the Nutrition Committee for South and East Asia*, Third Meeting, 1953. Rome: UN FAO, Apr. 1954.

————, *Report of the Nutrition Committee for South and East Asia, Fourth Session*, Tokyo, Japan, 1956. Rome: UN FAO, 1957.

Faulkner, F., "Key Issues in Infant Mortality", *Journal of Tropical Paediatrics and Environmental Child Health* 17, no. 1 (Mar. 1971).

Ferguson, J. P., "The Society and its Environments", in *Burma: A Country Study*, edited by Frederica M. Bunge, Area Handbook Series, 3rd edition. Washington, DC: US Government, 1983.

Fisher, Charles Alfred, "Some Comments on Population Growth in South-East Asia with Special Reference to the Period since 1830", in *The Economic Development of South-East Asia*, edited by Charles Donald Cowan. London: George Allen and Unwin, 1964.

Foll, C. V., "The Perils of Childhood in Upper Burma", *Journal of Tropical Paediatrics* 4, no. 3 (Dec. 1958).

————, "An Account of some of the Beliefs and Superstitions about Pregnancy, Parturition and Infant Health in Burma", *Journal of Tropical Paediatrics* 5, no. 1 (June 1959).

Foll, C. V. and Onmar Khin, "Perinatal Problems in Upper Burma", *Journal of Tropical Medicine and Hygiene* 61 (Sept. 1958).

Fox, D. G. R., "The Anopheline Mosquitoes of Burma". Thesis, Cambridge University, 1949.

Fox, John P., Carrie E. Hall and Lila R. Elveback, *Epidemiology, Man and Disease*. New York: Macmillan, 1970.

Francis, C. J. R. and Mamsa U. E. K., "Age of Puberty in the Burmese Male and Female", *Union of Burma Journal of Life Sciences* 3 (1970).

Furnivall, John Sydenham, *Colonial Policy and Practice: A Comparative Study of Burma and Netherlands India*. Cambridge: Cambridge University Press, 1948.

Fytche, Albert, *Burma Past and Present*, Vol. II. London: Kegan Paul and Co., 1878.

Gairdner, W. T., "On Infantile Death Rates, in their bearing on Sanitary and Social Science", in *Pamphlets PT.2348-57*, Secretary of State for India Library, 1861.

Gardiner, Peter and Mayling Oey, "Morbidity and Mortality in Java, 1880–1940: The Evidence of the Colonial Reports", in *Death and Disease in Southeast Asia*, edited by Norman G. Owen. Singapore: Oxford University Press, 1987.

Glass, R., S. Becker, M. Huq, B. Stoll, M. Khan, M. Merson, J. Lee and R. Black, "Endemic Cholera in Rural Bangladesh 1966–1980", *American Journal of Epidemiology* 116, no. 6 (1982).

Hall, Daniel George Edward, *A History of South-East Asia*, 4th edition. Basingstoke: Macmillan, 1981.

Hanley, Sarah B. and Kozo Yamamura, *Economic and Demographic Change in Pre-Industrial Japan 1600–1868*. Princeton: Princeton University Press, 1977.

Hehir, Patrick, *Prophylaxis of Malaria in India*. Allahabad: Pioneer Press, 1910.

Henry, Louis, *Population Analysis and Models*. Translated by Etienne van de Walle and Elise F. Jones. London: Edward Arnold, 1976.

Herbert, Patricia, *The Hsaya San Rebellion (1930–1932) Reappraised*. Working Paper No. 27. Melbourne: Monash University, Centre of Southeast Asian Studies, 1982.

HMSO, *Correspondence Regarding Measures for the Prevention of Plague: East India (Plague)*. London: HMSO, 1907.

_____, *Memorandum on Measures Adopted for Sanitary Improvements in India up to the end of 1867*. London: Eyre and Spottiswoode for HMSO, 1868.

_____, *Report of the Royal Commission on Labour in India*. London: HMSO, June 1931.

_____, *Statistical Report on the Sickness, Mortality and Invaliding Among Her Majesty's Troops Serving in Ceylon, the Tenasserim Provinces and the Burmese Empire*. London: HMSO, 1841.

Hoeprich, Paul D., ed., *Infectious Diseases: A Guide to the Understanding and Management of Infectious Processes*. Hagerstown, MD: Harper and Row, 1983.

Hull, Terence H., "Plague in Java", in *Death and Disease in Southeast Asia*, edited by Norman G. Owen. Singapore: Oxford University Press, 1987.

Imperial Gazetteer of India, Burma, Volume 1 and Volume 2. Calcutta: 1908.

Islam M. S., Rahaman M. M., Aziz K. M. S., Munshi M. H., Rahman M. and Patwari Y. P., "Birthcare Practice and Neonatal Tetanus in a Rural Area of Bangladesh", *Journal of Tropical Paediatrics* 28, no. 6 (Dec. 1982): 299–302.

Islam M. S., Rahaman M. M., Aziz, K. M. S., Rahman M., Munshi M. H. and Patwari, Y., "Infant Mortality in Rural Bangladesh: An Analysis of Causes During Neonatal and Postnatal Periods", *Journal of Tropical Paediatrics* 28, no. 6 (Dec. 1982): 294–8.

Jafar, M., "Malaria in Mingaladon Cantonment, Burma", *Indian Medical Gazette* 67 (Sept. 1932).

Jannetta, Ann Bowman, *Epidemics and Mortality in Early Modern Japan*. Princeton: Princeton University Press, 1987.

Jolly, G. G., "The Use of Germinated Pulse and Beans in the Natural Dietary of the Burmese", *Indian Medical Gazette* 58 (June 1923): 255–6.

_____, "Beri Beri in Cheduba Island, Arakan, Burma", *Indian Medical Gazette* 65 (July 1930): 383–6.

Journal of Tropical Medicine and Hygiene, "Infant Death Rate in Burma", 17 (1914). Notes and News.

Journal of Tropical Paediatrics, "Contraceptive Effect of Breast Feeding", 28, no. 1 (Feb. 1982). Editorial.

Kandiah, M., M. Lee, T. K. Ng, and Y. H. Chong, "Malnutrition in Malaria Endemic Villages of Bengkoka Peninsula, Sabah", *Journal of Tropical Paediatrics* 30, no. 1 (Feb. 1984).

Keeton, Charles Lee, *King Thebaw and the Ecological Rape of Burma*. New Delhi: Manohar Book Service, 1974.

Khin Maung Kyi U, "Rapid and Efficient Methods for Sampling Anopheline Populations in Insecticide Treated Areas", *Burma Medical Journal* 12 (Oct. 1964): 130–4.

Khin-Maung-Kyi, "Malaria Vectors in Burma. 1", *Union of Burma Journal of Life Sciences* (1970): 205–16.

_____, "Malaria Vectors in Burma. 2", *Union of Burma Journal of Life Sciences* 3 (1970): 217–25.

_____, "Malaria Vectors in Burma. 3", *Union of Burma Journal of Life Sciences* 5 (1972): 81–98.

————, "The Anopheline Mosquitoes of Burma. 1. Subgenus Anopheles Meigen Series Anopheles and Myzorhyneus Edwards", *Union of Burma Journal of Life Sciences* 4 (1971): 281–96.

————, "The Anopheline Mosquitoes of Burma. 3", *Union of Burma Journal of Life Sciences* 4 (1971): 473–83.

Khin-Maung-Naing, Tin-Tin-Oo, Kywe-Thein MS and Nwe-New-Hlaing, "Study on Lactation Performance of Burmese Mothers", *American Journal of Clinical Nutrition* no. 33 (Dec. 1980): 2265–8.

King, W. G. *Information Supplied for the Simla Anti-Malarial Conference of 1909.* Rangoon: Superintendent of Government Printing, 1909.

————, "Prevention of the Spread of Tuberculosis in Burma", *Indian Medical Gazette* 45, Supplement (1910): 5–9.

Ko Ko U and Khin May Khi, "Epidemiology of Tetanus Neonatorum in Rangoon", *Union of Burma Journal of Life Sciences* 3 (1970).

Koenig, William J., "The Early Konbaung Polity 1752–1819: A Study of Politics, Administration and Social Organisation in Burma". PhD dissertation, University of London, 1978.

Kunhikannan, N. K., "Infant Feeding in Burma", Current Topics, *Indian Medical Gazette* 55 (July 1920).

Kyaw Win, "A Report on Intestinal Helminthic Infections in Mon State", *Burma Medical Journal* 22, nos. 3 and 4 (July and Oct. 1976).

Kywe-Thein, Thane-Toe, Tin-Tin-Oo and Khin-Khin-Tway, "A Study of Infantile Beri-beri in Rangoon", *Union of Burma Journal of Life Sciences* 1 (1968).

Kywe-Thein, Tin-U, Tin-Tin-Oo and Khin-Kyi-Nyunt, "An Epidemiological Study of Protein Calorie Malnutrition in Rangoon", *Union of Burma Journal of Life Sciences* 4 (1971).

Laurie, William Ferguson Beaton, *Our Burmese Wars and Relations with Burma.* London: W. H. Allen and Co., 1880.

Lay Maung, "Methods of Obtaining Vital Statistics from Rural Areas with Particular Reference to Burma". Project report for Board of Examiners of the MSc Medical Demography Examination, London School of Hygiene and Tropical Medicine, University of London, August 1971.

Leach, Edmund Ronald, *Political Systems of Highland Burma: A Study of Kachin Social Structure.* London: Athlone Press, 1977.

League of Nations Epidemiological Reports, 1935/36, Volume 14/15.

League of Nations Health Organisation, *Intergovernmental Conference of Far-Eastern Countries on Rural Hygiene. Preparatory Papers, 2.* Geneva: 1937.

————, *Intergovernmental Conference of Far-Eastern Countries on Rural Hygiene. Preparatory Papers, 2. Note on Medical Organisation in Burma.* Geneva: 15 Mar 1937.

————, *Intergovernmental Conference of Far-Eastern Countries on Rural Hygiene. Preparatory Papers. Report of the Malayan Delegation.* Geneva: 1937.

————, *Intergovernmental Conference of Far-Eastern Countries on Rural Hygiene. Preparatory Papers. Report of the Philippines.* Geneva: Apr. 1937.

————, *Intergovernmental Conference of Far-Eastern Countries on Rural Hygiene. Report by the Preparatory Committee.* Geneva: League of Nations, 1937.

————, *Report of the Intergovernmental Conference of Far-Eastern Countries on Rural Hygiene, held at Bandoeng (Java), 3rd–13th August 1937.*

Lieberman, Victor B., *Burmese Administrative Cycles: Anarchy and Conquest c 1580–1760*. Princeton: Princeton University Press, 1984.

Lovric, Barbara, "Bali: Myth, Magic and Morbidity", in *Death and Disease in Southeast Asia*, edited by Norman G. Owen. Singapore: Oxford University Press, 1987.

MacDonald, Keith Norman, *The Practice of Medicine Among the Burmese*. Edinburgh: MacLachan and Stewart, 1879.

Ma Htay Nwe, "Malaria in Children in Lashio Township", *Burma Medical Journal* 26, no. 3 (Sept. 1980).

————, "Morbidity Pattern Seen in the Department of Child Health, General Hospital, Mandalay", *Burma Medical Journal* 20, no. 1 (Jan. 1972).

Mahajani, Usha, *The Role of Indian Minorities in Burma and Malaya*. Bombay: Vora and Co., 1960.

Ma Ma Tin, "Feeding Patterns of Infants and Young Children in Mandalay Region". Undated paper, probably 1970s. Burma Box, Nutrition Library of the London School of Hygiene and Tropical Medicine.

Mandell, Gerald L., Robert Gordon Douglas and John Eugene Bennett, eds., *Principles and Practice of Infectious Disease*. New York: J. Wiley and Sons, 1979.

Manderson, Lenore, "Blame, Responsibility and Remedial Action: Death, Disease and the Infant in Early Twentieth Century Malaya", in *Death and Disease in Southeast Asia*, edited by Norman G. Owen. Singapore: Oxford University Press, 1987.

Maung Ba Aung, "Why Burma is Sparsely Populated, a Suggestion", *Journal of the Burma Research Society* 4, Part 2 (1914).

Maung Tin, *Report on the Malaria Survey of Kya-in Township, Amherst District*. Rangoon: 1941.

May, Jacques Meyer, with the collaboration of Irma S. Jarcho, *The Ecology of Malnutrition in the Far and Near East: Food Resources, Habits and Deficiencies*. New York: Hafner Publishing Co., 1961.

McEvedy, Colin and Richard Jones, *Atlas of World Population History*. London: Penguin, 1978.

McNeill, William Hardy, *Plagues and Peoples*. Harmondsworth: Penguin, 1979.

Megau, J. W. D., S. P. Bhattacharji and B. K. Paul, "Further Observations on the Epidemic Dropsy Form of Beri Beri", *Indian Medical Gazette* 63 (Aug. 1928).

Meyer, E., "Depression et Malaria à Sri-Lanka 1925-1939", Vol. 1. Thesis, Écoles des Hautes Études en Science Sociales, 1980.

Miller, J., Richard G. Feachem and B. S. Drasar, "Cholera Epidemiology in Developed and Developing Countries", *Lancet* (2 Feb. 1985).

Mi Mi Khaing, *The World of Burmese Women*. London: Zed Books Ltd., 1984.

Mobsby, A., "The Nutrition Project, Burma. (WHO)", *Burma Weekly Bulletin* 5, no. 30 (Nov. 1956).

Mougne, C., "An Ethnography of Reproduction: Changing Patterns of Fertility in a Northern Thai Village" in *Nature and Man in South East Asia*, edited by P. A. Stott. London: School of Oriental and African Studies, 1978.

Mya Than (Dr), "Anti-Malaria Programme in Burma", Dissertation, D. P. and T. M., School of Preventive and Tropical Medicine, Rangoon, 1975.

Nash, June and Manning Nash, "Marriage, Family and Population Growth in Upper Burma", *Southwestern Journal of Anthropology* 19, no. 3 (1963).

Nokes, David, *Jane Austen: A Life*. London: Fourth Estate Ltd., 1997.

Notes on Sanitary Organisation and Development in Burma. Rangoon: Superintendent of Government Printing, 1915.

O'Gorman Lalor, N. P., *Spleen Census of the Province of Burma, with a Malarial Map of the Province and a Preliminary Note on Blackwater Fever*. Rangoon: Government Printing, 1912.

———, *Investigation of Malaria at Kyaukpyu*. Rangoon: Government Printing, 1912.

———, *Investigation of Malaria in the District of Katha*. Rangoon: Office of Superintendent of Government Printing, 1913.

Ohn Kyi (Dr Daw), "Beliefs and Practices about Foods and Feeding in Mon State (Moulmein)". Undated paper, probably 1970s. Burma Box, Nutrition Library, London School of Hygiene and Tropical Medicine.

Owen, Norman G., "Southeast Asia—The Paradox of Nineteenth Century Population Growth". Unpublished paper, March 1985.

———, "Measuring Mortality in the Nineteenth Century Philippines", in *Death and Disease in Southeast Asia*, edited by Norman G. Owen. Singapore: Oxford University Press, 1987.

———, "Toward a History of Health in Southeast Asia", in *Death and Disease in Southeast Asia*, edited by Norman G. Owen. Singapore: Oxford University Press, 1987.

Owen, Norman G., ed., *Death and Disease in Southeast Asia. Explorations in Social, Medical and Demographic History*. Singapore: Oxford University Press, 1987.

Paul, John Rodman, *Clinical Epidemiology*. Chicago: University of Chicago Press, 1958.

Pe Kyin, *The Nutritive Value of Burmese Foods*. Rangoon: Directorate of Health Services, 1967.

Peper, B., "Population Growth in Java in the Nineteenth Century", *Population Studies* 24 (1970).

Phayre, Arthur Purves, *Memorandum on the Sparseness of Population in British Burma*. Rangoon: Mission Press, 1862.

Po Po, "Nutritional Problems in Childhood", *Burma Medical Journal* 13, nos. 2 and 3 (Apr. and July 1965).

Postiglione, M. and V. Venkat Rao, "Malaria in Burma: A Review", *Indian Journal of Malariology* 10 (4 Dec. 1956).

Postmus, S., "Beri beri of Mother and Child in Burma", *Tropical and Geographical Medicine* 10 (1958).

———, "Diet and Nutritional Condition in Burma", *Burma Medical Journal* 5, no. 4 (Oct. 1957).

Pressat, Roland, *The Dictionary of Demography*, edited by Christopher Wilson. Oxford: Basil Blackwell, 1985.

Proceedings of the Chief Commissioner, Burma. In the General Department. No. 44.S. (Sanitary), (26/8/1891).

Proceedings of the Government of Burma in the Home (Medical) Department, Burma, (June 1911–Sept 1912), File 5/2, 11, Part B.

Pryer, Jane and Nigel Crook, *Cities of Hunger*. Oxford: Oxfam, 1988.

"Public Health and Births and Deaths 1867. British Burma". Extract from the *Proceedings of the Chief Commissioner in the Home Department*, No. 241. Rangoon: Rangoon Times Press, 1868. Abbreviated in text as PHBD.

Public Works Department, Burma, *Ye-u Canal Project Revised Estimate 1908*. Rangoon: Government Printing and Stationery, 1909.

Rahman S., "The Effect of Traditional Birth Attendants and Tetanus Toxoid in Reduction of Neonatal Mortality", *Journal of Tropical Paediatrics* 28, no. 4 (Aug. 1982): 163–5.

Reid, Anthony, "Low Population Growth and its Causes in Pre-Colonial Southeast Asia", in *Death and Disease in Southeast Asia*, edited by Norman G. Owen. Singapore: Oxford University Press, 1987.

————, *Southeast Asia in the Age of Commerce 1450–1680*, Vol. 1, "The Lands Below the Winds". New Haven: Yale University Press, 1988–93.

"Report of a Committee Convened for the Co-ordination of Policy Regarding the Prevention of Malarial Conditions Produced During the Construction of Roads and Railways", *Indian Journal of Malariology* 1 (2 June 1947): 253–63.

Report on the Public Health Administration of Burma. Rangoon: Government Press, 1921–1936. Abbreviated in text as *RPHAB*.

Report on Public Health and Vital Statistics for 1868. Rangoon: Chief Commissioner's Office Press, 1870. Written by J. McNeale Donnelly. Abbreviated in text as *RPHVS*.

Report on the Sanitary Administration of British Burma. Rangoon: Government Press, 1870–1889. Abbreviated in text as *RSABB*.

Report on the Sanitary Administration of Burma. Rangoon: Government Press, 1890–1920. Abbreviated in text as *RSAB*.

Report on the State of Public Health in Burma. Rangoon: Government Press, 1937– . Abbreviated in text as *RSPHB*.

Robequain, Charles, *The Economic Development of Indo-China*. Translated by Isabel A.Ward. Oxford: Oxford University Press, 1944.

Robertson, R. C., "A Malaria Survey on the China-Burman Highway", *Transactions of the Royal Society of Tropical Medicine and Hygiene* 34, no. 4 (Jan. 1941).

Ross, Ronald, *The Prevention of Malaria*. London: John Murray, 1910.

Ruzicka, Lado Theodor, "Mortality in India: Past Trends and Future Prospects", in *India's Demography: Essays on the Contemporary Population*, edited by Tim Dyson and Nigel Crook. New Delhi: South Asia Publishers Pvt. Ltd., 1984.

Sangermano, Father. *A Description of the Burmese Empire*. Translated by William Tandy. Originally published in 1833 in Rome for the Oriental Translation Fund of Great Britain and Ireland. Page references are based on the 1969 reprint edition by Augustus M. Kelley, New York.

Sao Yan Naing, "Beliefs and Practices in Nutrition in Northern Shan States". Undated paper, probably 1970s. Burma Box, Nutrition Library, London School of Hygiene and Tropical Medicine.

Sarin, B. P. "The Treatment of Acute Diarrhoea in Infants", *Burma Medical Journal* 4, No. 4 (Oct. 1956).

————, "Observations on 'Kwashiorkor' or Protein Undernutrition in Rangoon", *Burma Medical Journal* 5, no. 2 (Apr. 1957).

Schofield, F. D., V. M. Tucker and G. R. Westbrook, "Neonatal Tetanus in New Guinea", *British Medical Journal* (23 Sept. 1961): 785–9.

Scott, J. G. and J. P. Hardiman, *Gazetteer of Upper Burma and the Shan States. Part 2*, Vol. 2. Rangoon: Superintendent of Government Printing, 1900.

————, *Gazetteer of Upper Burma and the Shan States. Part 2*, Vol. 1. Rangoon: Superintendent of Government Printing, 1901.

Scrimshaw, Susan C. M., "Infant Mortality and Behaviour in the Regulation of Family Size", *Population and Development Review* 4, no. 3 (Sept. 1978).

Sein May Chit (Dr Daw), "Nutritional Problems in Burma". Undated paper, probably 1970s. Burma Box, Nutrition Library, London School of Hygiene and Tropical Medicine.

Sen, Amartya Kumar, *Poverty and Famines: An Essay on Entitlement and Deprivation*. Oxford: Clarendon Press, 1981.

Shorter Oxford English Dictionary on Historical Principles, Vol. II. Oxford: 1983.

Shryock, Henry S. and Jacob S. Siegal, *The Methods and Materials of Demography*, condensed and edited by Edward G. Stockwell. New York: Academic Press, 1976.

Shwe Oh, "Epidemiology of Neonatal Tetanus in Mandalay Division". Dissertation, Department of Preventive and Tropical Medicine, Institute of Medicine 1, Rangoon, 1973–4.

Singh, R. K., *Report on a Malaria Survey of Kengtung Town, Southern Shan States, Burma*. Rangoon: Government Press, 1940.

Sinton, John Alexander, *What Malaria Costs India*, Health Bulletin No. 26, Malaria Bureau No. 13. Simla: Government of India Press, 1939.

Smart, R. B., *Report on the Reclassification of the Soil in the Area Irrigated from the Shwebo Canal in the Shwebo District*. Rangoon: 1917.

Smith, P. C. and Shui-meng Ng, "The Components of Population Change in Nineteenth-century South-east Asia: Village Data from the Philippines", *Population Studies* 36, no. 2 (July 1982).

Snow John, monograph on cholera, in *Epidemiology, Man and Disease*, by John P. Fox, Carrie E. Hall and Lila R. Elveback. New York: Macmillan, 1970.

Soe Soe Aye, "Morbidity Pattern of Children at Rangoon Children Hospital", *Burma Medical Journal* 25, no. 1 (Jan. 1979).

Spiro, Melford E., *Kinship and Marriage in Burma*. Berkeley: University of California Press, 1977.

Stahlie, T. D., "The Role of Tetanus Neonatorum in Infant Mortality in Thailand", *Journal of Tropical Paediatrics* 6, no. 1 (June 1960).

Steel, Tom, *The Life and Death of St. Kilda*. UK: Fontana, 1975.

Steinberg, D. J., ed., *In Search of Southeast Asia*. Honolulu: University of Hawaii Press, 1985.

Steinberg, Sigfrid Henry, *The Thirty Years War and the Conflict for European Hegemony 1600–1660*. London: Edward Arnold, 1977.

Stephenson, L. S., David William T. Crompton, Michael C. Latham, S. E. Arnold and A. A. S. Jansen, "Evaluation of a Four Year Project to Control Ascaris Infection in Children in Two Kenyan Villages", *Journal of Tropical Paediatrics* 29, no. 3 (June 1983).

Sternstein, Larry, "The Growth of the World's Pre-eminent 'Primate City': Bangkok at its Bicentenary", *Journal of Southeast Asian Studies* 15, no. 1 (Mar. 1984).

Stewart, J. A., "Kyaukse Irrigation — A Side-light on Burmese History", *Journal of the Burma Research Society* 11, Part 1 (1921).

Strickland, G. Thomas, *Hunter's Tropical Medicine*. London: W. B. Saunders and Co., 1984.

Stuart, J., "Why Is Burma Sparsely Peopled?", *Journal of the Burma Research Society* 4, Part 1 (1914), and 5 (1915).

Sundrum, R. M., "Population Statistics of Burma", Economics Research Project, Statistical Paper No. 3. Rangoon: University of Rangoon, Dec. 1957.

Symes, Michael, *An Account of an Embassy to the Kingdom of Ava*. London: W. Bulmer and Co., 1800.

Symonds, B. E. R., "Clinical Studies on South Trinidadian Children. II. The Treatment of Neonatal Tetanus", *Journal of Tropical Paediatrics* 6, no. 1 (June 1960): 9–14.

Taeuber, Irene Barnes, *Population Growth and Development in Southeast Asia*, SEADAG Report, The Population Panels Seminar. New York: SEADAG, 1972.

Taylor, John, C. de C. Martin and U Thant, "Preliminary Enquiry into Beri-beri in Burma", *Indian Medical Research Memoirs*, Memoir No. 8 (Mar. 1928).

Terwiel, Barend Jan, "Asiatic Cholera in Siam: Its First Occurrence and the 1820 Epidemic", in *Death and Disease in Southeast Asia*, edited by Norman G. Owen. Singapore: Oxford University Press, 1987.

Thein Aung, "ARI in Childhood in Burma — What Happens Now?", in *Acute Respiratory Infections in Childhood*, edited by R. M. Douglas and E. Kerby-Eaton. Adelaide, SA: Department of Community Medicine University of Adelaide, 1985.

Tin E (Dr. Daw), "Beliefs and Practices about Foods and Feedings in Kachin State (Myitkyina)". Undated paper, probably 1970s. Burma Box, Nutrition Library, London School of Hygiene and Tropical Medicine.

Tin Tin Nyunt, "Estimation of Vital Rates for Burma and Their Effects on the Future Size of the Population". MA thesis, Australian National University, Department of Demography, Research School of Social Sciences, Canberra, Sept. 1978.

Tin Tin Oo and Khin Maung Naing, "A Comparison of Milk Output of Burmese Mothers by Three Different Methods", *Food and Nutrition Bulletin* 4, no. 4 (Dec. 1982).

————, "Breast Feeding and Weaning Practices for Infants and Young Children in Rangoon, Burma", *Food and Nutrition Bulletin* 7, no. 4 (Dec. 1985).

————, "Breast Feeding and Weaning Practices for Infants and Young Children in Rangoon". Summary in *DMR Bulletin* 1, no. 3 (Oct. 1986).

Tin U and Kyaw Myint, eds., "Report of the Peri-natal Mortality and Low Birth Weight Study Project — Burma", SEARO Inter-country Collaborative Project, WHO. Rangoon: Department of Medical Education, 1981.

Tomkins, A., G. Mann and S. Khanum, "New Approaches Toward the Prevention of Measles", *Postgraduate Doctor* 2, no. 1 (1986).

Trager, Frank N. and William J. Koenig, *Burmese Sit-tans 1764–1826*. Tucson: University of Arizona Press, 1979.

Tupasi, T. E., "Nutrition and Acute Respiratory Infection", in *Acute Respiratory Infections in Childhood*, edited by R. M. Douglas and E. Kerby-Eaton. Adelaide, SA: Department of Community Medicine University of Adelaide, 1985.

U Maung Gale, *Reports on the Dietary and Nutritional Surveys Conducted in Certain Areas of Burma*. Rangoon: Superintendent of Government Printing and Stationery, 1948.

Union of Burma Report by the Inter-Departmental Committee on Nutrition for National Defence (May 1963).

Vinijchaikul, K., "Pathological Studies of Acute Infantile Cardiac Beri-beri", *Journal of the Medical Association of Thailand* 47, no. 2 (Feb. 1964).

Visaria, Pravin M., "Provisional Population Totals of the 1971 Census", *Economic and Political Weekly* 6, no. 29 (1971).

Vyatkin, A. R., *The Population of Burma: Historio Demographic Outline*. Moscow: Chief Publishing House of Oriental Literature, 1979.

Warboys, Michael, "Science and British Colonial Imperialism 1895–1940". D.Phil. thesis, University of Sussex, 1979.

White, Herbert Thirkell, *A Civil Servant in Burma*. London: Edward Arnold, 1913.

WHO, "Control of Diarrhoeal Diseases", Interim Programme Report, 1986. WHO/CDD/87.26.

Whyte, Robert Orr, *Rural Nutrition in Monsoon Asia*. Kuala Lumpur: Oxford University Press, 1974.

Widjojo Nitisastro, *Population Trends in Indonesia*. Ithaca: Cornell University Press, 1970.

Williams, J. H., *Elephant Bill*. London: Penguin, 1964.

Wrigley, Edward Anthony, *Population and History*. London: Weidenfeld and Nicolson, 1969.

Wyler, David J. and Louis H. Miller, "Plasmodium Species (Malaria)", in *Principles and Practice of Infectious Disease*, edited by Gerald L. Mandell, R. Gordon Douglas and John E. Bennett. New York: J. Wiley and Sons, 1979.

Wyon, John Benjamin and John E. Gordon, *The Khanna Study: Population Studies in the Rural Punjab*. Cambridge, MA: Harvard University Press, 1971.

Yegar, Moshe, "The Panthay (Chinese Muslims) of Burma and Yunnan", *Journal of Southeast Asian History* 7, no. 1 (Mar. 1966).

Yule, Henry, *A Narrative of the Mission Sent by the Governor-General of India to the Court of Ava in 1855*. Originally published in 1858. Reprinted in Kuala Lumpur and New York by Oxford University Press in 1968.

Index